T0226963

Complementary and Alternative Medicine in Inflammatory Bowel Disease

Editors

ALI KESHAVARZIAN
ECE A. MUTLU

GASTROENTEROLOGY CLINICS OF NORTH AMERICA

www.gastro.theclinics.com

December 2017 • Volume 46 • Number 4

ELSEVIER

1600 John F. Kennedy Boulevard • Suite 1800 • Philadelphia, Pennsylvania, 19103-2899
http://www.theclinics.com

GASTROENTEROLOGY CLINICS OF NORTH AMERICA Volume 46, Number 4
December 2017 ISSN 0889-8553, ISBN-13: 978-0-323-55278-3

Editor: Kerry Holland
Developmental Editor: Casey potter

Gastroenterology Clinics of North America (ISSN 0889-8553) is published quarterly by Elsevier Inc., 360 Park Avenue South, New York, NY 10010-1710. Months of issue are March, June, September, and December. Business and Editorial Offices: 1600 John F. Kennedy Blvd., Suite 1800, Philadelphia, PA 19103-2899. Customer Service Office: 6277 Sea Harbor Drive, Orlando, FL 32887-4800. Periodicals postage paid at New York, NY and additional mailing offices. Subscription prices are $330.00 per year (US individuals), $100.00 per year (US students), $616.00 per year (US institutions), $361.00 per year (Canadian individuals), $220.00 per year (Canadian students), $756.00 per year (Canadian institutions), $458.00 per year (international individuals), $220.00 per year (international students), and $756.00 per year (international institutions). Foreign air speed delivery is included in all *Clinics* subscription prices. All prices are subject to change without notice. **POSTMASTER:** Send address changes to *Gastroenterology Clinics of North America*, Elsevier Health Sciences Division, Subscription Customer Service, 3251 Riverport Lane, Maryland Heights, MO 63043. **Telephone: 1-800-654-2452 (U.S. and Canada); 314-447-8871 (outside U.S. and Canada). Fax: 314-447-8029. E-mail: journalscustomerservice-usa@elsevier.com (for print support); journalsonlinesupport-usa@elsevier.com (for online support).**

Reprints. For copies of 100 or more, of articles in this publication, please contact the Commercial Reprints Department, Elsevier Inc., 360 Park Avenue South, New York, New York 10010-1710. Tel. 212-633-3874, Fax: 212-633-3820, E-mail: reprints@elsevier.com.

Gastroenterology Clinics of North America is also published in Italian by Il Pensiero Scientifico Editore, Rome, Italy; and in Portuguese by Interlivros Edicoes Ltda., Rua Commandante Coelho 1085, 21250 Cordovil, Rio de Janeiro, Brazil.

Gastroenterology Clinics of North America is covered in *MEDLINE/PubMed (Index Medicus), Excerpta Medica, Current Contents/Clinical Medicine, Science Citation Index, ISI/BIOMED*, and *BIOSIS*.

Contributors

EDITORS

ALI KESHAVARZIAN, MD, FRCP, FACP, AGAF, MACG
Josephine M. Dyrenforth Chair of Gastroenterology, Professor of Medicine, Pharmacology, Molecular Biophysics, and Physiology, Director, Division of Digestive Diseases and Nutrition, Director, Institute for Advanced Study of the Gut, Chronobiology and Inflammation, Rush University Medical Center, Chicago, Illinois, USA

ECE A. MUTLU, MD, MS, MBA, AGAF, FACG
Director, IBD Program, Director, Clinical Research, Professor of Medicine, Section of Gastroenterology and Nutrition, Rush University Medical Center, Chicago, Illinois, USA

AUTHORS

BINCY P. ABRAHAM, MD, MS, FACP
Associate Professor, Fondren Inflammatory Bowel Disease Program, Lynda K and David M Underwood Center for Digestive Disorders, Division of Gastroenterology and Hepatology, Houston Methodist, Weill Cornell Medical College, Houston, Texas, USA

SARAH BALLOU, PhD
Postdoctoral Fellow, Department of Medicine, Beth Israel Deaconess Medical Center, Boston, Massachusetts, USA

ABIGAIL R. BASSON, PhD, RD, LD
Digestive Health Research Institute, Department of Medicine, Case Western Reserve University, Cleveland, Ohio, USA

ALYSE BEDELL, MS
Graduate Student, Division of Gastroenterology, Northwestern University Feinberg School of Medicine, Chicago, Illinois, USA

CHARLES N. BERNSTEIN, MD
Distinguished Professor of Medicine, Director, University of Manitoba IBD Clinical and Research Centre, Bingham Chair in Gastroenterology, Max Rady College of Medicine, University of Manitoba, Winnipeg, Manitoba, Canada

DAVID G. BINION, MD
Professor of Medicine, Division of Gastroenterology, Hepatology and Nutrition, UPMC Presbyterian, University of Pittsburgh School of Medicine, Pittsburgh, Pennsylvania, USA

ALEXANDER S. BROWNE, MD
Department of Medicine, The Warren Alpert Medical School of Brown University, Providence, Rhode Island, USA

HELEN J. BURGESS, PhD
Professor, Biological Rhythms Research Laboratory, Department of Behavioral Sciences, Rush University Medical Center, Chicago, Illinois, USA

FABIO COMINELLI, MD, PhD
Digestive Health Research Institute, Professor, Departments of Medicine and Pathology, Case Western Reserve University, Cleveland, Ohio, USA

FAYEZ K. GHISHAN, MD
Professor, Department of Pediatrics, The University of Arizona, Tucson, Arizona, USA

BRUCE R. HAMAKER, PhD
Professor, Department of Food Science, Purdue University, West Lafayette, Indiana, USA

JANA G. HASHASH, MD, MSc
Assistant Professor of Medicine, Division of Gastroenterology, Hepatology and Nutrition, UPMC Presbyterian, University of Pittsburgh School of Medicine, Pittsburgh, Pennsylvania, American University of Beirut, Beirut, Lebanon, USA

MEGAN M. HOOD, PhD
Associate Professor, Department of Behavioral Sciences, Rush University Medical Center, Chicago, Illinois, USA

SHARON JEDEL, PsyD
Assistant Professor, Division of Digestive Diseases and Nutrition, Department of Internal Medicine, Rush University Medical Center, Chicago, Illinois, USA

SAMIR KAKODKAR, MD
Advanced Fellow in Inflammatory Bowel Disease Northwestern University, Feinberg School of Medicine, Chicago, IL, USA

COLLEEN R. KELLY, MD
Department of Medicine, The Warren Alpert Medical School of Brown University, Providence, Rhode Island, USA

PAWEL R. KIELA, DVM, PhD
Associate Professor, Departments of Pediatrics and Immunobiology, The University of Arizona, Tucson, Arizona, USA

JOSHUA R. KORZENIK, MD
Division of Gastroenterology, Hepatology and Endoscopy, Brigham and Women's Hospital, Crohn's and Colitis Center, Harvard Medical School, Boston, Massachusetts, USA

MINH LAM, PhD
Digestive Health Research Institute, Department of Medicine, Case Western Reserve University, Cleveland, Ohio, USA

ERIN R. LANE, MD
Department of Pediatrics, Division of Gastroenterology, Seattle Children's Hospital, University of Washington, Seattle, Washington, USA

DALE LEE, MD
Department of Pediatrics, Division of Gastroenterology, Seattle Children's Hospital, University of Washington, Seattle, Washington, USA

DEVIN LINCENBERG, PsyD
Postdoctoral Fellow, Oak Park Behavioral Medicine LLC, Oak Park, Illinois, USA

ECE A. MUTLU, MD, MS, MBA, AGAF, FACG
Director, IBD Program, Director, Clinical Research, Professor of Medicine, Section of Gastroenterology and Nutrition, Rush University Medical Center, Chicago, Illinois, USA

GEOFFREY C. NGUYEN, MD, PhD, FRCPC
Mount Sinai Hospital Centre for Inflammatory Bowel Disease, Institute of Health Policy, Management and Evaluation, University of Toronto, Toronto, Ontario, Canada

EAMONN M.M. QUIGLEY, MD, FRCP, FACP, MACG, FRCPI
Professor of Medicine Lynda K and David M Underwood Center for Digestive Disorders, Division of Gastroenterology and Hepatology, Houston Methodist, Weill Cornell Medical College, Houston, Texas, USA

DAVID S. RAMPTON, PhD, FRCP
Professor of Clinical Gastroenterology, Centre for Immunobiology, Blizard Institute, Barts and The London School of Medicine and Dentistry, Queen Mary University of London, London, United Kingdom

HEATHER E. RASMUSSEN, PhD, RDN
Associate Professor, Department of Clinical Nutrition, Rush University Medical Center, Chicago, Illinois, USA

GREGORY M. SEBEPOS-ROGERS, MRCP
Specialist Registrar in Gastroenterology, Department of Gastroenterology, Royal London Hospital, Barts Health NHS Trust, London, United Kingdom

DANIEL J. STEIN, MD
Medical Director of the Inflammatory Bowel Disease Program, Associate Professor of Medicine, Division of Gastroenterology and Hepatology, Medical College of Wisconsin, Milwaukee, Wisconsin, USA

DAVID L. SUSKIND, MD
Department of Pediatrics, Division of Gastroenterology, Seattle Children's Hospital, University of Washington, Seattle, Washington, USA

GARTH R. SWANSON, MD
Associate Professor, Department of Digestive Diseases, Rush University Medical Center, Chicago, Illinois, USA

TIFFANY H. TAFT, PsyD
Research Assistant Professor, Licensed Clinical Psychologist, Division of Gastroenterology, Northwestern University Feinberg School of Medicine, Chicago, Illinois, USA

RACHEL W. WINTER, MD, MPH
Division of Gastroenterology, Hepatology and Endoscopy, Brigham and Women's Hospital, Crohn's and Colitis Center, Harvard Medical School, Boston, Massachusetts, USA

PETROS ZEZOS, MD, PhD
Mount Sinai Hospital Centre for Inflammatory Bowel Disease, University of Toronto, Toronto, Ontario, Canada

Contents

Preface: Complementary and Alternative Treatments Are Needed to Enhance the Care of the Inflammatory Bowel Disease Patient   xiii

Ali Keshavarzian and Ece A. Mutlu

Use of Complementary and Alternative Medicine in Inflammatory Bowel Disease Around the World   679

Petros Zezos and Geoffrey C. Nguyen

> Use of complementary and alternative medicine (CAM) is common among patients with inflammatory bowel disease (IBD). CAM can be broadly categorized as whole medical systems, mind-body interventions, biologically based therapies, manipulative and body-based methods, and energy therapies. Most do not use it to treat IBD specifically, and most take it as an adjunct to conventional therapy not in place of it. However, patients are frequently uncomfortable initiating a discussion of CAM with their physicians, which may affect adherence to conventional therapy. A greater emphasis on CAM in medical education may facilitate patient-physician discussions regarding CAM.

Complementary and Alternative Medicine Strategies for Therapeutic Gut Microbiota Modulation in Inflammatory Bowel Disease and their Next-Generation Approaches   689

Abigail R. Basson, Minh Lam, and Fabio Cominelli

> The human gut microbiome exerts a major impact on human health and disease, and therapeutic gut microbiota modulation is now a well-advocated strategy in the management of many diseases, including inflammatory bowel disease (IBD). Scientific and clinical evidence in support of complementary and alternative medicine, in targeting intestinal dysbiosis among patients with IBD or other disorders, has increased dramatically over the past years. Delivery of "artificial" stool replacements for fecal microbiota transplantation (FMT) could provide an effective, safer alternative to that of human donor stool. Nevertheless, optimum timing of FMT administration in IBD remains unexplored, and future investigations are essential.

Dietary Therapies in Pediatric Inflammatory Bowel Disease: An Evolving Inflammatory Bowel Disease Paradigm   731

Erin R. Lane, Dale Lee, and David L. Suskind

> Nutrition has long been recognized as a critical component in the treatment of pediatric inflammatory bowel disease (IBD). Formerly, nutritional interventions have focused on targeting improved weight gain and linear growth, as well as correction of micronutrient deficiencies. Recently, there has been growing interest and study of dietary interventions for induction and maintenance of remission. In addition to exclusive enteral nutrition, successes have been achieved with specific exclusion diets. This article evaluates the current literature regarding the role of diet and nutrition in

the pathogenesis of disease, as well as the role of diet as primary therapy for pediatric IBD.

Diet as a Therapeutic Option for Adult Inflammatory Bowel Disease   745

Samir Kakodkar and Ece A. Mutlu

There are many mechanisms to explain how food may drive and ameliorate inflammation. Although there are no consistent macronutrient associations in inflammatory bowel disease (IBD) development, many exclusion diets have been described: IgG-4 guided exclusion diet; semivegetarian diet; low-fat, fiber-limited exclusion diet; Paleolithic diet; Maker's diet; vegan diet; Life without Bread diet; exclusive enteral nutrition (EEN), the Specific Carbohydrate Diet (SCD), and the low FODMAP diet. The literature on diet and IBD is reviewed with a particular focus on EEN, SCD, and low FOD-MAP diets. Lessons learned from the existing observations and strengths and shortcomings of existing data are presented.

Probiotics in Inflammatory Bowel Disease   769

Bincy P. Abraham and Eamonn M.M. Quigley

Evidence indicates that the gut microbiota and/or interactions between the microbiota and the host immune system are involved in the pathogenesis of inflammatory bowel disease (IBD). Strategies that target the microbiota have emerged as potential therapies and, of these, probiotics have gained the greatest attention. Data derived from animal models of IBD have revealed the potential of several bacterial strains to modify the natural history of IBD. However, although there is some evidence for the efficacy of probiotics in ulcerative colitis and in pouchitis, in particular, there has been little indication that probiotics exert any benefit in Crohn disease. More targeted approaches involving live bacteria, genetically modified bacteria, and bacterial products are now being evaluated.

Prebiotics and Inflammatory Bowel Disease   783

Heather E. Rasmussen and Bruce R. Hamaker

Dietary fiber, specifically prebiotics, is the primary source of energy for the gut microbiota and thus has the potential to beneficially modify microbiota composition. Prebiotics have been used in in vitro studies and with animal models of colitis with largely positive results. Human studies are few and have been conducted with only a few select prebiotics, primarily fructan-containing fibers. Although disease activity and inflammatory markers have improved, more needs to be learned about the specific prebiotic compounds and how they can be used to best improve the gut microbiota to counter changes induced by inflammatory bowel disease.

Vitamins and Minerals in Inflammatory Bowel Disease   797

Fayez K. Ghishan and Pawel R. Kiela

Indiscriminate use of multivitamin/mineral supplements in the general population may be misguided, but patients with chronic Inflammatory Bowel Diseases (IBD) should be monitored and compensated for nutritional deficiencies. Mechanistic links between vitamin/mineral deficiencies and IBD pathology has been found for some micronutrients and normalizing their levels is clinically beneficial. Others, like vitamin A, although instinctively desirable, produced disappointing results. Restoring normal levels of the selected micronutrients requires elevated doses to compensate for defects in absorptive or signaling mechanisms. This article describes some aspects of vitamin and mineral deficiencies in IBD, and summarizes pros and cons of supplementation.

Herbs and Inflammatory Bowel Disease   809

Gregory M. Sebepos-Rogers and David S. Rampton

Although herbal preparations are widely used by patients with inflammatory bowel disease (IBD), evidence for their efficacy is limited and they may not always be safe. Mainly small studies of varying quality have suggested that several herbal preparations could be of benefit in IBD, but larger better-designed trials are needed to establish their place in inducing and maintaining remission. Patients and health care workers need to be made more aware of the limitations and risks of using herbal products for IBD.

Fecal Transplant in Inflammatory Bowel Disease   825

Alexander S. Browne and Colleen R. Kelly

Patients with inflammatory bowel disease (IBD) have differences in their gastrointestinal microbiome compared with healthy individuals, although it is unclear whether this is a cause or consequence of chronic inflammation. There is hope that manipulation of the gut microbiome through fecal microbiota transplant (FMT), commonly used to treat patients with *Clostridium difficile* infection, may also be an effective therapy in IBD. This article reviews the evidence supporting FMT in IBD, including case reports, case series, and randomized controlled trials. The article also focuses on questions of safety and speculates on the future of this therapy.

The Brain-Gut Axis and Stress in Inflammatory Bowel Disease   839

Charles N. Bernstein

The brain-gut axis serves as a circuit that incorporates the human experience, the state of mind, the gut microbiome, and the immune response that ultimately drives the phenotypic expression of inflammatory bowel disease (IBD). There are several biological pathways through which stress can play a deleterious role, including through increasing intestinal permeability, which can facilitate intestinal translocation of bacteria. Stress has an impact on symptoms in IBD; however, there is limited evidence that stress triggers increased intestinal inflammation. Although attention to stress and psychiatric comorbidity is important in the management of IBD, there are few clinical trials to direct management.

Psychological Considerations and Interventions in Inflammatory Bowel Disease Patient Care   847

Tiffany H. Taft, Sarah Ballou, Alyse Bedell, and Devin Lincenberg

The presence of psychological comorbidities, specifically anxiety and depression, is well documented in inflammatory bowel disease (IBD).

The drivers of these conditions typically reflect 4 areas of concern: disease impact, treatment concerns, intimacy, and stigma. Various demographic and disease characteristics increase the risk for psychological distress. However, the risk for anxiety and depression is consistent throughout the IBD course and is independent of disease activity. Early intervention before psychological distress becomes uncontrolled is ideal, but mental health often is unaddressed during patient visits. Understanding available psychological treatments and establishing referral resources is an important part of the evolution of IBD patient care.

Mindfulness-Based Interventions in Inflammatory Bowel Disease   859

Megan M. Hood and Sharon Jedel

Mindfulness-based interventions may be beneficial psychosocial treatments for improving the health and well-being of patients with inflammatory bowel disease. This article reviews 8 studies, assessing 7 psychosocial interventions, which include mindfulness and/or meditation components. The strongest effects of the interventions were found in quality of life and anxiety/depression, with inconsistent or minimal changes in other psychosocial areas, such as perceived stress and in disease-related outcomes and other physiologic functioning. Mindfulness interventions for patients with inflammatory bowel disease may be a supplemental treatment option to improve quality of life and distress in this population, although results are preliminary and interventions require additional testing.

Massage Acupuncture, Moxibustion, and Other Forms of Complementary and Alternative Medicine in Inflammatory Bowel Disease   875

Daniel J. Stein

Complementary and alternative medicine is frequently used by patients with inflammatory bowel disease (IBD); the most common are massage, acupuncture, and moxibustion therapy. Massage therapy is poorly studied in patients with IBD; therefore, its benefits remain unknown. Acupuncture and moxibustion therapy have been shown to improve inflammation and symptoms in animal and human studies. However, current clinical trials of acupuncture and moxibustion are of insufficient quality to recommend them as alternative therapy. Nonetheless, because these therapies seem generally to be safe, they may have a role as complementary to conventional therapy.

Sleep and Circadian Hygiene and Inflammatory Bowel Disease   881

Garth R. Swanson and Helen J. Burgess

There is increasing evidence that sleep and circadian disruption can worsen the disease course in inflammatory bowel disease (IBD). Sleep and circadian disruption are prevalent in society and are associated with worse outcomes in IBD. Emerging research suggests sleep and circadian disruption can affect key components in IBD disease flares, including intestinal permeability, translocation of bacterial endotoxins, intestinal dysbiosis, and proinflammatory cytokines. Much of this research has been conducted in animal models. There is a clear need for large randomized controlled trials in human patients with IBD, where the potential for chronotherapeutic strategies to improve disease course can be tested.

Exercise and Inflammatory Bowel Disease: Insights into Etiopathogenesis and Modification of Clinical Course   **895**

Jana G. Hashash and David G. Binion

There is sparse information regarding exercise and inflammatory bowel disease (IBD). Furthermore, the importance of regular exercise in the optimal management of IBD has not received attention in guidelines and is often overlooked by practitioners. This article summarizes evidence regarding the health benefits of exercise, guidelines regarding exercise in the general population and populations with chronic inflammatory disorder, limitations regarding exercise capacity in patients with IBD, the association of lack of exercise with IBD pathogenesis, the role of exercise in beneficially modulating the IBD clinical course, and extraintestinal benefits of exercise in patients with IBD.

The Practical Pros and Cons of Complementary and Alternative Medicine in Practice: Integrating Complementary and Alternative Medicine into Clinical Care   **907**

Rachel W. Winter and Joshua R. Korzenik

Complementary and alternative medicine (CAM) is changing health care for individuals with inflammatory bowel disease. The move toward increasing patient autonomy and addressing lifestyle and psychosocial factors contributes to this shift. Numerous clinics and centers are offering new models to incorporate these elements. There is need for better and more robust data regarding CAM efficacy and safety. CAM offers a test kitchen for new approaches to care and care delivery, which are now being developed and studied, and has the possibility to affect patient quality of life, disease morbidity, cost, and use of health care.

GASTROENTEROLOGY
CLINICS OF NORTH AMERICA

FORTHCOMING ISSUES

March 2018
Nutritional Management of Gastrointestinal Disease
Andrew Ukleja, *Editor*

June 2018
Gastrointestinal Transplantation
Enrico Benedetti and Ivo G. Tzvetanov, *Editors*

September 2018
Gastrointestinal Imaging
Perry J. Pickhardt, *Editor*

RECENT ISSUES

September 2017
Crohn's Disease
Edward V. Loftus, *Editor*

June 2017
Liver Pathology
Jay H. Lefkowitch, *Editor*

March 2017
The Gut Microbiome
Eamonn M.M. Quigley, *Editor*

Preface

Complementary and Alternative Treatments Are Needed to Enhance the Care of the Inflammatory Bowel Disease Patient

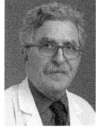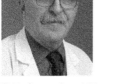

Ali Keshavarzian, MD   Ece A. Mutlu, MD, MS, MBA
Editors

Inflammatory bowel disease (IBD) is a complex chronic disorder with a rising number of patients in the United States and worldwide. Those of us who are taking care of the IBD patient recognize daily the limitations of standard medical therapies that we have to treat this disease. Current therapies are only partially effective even when it comes to controlling patient symptoms, targeting primarily one aspect of the disease pathogenesis (ie immune activation). They are also woefully inadequate in inducing mucosal healing and eliminating the inflammatory ulcerations in the gastrointestinal track in a significant majority. As such, flares of the disease are common especially in those with subclinical inflammation of the gastrointestinal tract. The causes of many of the IBD flares are unknown, but seem to be related to modifiable lifestyle factors. Currently, there are few traditional treatments that may address such lifestyle factors, if any. Therefore, additional approaches to IBD care are much needed to assure the long-term well-being of our patients for this lifelong disease, until a permanent cure for IBD can be found.

Complementary and alternative treatments have the potential to help improve symptoms, quality of life, as well as in some instances, make an impact in inducing or maintaining remission in IBD. Such treatments can not only address immune activation but also target additional mechanisms that have been purported to play a role in the disease pathogenesis. In this issue of the *Gastroenterology Clinics of North America*, we have gathered a large number of experts in their respective fields to answer the

Gastroenterol Clin N Am 46 (2017) xiii–xiv
https://doi.org/10.1016/j.gtc.2017.09.001
0889-8553/17/© 2017 Published by Elsevier Inc.

question of what complementary or alternative approaches can be helpful in management of the IBD patient. Together with these experts, we hereby present you the latest data on such treatments for IBD, in an effort to fill a large gap in patient care. These data are presented in the form of short reviews, and many carefully selected, pertinent publications are also given as references and can be the basis of additional reading, for those who are interested in further expanding their knowledge. Since it is not possible to cover any- and- all imaginable therapies within the complementary and alternative realm, we have limited our topics to those most frequently asked about by our own patients. They still cover a wide range from dietary options and nutraceuticals, to fecal transplant to probiotics and probiotics, and treatments that make use of the mind-body connection as well as herbs, vitamins, minerals, and other therapies such as acupuncture and moxibustion. We also present tips on how to begin implementing such therapies in a gastroenterology practice.

We hope that this issue of the journal will be useful for every gastroenterologist in considering the addition of such therapies to his/her practice. In addition to the knowledge provided, we also hope that this issue enhances and expands communication between traditional care providers practicing at all levels (such as primary care physicians, gastroenterologists, physician extenders, nurses, and trainees and medical students) and alternative providers thereby strengthening the bond between them in patient care. We expect that nurturing such bonds can also be expected to improve IBD research by generating novel hypotheses and thereby developing or enriching the direction of research. Only then, we can expect that our IBD patients will have all the options to pick and choose from, when it comes to enhancing their health and well-being.

Sincerely,

Your editors,

Ali Keshavarzian, MD
Rush University Medical Center
Division of Digestive Diseases & Nutrition
1725 West Harrison Street
Suite 206
Chicago, IL 60612, USA

Ece A. Mutlu, MD, MS, MBA
Rush University Medical Center
Division of Digestive Diseases & Nutrition
1725 West Harrison Street
Suite 206
Chicago, IL 60612, USA

E-mail addresses:
ali_keshavarzian@rush.edu (A. Keshavarzian)
Ece_Mutlu@rush.edu (E.A. Mutlu)

Use of Complementary and Alternative Medicine in Inflammatory Bowel Disease Around the World

 CrossMark

Petros Zezos, MD, PhD[a], Geoffrey C. Nguyen, MD, PhD, FRCPC[a,b,*]

KEYWORDS

- Complementary and alternative medicine • Traditional medicine
- Inflammatory bowel disease

KEY POINTS

- Worldwide, the use of complementary and alternative medicine (CAM) is common in the general population and is especially used by patients with chronic diseases or conditions, including ulcerative colitis and Crohns disease.
- Patients with IBD are frequently using or have used a wide variety of CAM practices and products to treat their disease, ameliorate their symptoms, or just to feel better.
- This is a global phenomenon with geographic and local diversity of the CAM practices and products influenced by cultural factors.
- The main reasons for CAM use include conventional treatment failure or side effects and patients' wish to gain greater control over their disease with more "natural" and "safer" products or practices.

INTRODUCTION

Worldwide, the use of complementary and alternative medicine (CAM) is common in the general population and is especially used by patients with chronic diseases or conditions, including ulcerative colitis and Crohn disease. Because many patients are showing increasing interest in CAM use and seeking information and advice from their health practitioners, it is important that gastroenterologists and other physicians who are involved in the care of patients with inflammatory bowel diseases (IBDs) become

Financial Conflicts of Interest: None.
[a] Department of Medicine, Mount Sinai Hospital Centre for Inflammatory Bowel Disease, University of Toronto, 600 University Avenue, Suite 437, Toronto, Ontario M5G 1X5, Canada; [b] Institute of Health Policy, Management and Evaluation, University of Toronto, 600 University Avenue, Suite 437, Toronto, Ontario M5G 1X5, Canada
* Corresponding author. Mount Sinai Hospital, 600 University Avenue, Suite 437, Toronto, Ontario M5G 1X5, Canada.
E-mail address: geoff.nguyen@utoronto.ca

more familiar with CAM therapies, including the spectrum of CAM practices and products, the potential for combination with conventional therapies, and finally, the risks and benefits of CAM use.[1–3]

In this article, the authors provide details for CAM use among patients with IBD around the world over the last decade, focusing on the geographic variations regarding the prevalence of CAM use, the common CAM practices and products used, the reasons for CAM use, and the factors associated with their use. Details of individual CAM therapies used in IBD are covered in other reviews included in this issue.

TERMINOLOGY AND DEFINITIONS

There is heterogeneity in CAM terminology because of different traditions and cultures across the world. The World Health Organization (WHO) provides the definitions for traditional medicine (TM) and CAM.[4] TM is the total of the knowledge, skill, and practices based on the theories, beliefs, and experiences indigenous to different cultures, whether explicable or not, used in the maintenance of health as well as in the prevention, diagnosis, improvement, or treatment of physical and mental illness. CAM refers to a broad set of health care practices that are not part of that country's own tradition or conventional medicine and are not fully integrated into the dominant health care system. They are used interchangeably with TM in some countries. The use of TM remains widespread in developing countries, whereas the use of CAM is increasing in developed countries.[4] The term complementary medicine (CM) implies that CAM is used in combination with conventional medicine, whereas in alternative medicine, CAM is used in place of conventional medicine.

The National Center for Complementary and Alternative Medicine (NCCAM), which is part of the National Institutes for Health in the United States, characterizes the term integrative medicine as the incorporation of complementary approaches into mainstream health care in an evidence-based and coordinated way.[5] The WHO Traditional Medicine Strategy 2014 to 2023 includes the integration, where feasible, of TM/CM within national health care systems.[4]

The NCCAM groups CAM into 5 broad categories (**Table 1**): (1) Whole medical systems: theories and practices such as homeopathic medicine, traditional Chinese medicine, and traditional Indian Ayurveda medicine; (2) Mind-body interventions: strengthen communication between the mind and body; (3) Biologically based therapies; (4) Manipulative and body-based methods; (5) Energy therapies: use of energy fields in the body to promote health and healing, for example, qi gong, tai chi, and magnet therapy.

Table 1	
Types of complementary and alternative medicine	
Whole medical systems	Homeopathic medicine, naturopathic medicine, traditional Chinese medicine/acupuncture, Ayurveda
Mind-body medicine	Meditation, prayer, mental healing, yoga, relaxation techniques, hypnotherapy
Biologically based therapies	Herbal products, dietary supplements (vitamins, minerals), probiotics
Manipulative and body-based practices	Chiropractic, osteopathy, massage
Energy medicine	Qi gong, tai chi, magnet therapy, movement therapies

USE OF COMPLEMENTARY AND ALTERNATIVE MEDICINE IN GENERAL POPULATION

Economic and sociocultural factors influence the use of TM and CAM. According to WHO, in Africa up to 80% of the population uses TM for its health care needs, whereas in China, TM accounts for around 40% of all health care delivered. Moreover, in Latin America, populations continue to use TM. In the following Western countries, the proportion of the population that has used CAM at least once were the following: 48% in Australia, 70% in Canada, 42% in United States, 38% in Belgium, and 75% in France.[6]

In a recent systematic review, Harris and colleagues[7] explored the prevalence of CAM use by the general population across 15 countries throughout the world. The prevalence of CAM use ranged from 9.8% to 76% across the 15 countries, with more frequent use by adults. East Asian countries, including Japan (76%), South Korea (75%), and Singapore (76%), were among the countries with the highest CAM use, whereas high percentages were also found in Australia (69%) and United States (40%). However, the frequency of CAM use did not seem to have increased compared with prior published reviews in 2000.[1,8]

USE OF COMPLEMENTARY AND ALTERNATIVE MEDICINE IN GASTROINTESTINAL DISEASES

CAM use is common among patients suffering from gastrointestinal diseases. Recently, Hung and colleagues[9] reported a survey study on the prevalence, the demographic predictors, and the reasons for CAM use in patients with all types of gastrointestinal disease contacted in a single large US academic institution. They reported an overall 44% prevalence of CAM use. Supplements or diets were used by 98% of the patients, including probiotics (64%), fish oil (36%), and gluten-free diet (26%). CAM therapies were used by 46% of the patients, including massage therapy (56%), meditation (33%), and acupuncture (31%). CAM users were predominantly women (81%), and the most common symptoms leading to CAM use were constipation (44%), diarrhea (47%), and bloating (59%). The most frequent reason for CAM use was the wish to feel generally better (68%). Finally, most of the patients reported better physical well-being (57%) and improved gastrointestinal symptoms (62%) with CAM use.

USE OF COMPLEMENTARY AND ALTERNATIVE MEDICINE IN INFLAMMATORY BOWEL DISEASES

CAM use is common among patients with IBD. Between 1998 and 2011, Hilsden and colleagues[10] reported that 21% to 60% of North Americans and Europeans had tried CAM and 11% to 34% were currently using it.

Frequency of Complementary and Alternative Medicine Use Around the World in Inflammatory Bowel Diseases

The authors conducted a literature search in PubMed and focused on articles describing epidemiologic studies of CAM use in IBD around the world published during the last decade (2006–2017).[11–27] Most of the studies were clinical and cross-sectional and were conducted during the last decade. There was wide variation in the reported prevalence of CAM use among different countries and geographic regions around the world. The results of the studies are summarized in **Table 2**.

Throughout the studies, the definition of CAM varied greatly as did the number and types of CAMs described, investigated, and included. Discrepancy was also observed across the studies in reporting current or past or overall CAM use among

Table 2
Prevalence of complementary and alternative medicine use in patients with inflammatory bowel diseases around the world (2006–2016)

Author, Year	N	Country	Sample	Current CAM Use, %	Current or Past CAM Use, %
Bensoussan et al,[11] 2006	325	France	Clinic, postal survey 2001–2003	11	21
Joos et al,[12] 2006	413	Germany	Clinic 1998–2000	—	52
D'Inca et al,[13] 2007	552	Italy	Clinic	—	28
Langhorst et al,[14] 2007	112/994	Germany	National	9.8	47.3/51
Lakatos et al,[15] 2010	655	Hungary	Clinic	—	31
Bertomoro et al,[16] 2010	2011	Italy	Clinic 2006–2007	—	23.6
Fernánadez et al,[17] 2012	705	Spain	Clinic 2010–2011	—	23
Weizman et al,[18] 2012	380	Canada	Clinic 2010–2011	—	56
Rawsthorne et al,[19] 2012	309	Canada	Clinic 2002–2006	40	74
Opheim et al,[20] 2012	430	Norway	Clinic 2009–2011	—	49 (past 12 mo)
Park et al,[21] 2013	366	South Korea	Clinic 2012–2013	—	29.5
Koning et al,[22] 2013	1370	New Zealand	Clinic 2003–2005	—	44 (past 12 mo)
Abitbol et al,[23] 2014	767	France	Internet 2011–2012	65	77
Mountifield et al,[24] 2015	473	Australia	Clinic	—	45.4
Nguyen et al,[25] 2016	392	Canada	Clinic 2010–2012	—	62
Oxelmark et al,[26] 2016	648	Sweden	Clinic 2008–2009	—	48 (past 12 mo)
Portela et al,[27] 2017	442	Portugal	Clinic, postal survey 2011–2012	12	31

patients with IBD. A few studies explored current CAM use separately and reported a range from 7.5% to 65%.[11,14,19,23,27] Abitbol and colleagues[23] reported a high prevalence of current CAM use (65%) in their IBD cohort compared with the other studies. The investigators cautioned that there may have been selection bias because their study targeted the recruitment of patients with IBD with an interest in CAM. Rawsthorne and colleagues[19] performed the only prospective longitudinal study in CAM use over 54 months in patients with IBD in Manitoba, Canada. Overall, 74% of the IBD cohort had used CAM during that period. At any time point, approximately 40% were using some type of CAM and 14% were using CAM consistently over the entire study period. The latter finding underlines the importance of incorporating a discussion about CAM use between patients with IBD and their attending physicians during follow-up visits.

All studies reported current or past CAM use together, with a prevalence ranging from 21% to 77%.[11–27] Higher prevalence of CAM use was observed in Northern America[18,19,25] (44%–74%) and Northern Europe[12,14,20,26] (44%–77%). Interestingly, studies from Central and Southern Europe[13–17,27] reported lower prevalence of CAM use (23%–31%). In Australia[24] and New Zealand,[22] the prevalence was similar to that in Northern America and Europe (45%). Finally, Park and colleagues[10] reported 28% CAM use in Korean patients with IBD. In general, the above observations from the Western countries were similar to those of Hilsden and colleagues.[10]

Complementary or Alternative Use?

In the few studies that investigated whether CAM was being used as a complementary or alternative treatment to conventional therapy, it was clear that most patients with IBD used CAMs together with their conventional treatment. The use of CAMs as an alternative treatment ranged from 10% to 25%.[13,14,16,20] An interesting finding by Langhorst and colleagues[14] in their study is that although most of the patients were interested in treatment with CAM and felt that they were insufficiently informed about CAMs, they did not regard the scientific evidence as an important factor for their use.

Complementary and Alternative Medicine Use for Inflammatory Bowel Disease Treatment?

In most of the studies, it is not clear if patients used CAM for their IBD, other health issues, for improving their general well-being, or to prevent disease or its complications. In the Manitoba study, only 18% of the consumers used CAM for their IBD.[19] Similarly, another study from Canada reported that only one-third of the patients with IBD used CAM for the treatment of IBD, and the remaining two-thirds used it for general health.[25] In France, Bensoussan and colleagues[11] reported similar prevalence of CAM use (21%) to treat IBD. Park and colleagues[21] reported that approximately half of patients with IBD in their cohort used CAM to improve their general health and not IBD itself. Because most of the patients with IBD use CAMs not specifically for their disease treatment, it is possible that they will not discuss it with their IBD provider.

Complementary and Alternative Medicine Types Used Around the World

A wide geographic variation has been observed in the types of CAM used around the world (**Table 3**). This diversity may reflect a real local pattern or may be due to study methodology. Homeopathy (44%–55%),[11–14,16,23,27] probiotics (37%–43%),[12,23] and herbal products (19%–54%)[14–16,23,26,27] are the preferred CAM types in both Northern and South Europe. In Canada, the most common CAM types used by patients with IBD were probiotics (65%), fish oil (49%), massage therapy (43%), and naturopathy

Table 3 Types of complementary and alternative medicine used around the world		
Therapy	**Proportion of CAM Users, %**	**Studies**
Massage	21–40	18,25,26
Herbal products	19–54	12,14–16,22–24,26,27
Relaxation	10	26
Homeopathy	38–55	11–14,16,23,27
Probiotics	37–65	12,18,23–25
Fish oil	49–50	18,25
Classical naturopathy	38–44	12,18,25
Acupuncture/traditional Chinese medicine	33	12

(39%).[25] Nguyen and colleagues[25] reported that the pattern of CAM types used for IBD did not differ significantly from those used for general health except for more common use of probiotics for IBD. In the Manitoba study, massage therapy and chiropractic services were the most commonly used CAM types, whereas a wide range of CAM products were used with a prevalence no more than 8% each.[19] In Australia and New Zealand, oral CAM products were most commonly used, including herbal medicine, vitamins, supplements, and probiotics.[22,24]

CAM users report frequent concurrent use of multiple CAM products.[11,13] Mountifield and colleagues[24] reported that 65% of the CAM users regularly used more than one CAM type.

THE COMPLEMENTARY AND ALTERNATIVE MEDICINE USER PROFILE
Reasons and Predictors for Complementary and Alternative Medicine Use

Some studies investigated the reason for CAM use among patients with IBD, whereas others tried to identify the factors (predictors) associated with CAM use in their IBD cohort. The most common reasons (**Table 4**) for CAM use among patients with IBD included lack of efficacy of conventional IBD therapy,[14,18,25,27] experienced or perceived side effects of conventional treatments,[14,18,24,25,27] the belief that CAM use is more natural and therefore safer,[16,18,24,25] and the wish for greater control over the disease.[14,18,25] Factors independently associated with CAM use included female gender,[16,19,20,22] younger age,[18,20,22] higher educational level,[16,18,20,22] side effects with conventional treatment,[18,20,21] and longer disease duration.[21]

Satisfaction and Adverse Events with Complementary and Alternative Medicine Use

Overall, most patients with IBD reported satisfaction with CAM use (67%–83%),[18,26,27] improvement in general well-being (30%–45%),[13,16] IBD symptoms improvement (40%),[13] and fewer disease relapses (16%–22%).[13,16] On the contrary, Fernández and colleagues[17] in their study reported that most of the CAM users (63%) did not observe benefit with CAM, whereas Park and colleagues[21] reported that only 4% of CAM users stated better outcomes. A few studies reported side effects due to CAM use ranging from 12% to 15% without detailing which side effects were associated with which specific CAM modalities.[12,21,26]

Table 4
Common reasons for complementary and alternative medicine use by patients with inflammatory bowel disease

Reason	Studies
Conventional treatment failure	14,18,25,27
Side effects of conventional therapy (experienced or perceived)	14,18,24,25,27
Stress	14
Holistic approach	14,24
Greater control over disease	14,18,25
Search for "optimal" therapy	14
To ameliorate symptoms	16,26
Hope to cure	16,27
Reduce no of drugs	16
More natural and safer	16,18,24,25

Adherence to Conventional Treatment

Most of the studies found that patients with IBD were highly adherent to conventional therapy while using concurrent CAM (80%–90%).[16,18,21,24,25,27] In contrast, Bertomoro and colleagues[16] in their IBD cohort reported that nonadherence to conventional therapy was associated with CAM use in 46% of users, whereas Abitbol and colleagues[23] in their study found that CAM users stopped their conventional treatment more often (odds ratio = 9.3, $P<.0001$).

Recently, Nguyen and colleagues,[25] in the COMPLIANT study, reported that although most of CAM users (90%) expressed the intention to continue taking their conventional medications, CAM use was associated with less favorable adherence to conventional therapy. Interestingly, it was only individuals using CAM specifically for IBD who had lower adherence, whereas those who used CAM for general health had similar adherence patterns as non-CAM users. In their analysis, the investigators found that 97% of the nonadherent individuals reported that it was unintentional, because of either carelessness or forgetfulness.

Physician Awareness

Current studies support the belief that CAM users frequently (30%–75%)[11–13,16,21,23,24] do not discuss or inform the use of CAM with their IBD physician because of various reasons, including fear of disapproval by them, feeling that they lack knowledge about CAM, or thinking that this is not necessary because CAM therapies are a different treatment.

Weizman and colleagues[18] reported that among CAM users, 91% would feel comfortable discussing CAM use with their gastroenterologist; however, only 34% consulted with the gastroenterologist before starting CAM therapies. Mountifield and colleagues[24] found that only half of the patients (54%) discussed their CAM treatment with their physician. They would be more comfortable discussing CAM use with their attending physician (87%) than discussing conventional therapy with their alternative practitioner (62%). More recently, Portela and colleagues[27] reported that 59% of CAM users avoided informing their treating physician about CAM use primarily because they were afraid of the physician's reaction (71%). However, a majority (85%) indicated that they would like to have the chance to discuss about CAM use with their physician.

Lindberg and colleagues[28] performed a qualitative study with significant observations. They found that patients with IBD would like to discuss CAM use with their physician, but they would prefer to be asked about CAM to be able to start a dialogue. The patients' reluctance to initiate discussion about CAM was related to fear that they would not be taken seriously by their physician. On the other hand, the patients stated that they would be more comfortable in discussing CAM use with the IBD nurses.

Gallinger and Nguyen[29] performed a Web survey among gastroenterologists with an interest in IBD, members of the American Gastroenterological Association, and reported that 68% of the responders to the survey considered CAM a good adjuvant to IBD therapy, and 72% were comfortable discussing with their patients. Nearly a third reported initiating conversations on CAM with their patients, whereas 90% agreed that their patients were reluctant to start a discussion about this topic. More than half (55%) stated they had no systematic approach to discussing CAM, and 65% reported no formal educational training in CAM therapies.

All the above indicate that actions should be taken with the implementation of CAM-related topics in medical schools, in the gastroenterology residency curriculum, and in the continuing medical education programs for specialists to cover this gap of knowledge among gastroenterologists.

In conclusion, physicians treating patients with IBD should be well informed and educated about CAM and should incorporate the use of CAM in the discussion with their patients. Many patients with IBD use CAM occasionally or even continuously, and this might affect the adherence to conventional treatment, cause side effects with the concurrent use of conventional treatment, and lead to poor disease outcomes and quality of life.[25] Therefore, it is important for physicians to inquire about CAM use among their patients.

Furthermore, the development of an international survey of CAM use among patients with IBD would be a valuable tool, both in clinical practice and in studies, to serve as a template and to enable the acquisition of more standardized and comparable data.[30]

SUMMARY

Patients with IBD are frequently using or have used a wide variety of CAM practices and products to treat their disease, to ameliorate their symptoms, or just to feel better. This trend is a global phenomenon with geographic and local diversity of the CAM practices and products influenced by cultural factors. The main reasons for CAM use include conventional treatment failure or side effects and patients' wish to gain greater control over their disease with more "natural" and "safer" products or practices. The above behavior is not different from the general population or patients with other chronic diseases. Most of patients with IBD remain adherent to the conventional treatment, use CAM in a complementary fashion, and feel satisfied with CAM therapies. Obviously, there are communication barriers between patients and physicians about CAM use, and patients often do not disclose CAM use to their physicians because of the fear of disapproval. On the other hand, the lack of physician's formal education on CAM therapies and the insufficient evidence-based data of CAM use often make physicians uncomfortable to discuss CAM with their patients.

Incorporating an educational curriculum about CAM therapies during medical school training and in postgraduate programs would be of great value. Physicians should involve their patients in disease management decisions, discuss the integration of CAM with the conventional treatments, and assess the safety of CAM modalities by determining if CAM use would adversely interact with traditional IBD therapies. Education of the public and the patients about CAM therapies, their benefits and their risks, is also important. Online educational tools on CAM that have been vetted by medical experts would be a valuable resource for both patients and physicians. In addition, well-designed epidemiologic studies with a standardized questionnaire will improve knowledge about the epidemiology of CAM use, whereas well-designed clinical studies would provide solid evidence for integration of CAM therapies in clinical practice.

REFERENCES

1. Harris P, Rees R. The prevalence of complementary and alternative medicine use among the general population: a systematic review of the literature. Complement Ther Med 2000;8(2):88–96.
2. Mongiovi J, Shi Z, Greenlee H. Complementary and alternative medicine use and absenteeism among individuals with chronic disease. BMC Complement Altern Med 2016;16:248.

3. Barnes PM, Bloom B, Nahin RL. Complementary and alternative medicine use among adults and children: United States, 2007. Natl Health Stat Rep 2008;12: 1–23.
4. World Health Organization. WHO traditional medicine strategy 2014–2023. Geneva (Switzerland): World Health Organization; 2013. Available at: www.who. int/medicines/publications/traditional/trm_strategy14_23/en/.
5. Complementary, alternative, or integrative health: what's in a name? Available at: https://www.nccam.nih.gov/health/whatiscam. Accessed March 15, 2017.
6. World Health Organization. WHO traditional medicine strategy 2002-2005. Geneva (Switzerland): World Health Organization; 2003. Available at: www.who. int/medicines/publications/traditionalpolicy/en/.
7. Harris PE, Cooper KL, Relton C, et al. Prevalence of complementary and alternative medicine (CAM) use by the general population: a systematic review and update. Int J Clin Pract 2012;66(10):924–39.
8. Ernst E. Prevalence of use of complementary/alternative medicine: a systematic review. Bull World Health Organ 2000;78:252–7.
9. Hung A, Kang N, Bollom A, et al. Complementary and alternative medicine use is prevalent among patients with gastrointestinal diseases. Dig Dis Sci 2015;60(7): 1883–8.
10. Hilsden R, Verhoef M, Rasmussen H, et al. Use of complementary and alternative medicine by patients with inflammatory bowel disease. Inflamm Bowel Dis 2011; 17(2):655–62.
11. Bensoussan M, Jovenin N, Garcia B, et al. Complementary and alternative medicine use by patients with inflammatory bowel disease: results from a postal survey. Gastroenterol Clin Biol 2006;30(1):14–23.
12. Joos S, Rosemann T, Szecsenyi J, et al. Use of complementary and alternative medicine in Germany - a survey of patients with inflammatory bowel disease. BMC Complement Altern Med 2006;6:19.
13. D'Inca R, Garribba AT, Vettorato MG, et al. Use of alternative and complementary therapies by inflammatory bowel disease patients in an Italian tertiary referral centre. Dig Liver Dis 2007;39(6):524–9.
14. Langhorst J, Anthonisen IB, Steder-Neukamm U, et al. Patterns of complementary and alternative medicine (CAM) use in patients with inflammatory bowel disease: perceived stress is a potential indicator for CAM use. Complement Ther Med 2007;15(1):30–7.
15. Lakatos P, Czegledi Z, David G, et al. Association of adherence to therapy and complementary and alternative medicine use with demographic factors and disease phenotype in patients with inflammatory bowel disease. J Crohns Colitis 2010;4(3):283–90.
16. Bertomoro P, Renna S, Cottone M, et al. Regional variations in the use of complementary and alternative medicines (CAM) for inflammatory bowel disease patients in Italy: an IG-IBD study. J Crohns Colitis 2010;4(3):291–300.
17. Fernández A, Acosta M, Vallejo N, et al. Complementary and alternative medicine in inflammatory bowel disease patients: frequency and risk factors. Dig Liver Dis 2012;44(11):904–8.
18. Weizman AV, Ahn E, Thanabalan R, et al. Characterisation of complementary and alternative medicine use and its impact on medication adherence in inflammatory bowel disease. Aliment Pharmacol Ther 2012;35(3):342–9.
19. Rawsthorne P, Clara I, Graff LA, et al. The Manitoba inflammatory bowel disease cohort study: a prospective longitudinal evaluation of the use of complementary and alternative medicine services and products. Gut 2012;61(4):521–7.

20. Opheim R, Bernklev T, Fagermoen M, et al. Use of complementary and alternative medicine in patients with inflammatory bowel disease: results of a cross-sectional study in Norway. Scand J Gastroenterol 2012;47(12):1436–47.

21. Park DI, Cha JM, Kim HS, et al. Predictive factors of complementary and alternative medicine use for patients with inflammatory bowel disease in Korea. Complement Ther Med 2014;22(1):87–93.

22. Koning M, Ailabouni R, Gearry R, et al. Use and predictors of oral complementary and alternative medicine by patients with inflammatory bowel disease: a population-based, case-control study. Inflamm Bowel Dis 2013;19(4):767–78.

23. Abitbol V, Lahmek P, Buisson A, et al. Impact of complementary and alternative medicine on the quality of life in inflammatory bowel disease: results from a French national survey. Eur J Gastroenterol Hepatol 2014;26(3):288–94.

24. Mountifield R, Andrews JM, Mikocka-Walus A, et al. Doctor communication quality and friends' attitudes influence complementary medicine use in inflammatory bowel disease. World J Gastroenterol 2015;21(12):3663–70.

25. Nguyen GC, Croitoru K, Silverberg MS, et al. Use of complementary and alternative medicine for inflammatory bowel disease is associated with worse adherence to conventional therapy: the COMPLIANT study. Inflamm Bowel Dis 2016;22(6):1412–7.

26. Oxelmark L, Lindberg A, Löfberg R, et al. Use of complementary and alternative medicine in Swedish patients with inflammatory bowel disease: a controlled study. Eur J Gastroenterol Hepatol 2016;28(11):1320–8.

27. Portela F, Dias CC, Caldeira P, et al. The who-when-why triangle of CAM use among Portuguese IBD patients. Dig Liver Dis 2017;49(4):388–96.

28. Lindberg A, Fossum B, Karlen P, et al. Experiences of complementary and alternative medicine in patients with inflammatory bowel disease - a qualitative study. BMC Complement Altern Med 2014;14:407.

29. Gallinger ZR, Nguyen GC. Practices and attitudes toward complementary and alternative medicine in inflammatory bowel disease: a survey of gastroenterologists. J Complement Integr Med 2014;11(4):297–303.

30. Quandt S, Verhoef M, Arcury T, et al. Development of an International questionnaire to measure use of complementary and alternative medicine (I-CAM-Q). J Altern Complement Med 2009;15(4):331–9.

Complementary and Alternative Medicine Strategies for Therapeutic Gut Microbiota Modulation in Inflammatory Bowel Disease and their Next-Generation Approaches

Abigail R. Basson, PhD, RD, LD[a,b], Minh Lam, PhD[a,b],
Fabio Cominelli, MD, PhD[a,b,c],*

KEYWORDS

- Inflammatory bowel disease • Crohn disease • Ulcerative colitis • Gut microbiota
- Complementary and alternative medicine • Nutraceuticals • Next-generation

KEY POINTS

- The human gut microbiome exerts a major impact on human health and disease, and therapeutic gut microbiota modulation is now a well-advocated strategy in the management of many diseases, including inflammatory bowel disease (IBD).
- Scientific and clinical evidence in support of complementary and alternative medicine (CAM), in targeting intestinal dysbiosis among patients with IBD, or other disorders, has increased dramatically over the past years.
- Delivery of "artificial" stool replacements for fecal microbiota transplantation (FMT) could provide an effective, safer alternative to that of human donor stool. Nevertheless, optimum timing of FMT administration in IBD remains unexplored, and future investigations to this end are essential.

Continued

Conflict of Interest: All authors declare no conflict of interest.
Financial research support for this publication comes from the National Institute of Diabetes and Digestive and Kidney Diseases of the National Institutes of Health (NIH) under Award number P30DK097948 as part of the Digestive Diseases Research Core Centers program as well as NIH awards DK091222, DK042191, DK055812, and DK097948 to F. Cominelli.
[a] Digestive Health Research Institute, Case Western Reserve University, Cleveland, OH, USA;
[b] Department of Medicine, Case Western Reserve University, Cleveland, OH, USA; [c] Department of Pathology, Case Western Reserve University, Cleveland, OH, USA
* Corresponding author. Case Western Reserve University, School of Medicine, University Hospitals Cleveland Medical Center, 11100 Euclid Avenue, Cleveland, OH 44106-5066.
E-mail address: Fabio.Cominelli@uhhospitals.org

Continued

- As a prerequisite, future studies must consider host initial microbiome, because baseline composition of gut microbiota plays a key role in an individual responsiveness to nutrition modulation.
- Animal and human studies continue to uncover the Pandora of interactions that endure between members of gut microbiome, their associated metabolites, dietary compounds, as well as the neurologic and immune systems of the host, all of which are characteristic to each individual.

INTRODUCTION

Crohn disease (CD) and ulcerative colitis (UC), both subtypes of inflammatory bowel disease (IBD), are chronic relapsing-remitting inflammatory disorders of the gastrointestinal tract associated with a deregulation of the T-cell–mediated immune responses toward intestinal bacteria.[1–3] Disease pathogenesis is thought to reflect a complex interaction between genetic susceptibility, a defective immune system, host intestinal microbiota, and environmental factors.[4] Despite substantial progress in the mechanistic understanding of chronic intestinal inflammation, including the integral role of enteric bacteria in disease pathogenesis, the precise cause of IBD is still unknown, and available treatment modalities for CD are not curative. Therefore, effective control of IBD, especially CD, is a realistic goal, and an ideal therapy is one that can alter the natural history of the disease in preventing complications while featuring a safe side-effect profile and acceptable methods of delivery.

Intestinal bacteria are now considered to be a metabolically active "organ," and the immunologic tone within the intestine should be that of tolerance toward the commensal bacteria, a balance maintained by the innate immune systems' ability to recognize intestinal antigens and appropriately activate or suppress T-cell reactivity to these antigens. It is now recognized that primary colonization of the gut begins in utero, via the umbilical cord, introducing members of the genera *Enterocuccus*, *Streptococcus*, *Staphlococcus*, and *Propinibacterium*,[5] and possibly also via the placenta, introducing maternally derived microbes.[6] Further colonization, associated with infant delivery (ie, vaginal vs cesarean),[7] is followed by a rapid escalation in gut microbial diversity during infancy, consisting of bacteria, archaea, viruses, and fungi.[8,9] 16S-ribosomal RNA and whole-genome sequencing have revealed microbial succession during these early years is nonrandom, potentially implying that early colonization patterns set the stage for bacterial community structures later in life.[9] Age-related factors associated with microbiota composition are of particular interest in IBD, considering the variability in age of onset,[10] the phenotypic differences noted between early and late onset,[10,11] and the reality that efficacy in terms of optimum timing for fecal microbiota transplantation (FMT) is not understood.

Despite the fact that more than 60 bacterial phyla exist in the world, the gut microbiome of a healthy human primarily consists of bacterial members belonging to 2 phyla: Firmicutes (~65%) and Bacteroidetes (~25%), thus implying strong underlying constraints in patterns of microbial colonization and succession.[8,12] The remaining bacterial species are typically distributed among the phyla Actinobacteria (eg, *Bifidobacterium* spp), Proteobacteria (eg, *Escherichia coli*), and Verrucomicrobacteria (eg, *Akkermansia muciniphilia*), with a possible smaller presence of Fusobacteria and Cyanobacteria.[13] Nonbacterial species, such as archaea, fungi (ie, mycobiota), and viruses (ie, virome), also inhabit the human intestinal tract,[14] with the human virome largely consisting of bacteriophages, which are numerous, and far more diverse than their bacterial counterparts.[8] Certain viral[15] and fungal species (eg, *Candida albicans*)[16–19] identified within the human virome and mycobiota are shown to directly interact with the intestinal immune system and have been portrayed for their role in IBD pathogenesis.[20] Other species, such as the yeast *Saccharomyces boulardii*, appear protective against intestinal inflammation.[21–24] Notably, intestinal organisms survive in a community governed by a robustness of symbiotic and highly competitive relationships between, and within, host commensals and pathogenic populations. Current research to elucidate these mechanisms takes advantage of the significant, yet fairly recent, technological advancements in next-generation sequencing, synthetic biology, and genetic engineering techniques that are available.

Decades of literature have proposed the concept that gastrointestinal colonization, particularly early in life, plays a key role in development of immune systems and host tolerance to antigens, and it is only over recent years studies have revealed specific microorganisms can directly influence T-cell development and maintenance as well as downstream responses.[25–29] T-regulatory cells (Tregs) play an essential role in maintaining gastrointestinal homeostasis through suppression of responses to pathogenic bacteria[30] and food antigens.[31] For example, specific bacterial members belonging to Clostridia,[32,33] and potentially *Parabacteroides*,[34] have been identified to induce Tregs, possibly through production of the short-chain fatty acid (SCFA) butyrate.[35,36] There are also data demonstrating the induction of interleukin-10 (IL-10)-producing Tregs, via polysaccharide A, a *Bacteroides fragilis*–generated metabolite.[37] More recently, specific microbial populations *Clostridium ramosum*, *Bacteroides thetaiotaomicron*, *Peptostreptococcus magnus,* and *B fragilis* were identified to control expression of a distinct Rory-expressing Treg subset population.[38] Animal studies have revealed segmented filamentous bacteria mediate dendritic cell activity, via production of serum amyloid A, leading to a downstream Th17 response.[32,39,40] At present, clinical application of microbiota modulation strategies that can target specific immune mechanisms remain forthcoming. Additional studies are essential to delineate the mechanisms by which specific microbiota and their metabolites affect immune cell subtypes as well as the potential for other factors, such as diet and medication, to influence these intricate interactions.

COMPLEMENTARY AND ALTERNATIVE MEDICINE

Complementary and alternative medicine (CAM) refers to health care strategies developed separately to that of Western or conventional mainstream medicine, with the term "complementary" implying usage of these therapies in addition to conventional medicine.[41] In the past, many IBD professionals have avoided CAM because of a lack in supporting scientific evidence, despite reports indicating that upwards of 50% of IBD patients use nonconventional therapies (ie, CAM) at some point during their disease course.[42–45] Over recent years, however, the body of scientific and clinical evidence in support of CAM has increased dramatically, resulting in a high level of acceptance among medical professionals. Moreover, advanced research technologies are working to reshape the face of many CAM strategies (eg, genetically engineered probiotics) into those of precise, next-generation CAM (NG-CAM) systems, designed for treatment of specific disease states, including IBD. Still, the integration of CAM/NG-CAM into any medical management plan, whether intended as short or long term, should be tailored to each individual patient and performed by an experienced practitioner capable of evaluating all facets of the available evidence with regard to benefits, safety, and cost.[41]

In terms of gut microbiota modulation, CAM/NG-CAM approaches can be classified into 1 of 4 major groups: (1) nutraceuticals, (2) mind-microbe balance, (3) dietetic management, and (4) microbiome therapy. Nutraceuticals refers to an unsuccessfully regulated group of food products ranging from herbals, botanicals, phytochemicals, and isolated nutrients to certain foods and beverages (ie, "functional foods") stocking specific health benefits based on their ingredients. Recent efforts to overcome the issue of nutraceutical bioavailability have led to advanced microbiome-triggered delivery systems and development of nutraceutical-producing bio-organisms. A growing body of evidence suggests that stress profoundly impacts gut microbiota composition and that the converse is also true, intestinal microorganisms are capable of altering host behavior. Conventionally known as the "gut-brain axis," the mind-microbe balance infers that, to achieve optimal host response from any therapeutic agent, necessitates full consideration of the intimate communication bond between both mind and microbe. Dietetic management encompasses a wide spectrum of dietary regimes characterized by their macronutrient profiles, the nutrient composition or origin of specific foods (eg, fiber type, gluten-free, saturated vs unsaturated fatty acids), or a combination of these. For example, elimination diets, individual fatty acids, high-fat (HF) diets differing in fat source (animal vs plant), and a range of dietary plant fibers have all been shown to impact gut microbial communities. Microbiome therapy is primarily gathered into 3 major paradigms: additive, transformative, and subtractive. Additive therapy involves supplementing gut microbiota with individual, or combinations of, bacterial strains (ie, probiotics), whereas transformative therapy entails modulation of the gut microbial community as a whole through FMT. These strategies are now evolving toward genetically engineered probiotic strains designed for specific mechanisms of disease, and the use of "artificial" stool products in FMT. Subtractive therapy refers to selective elimination of pathogenic members of the gut microbiome, with recent studies exploring bacteriophages, a viral species able to kill a precise gamut of bacteria with exquisite specificity, as a potential therapeutic modality for shaping microbiota populations in IBD. Notably, specific dietary compounds have been an important tool for managing activation and biosafety of engineered organisms. Because it is impossible to cover the spectrum of CAM therapies held within the aforementioned groups, this review focuses on CAM and recent NG-CAM that interact with the gut microbiota in

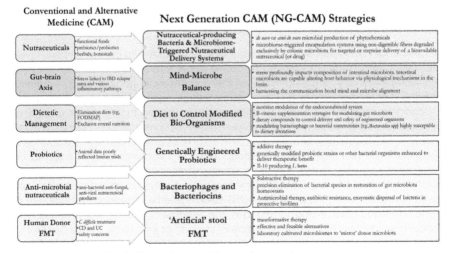

Fig. 1. Conventional and alternative medicine and strategies.

context to IBD. **Fig. 1** provides an overview of the CAM and NG-CAM strategies discussed in this review.

One of the challenges drawing particular attention in the current literature is that baseline (ie, pretreatment) composition of host intestinal microbiota, namely bacterial diversity, abundance, and their functionality, may in fact predict individual responsiveness to therapeutic interventions.[46–49] For instance, one study identified microbiota gene richness at baseline as predictive of inflammatory and metabolic response, following a low-calorie diet intervention.[50] In another diet study involving caloric restriction in obese individuals, preintervention abundance of A muciniphila was found inversely related to degree of responsiveness for fasting glucose, body composition, and subcutaneous adipocyte diameter.[51] However, further studies are required before individual bacterial species (or microbiome profiles) can be applied as predictive tools for treatment success.

NUTRACEUTICALS

Nutraceuticals are foods, or food products, that provide health and medical benefits in the prevention or treatment of disease.[52] Chemically, nutraceuticals include a range of bioactive substances classified as polyphenolic compounds (eg, curcumin, resveratrol, ellagitannins, flavenoids), isoprenoids (eg, terpenoids, carotenoids), minerals (eg, calcium, zinc), amino acid derivatives (eg, indoles, choline), carbohydrate derivatives (eg, oligosaccharides, polysaccharides), fatty acid and structural lipids (eg, n-3 polyunsaturated fatty acids [PUFAs]), and prebiotics.[53] In the United States, there is no specific regulatory framework for nutraceuticals or functional foods,[54] and most marketed nutraceuticals do not require clinical trials to support efficacy claims.[55,56] Although recognized as nutraceuticals, the probiotic arena of today has transcended as an NG-CAM in microbiome therapy through genetic engineering technology, and thus, is presented accordingly in this review.

Prebiotics

Prebiotics typically refer to selectively fermented nondigestible compounds that foster growth and activity of health-promoting intestinal microbiota.[57] A review of prebiotic fibers is available elsewhere.[58] Intestinal bacteria rapidly ferment these nondigestible fibers, producing metabolites central to gastrointestinal health, such as n-3 fatty acids, metabolic derivatives of tryptophan, and the SCFAs acetate, butyrate, and propionate.[36,59] Ingestion particularly favors growth of beneficial species *Lactobacillus* and *Bifidobacterium*, contributing to SCFAs.[60,61] Gastrointestinal benefits associated with prebiotics have included enhanced mucosal immunity, gut barrier integrity, and epithelial protection from pathogenic bacteria and other metabolites.[60,61] Bacteria-derived butyrate supports barrier function through 2 distinct mechanisms, namely, hypoxia-inducible factor activity via increased colonic epithelial cell oxygen consumption[62,63] and suppression of histone deacetylases butyrate that can increase tight junction proteins.[64]

Dietary components, such as fructo-oligosaccharides (FOS), galacto-oligosaccharides (GOS), soya-oligosaccharides, xylo-oligosaccharides, and pyrodextrins, have been proposed to increase bacterial diversity[60,65] as well as selectively enrich *Bifidobacterium* spp in the gut.[58] During growth, intake of prebiotic fibers FOS, GOS, and soluble corn fiber have been shown to increase absorption of calcium in humans and rats, enhancing bone properties through shifts in gut microbiota.[66–69] There is also evidence that soluble corn fiber increases calcium retention in older individuals who have reached peak bone mass[69] and is capable of altering functional pathways associated with macronutrient and vitamin metabolism.[70] The dietary prebiotic thus holds potential clinical utility in IBD considering the high prevalence of suboptimal bone density among patients.[71–73] Both animal and human studies demonstrate increased SCFAs with selective enrichment of *Bifidobacterium* following ingestion of resistant starches (RS), specifically RS1 and RS2.[74–76] In humans, RS appears to predominantly elicit colonization by *Ruminococcus bromii* and promote butyrogenic species *Faecalibacterium prausnitzii* and *Eubacterium rectale*.[77,78] Another prebiotic dietary fiber, germinated barley foodstuff, provides a glutamine-rich insoluble protein[79] identified to effectively increase luminal butyrate, lactate, and acetate production via expansion of *Bifidobacterium* and *Lactobacillus*.[80] Clinical studies suggest germinated barley foodstuff may exert therapeutic benefit in UC patients with mild to moderate disease activity, attenuating clinical activity index and mucosal damage, through promotion of *Bifidobacterium* and butyrate-producing *Eubacterium limosum*.[81–84]

Human prebiotic clinical intervention trials and effects on gut microbiota support the concept that prebiotic feeding increases abundance of certain bacteria and the production of various dietary metabolites. However, strong individuality in responsiveness is observed, underscoring the likelihood that initial composition of host microbiota can mediate effects of nutrition modulation.[47] There is also the possibility that the structural variations found to exist between a single plant species[85] could prevent *Bifidobacterium* from degrading certain fiber structures, because bacterium may not possess the appropriate enzymes. Even so, considering the high capacity for microbial horizontal gene transfer in the human gut,[86,87] interindividual differences would likely persist. Recently, Bindels and colleagues[65,88] proposed that prebiotics be redefined as nondigestible compounds that, through its metabolization by microorganisms in the gut, modulates composition and activity of the gut microbiota, thus conferring a beneficial physiologic effect on the host.

Polysaccharides

Polysaccharides refers to a heterogeneous group of structurally diverse carbohydrate molecules, many of which are used by the food industry as additives to enhance viscosity and texture of foods. Carrageenans, one of the more widely used food additives, derive from several species of red seaweed (*Rhodophyceae*) and are unique in cellular structure. Microbial fermentation of carrageenans requires specific gut microbiome-encoded enzymes, known as carbohydrate active enzymes ("CAZymes").[89] CAZymes have been identified in genomes of marine microbes, but are absent in the human microbiome genome; thus, humans are unable to digest carrageenan.[86,87,90] Interestingly, metagenomic studies have now uncovered bacterial members of the human gut belonging to the genus *Bacteroides* (eg, *Bacteroides plebeius*) that possess CAZyme encoding genes, thus allowing breakdown of specific carbohydrates, and in turn, an additional energy source.[87,91] This evolutionary adaptation is thought to reflect a natural horizontal gene transfer, in that, bacterial taxa, native to the human gut, have the ability to acquire genes from other microbes typically found outside of the human gut.[86,87] The extent to which extrinsically acquired genes could influence microbial ecology of the human gut warrants further investigation, especially considering the rising consumption of various traditional seaweeds, such as nori (species of red algae genus *Porphyra*), traditionally used to prepare sushi throughout many nations outside of Asia.

Squid ink polysaccharide

Mouse models of chemotherapy have reported biological activities of squid ink polysaccharide to include antitumor, antioxidant, and anticoagulation effects, as well as enhancement of both immunoglobulin A (IgA) secretion and gut barrier integrity.[92-96] These models suggested that the polysaccharide induced beneficial effects through reversal of chemotherapy-related dysbiosis. One recent animal study reported squid ink polysaccharide decreased abundance of *Ruminococcus*, *Bilophila*, *Oscillospira*, *Dorea*, and *Mucispirillum*, bacterium known to thrive during early disruption of the colonic mucosal surface layer.[97]

Casein Glycomacropeptide

Glycomacropeptide (GMP), a sialic acid–rich peptide, releases in whey during cheese making, and from bovine milk, releasing approximately 10 times higher amounts in the casein component of whey (ie, casein GMP).[98] GMP is significantly rich in amino acids proline, glutamine, serine, and threonine, as well as the branched chain amino acids isoleucine and valine. There is evidence that certain amino acids act as precursors to SCFA synthesis.[99-103] Specifically, anaerobic bacteria have the ability to metabolize glycine, threonine, glutamate, lysine, ornithine, and aspartate, into acetate, which other gut microbiota use to generate butyrate.[99] Threonine appears to be the most versatile because it also used to generate propionate.[104,105]

Animal models of induced colitis suggest that casein GMP may attenuate intestinal damage (morphologic/histologic) via NF-KB/p65 pathway inhibition.[106] Animal models also indicate that Casein GMP could mediate intestinal inflammation via the gut microbiota,[107-109] with administration associated with reductions in Proteobacteria and genera *Desulfovibrio* (from 30%–35% to 7%), and increases in acetate, propionate, and butyrate levels (cecum).[110] Recent data proposed that GMP exerts antiallergenic activity via modulation of gut microbiota.[111] Specifically, the GMP-induced increase in *Lactobacillus*, *Bifidobacterium*, and *Bacteroides*, was attributed to increased TGF-β production and reductions in mast cells.[111] Clinical trials for active distal colitis in UC patients have reported casein GMP is well tolerated, exerting similar disease-modifying effects to that of mesalazine.[112,113]

Mushroom Extracts

Mushrooms are recognized for their nutritional value and insoluble fiber content, with evidence supporting their unique range of bioactive metabolite substances.[114] Other compounds include mushroom polysaccharides, all of which with prebiotic properties, such as β-D-glucan polymers, polysaccharopeptides, polysaccharide proteins (eg, Polysaccharide K), chitin, mannans, galactans, and xylans.[115] Isolation of bioactive substances requires the young fruiting body (mycelium with primordia), thus extracted before the mushroom blooms,[114] with triterpenes, lipids, and phenols depicted for their immunomodulatory properties.[114,116] Mushroom bioactive metabolites are shown to stimulate different cells in the immune system, albeit that the ability of certain metabolites promote or suppress immune systems depends on dosage, route, and timing of administration, as well as how the mushroom is cultivated (ie, soil, harvesting, geography).[114] Nevertheless, various bioactive metabolites are in use clinically[117,118] and are available commercially worldwide in the form of capsules, food additives, syrups, or teas.[117]

In a mouse model of diet-induced obesity, administration of a water extract of *Ganoderma lucidum* mycelium (WEGL) was found to reverse HF diet–induced gut dysbiosis, noted by decreased *Firmicutes*-to-*Bacteroidetes* ratio and *Proteobacteria* levels, with a 10-fold increase in butyrate-producing species *Roseburia*.[119] The anti-inflammatory and gastroprotective effects identified were recapitulated following FMT (WEGL microbiota inoculum) into WEGL-naïve recipients fed an HF diet.[119] In a recent report, administration of *G lucidum* (100 mg/kg rat body weight, as oral suspension) improved barrier function via upregulation of occludin expression and increased ileal IgA.[120] Change in immune function correlated with improved microbiota richness, decreased *Firmicutes-to-Bacteroidetes* ratio, and reduced relative abundance of *Proteobacteria* (cecal content). However, a 2015 *Cochrane Review* of randomized controlled clinical trials (5 trials, N = 398) investigating effectiveness of WEGL (as antiobesity) and *G lucidum* for treatment of pharmacologically modifiable risk factors of cardiovascular disease (CVD) did not support use in CVD or type 2 diabetes.[121] In addition, participants who took *G lucidum* for 4 months were 1.67 times (RR = 1.67; 95%CI 0.86–3.24) more likely to experience an adverse event versus placebo. Adverse effects included nausea, diarrhea, or constipation.

Phytochemicals

Phytochemicals are naturally occurring plant chemicals that provide plants with color, odor, and flavor. Thousands of structurally heterogeneous phytochemical compounds have been identified thus far, many of which are shown to influence chemical processes of the host, including several pathways related to IBD pathogenesis.[122] Supplementation strategies in animal models of IBD seem to ameliorate intestinal inflammation, with or without changes to gut microbiota; however, data have poorly reflected in human clinical trials.[123] Differences in study design and reports of conflicting or harmful effects have limited generalization of findings. Details of this are outside the scope of the present review and are discussed extensively elsewhere.[124–126]

Approximately 90% to 95% of total dietary polyphenols reach the colon unabsorbed.[127] Microbial modulation has been reported in animal or human studies, or both, by epigallocatechin gallate (EGCG, main catechin of green tea),[128–131] ellagic acid and ellagitannis (pomegranate, raspberries, blackberries, strawberries, and chestnuts),[132,133] ginseng saponins (ginsenodises),[134,135] and resveratrol (red wine).[136,137] In vitro evidence has shown that naringenin (a flavone) can inhibit growth and adhesion of the gram-negative pathogen *Salmonella typhimurium*, yet enhance proliferation of the anti-inflammatory probiotic strain *Lactobacillus rhamnosus*.[138,139] Recently, EGCG supplementation was shown to decrease DNA damage in mice fed an HF diet, with reversal of tissue-specific gene expression and methylation patterns of *DNA methyltransferase 1* and *MutL homologue 1*, implying potential for epigenetic consequences.[140] The ratio of *Firmicutes* to *Bacteroidetes* in supplemented mice was also significantly lower than that of controls.

The ability for phytochemicals to influence composition and metabolic activity of colonic bacteria definitely exists, but efficacy intimately reflects dosage, timing, and route of administration. Bioavailability is also an important issue and depends on phytochemical origin (whole food vs extract), overall diet composition,[141] as well as host colonic microbiome via bacterial metabolism of dietary polyphenols, in turn affecting bioavailability and derived metabolites.[122,142,143] Although certain colonic bacteria can enhance bioavailability of dietary,[124,143–147] recent data revealed microbial metabolism of certain phytochemicals (eg, quercetin) could indirectly influence the effects (enhance or suppress) of other dietary compounds, such as *n*-3 PUFAs.[148]

Microbiome triggered delivery

In an effort to overcome bioavailability issues, several groups have focused on colon-targeted delivery systems, using nondigestible fibers (eg, RS) degraded exclusively by colonic microbiota, for encapsulation and delivery of bioavailable nutraceuticals.[149–151] This method of encapsulation has proven clinically effective for delivery of 1, 25-dihydroxyvitamin D3-25-b-glucuronide (hormonally active vitamin D) in treating localized colonic inflammation, without risk of hypercalcemia or intestinal loss.[152,153] In another study, mesalamine linked with L-glutamine via azo linkage, a bond specifically cleaved by the colonic microbiome, was reported to reach 84.7% targeted drug and nutraceutical delivery in the colon.[154]

Colon-targeted drug delivery systems intended for IBD patients have implemented food grade materials, including soy protein, β-lacto globulin (whey), chitosan, and zein.[126] To improve encapsulation and pH controlled release of nutraceuticals, smart pH nanoparticles, namely carboxymethyl chitosan and calcium pectinate cross-linked with polyethyleneimine (PEI), a promising synthetic vector, have also been established.[155] The latter coating method is degraded only by pectinases in the colonic environment and was reported to protect resveratrol activity until desired release into the lower bowel.[156] Other colon-targeted carrier systems of curcumin have proven successful in vivo.[157–159] Several groups have effectively implemented coencapsulation, essentially 2 nutraceuticals in a single carrier. Nutraceutical coencapsulations comprise the following: curcumin/resveratrol,[160] curcumin/catechin,[161] curcumin/piperine,[162] gallic acid/curcumin coadministered with ascorbic acid/quercetin,[163] curcumin/flax seed oil,[164] and prebiotic/probiotic codelivery.[165] Efforts to develop multilayered particulate drug delivery systems for controlled, sustained drug release, including coencapsulation of drug and nutraceutical while preventing pharmacologic cross-reactivity, has shown immense promise as an NG-CAM approach in nutraceutical and drug delivery.[126,166]

Medical Cannabis

Cannabinoids, derived from the cannabis plant *Cannabis sativa*, include more than 60 aromatic hydrocarbons, of which Δ^9-tetrahydrocannabinol is the primary psychoactive component. The endocannabinoid system is ubiquitously expressed throughout the human and rodent body, modulating intestinal peristalsis, gastric acid secretion, hunger (including fat-rich intake),[167–169] gut barrier integrity, and intestinal inflammation, with gut microbiota interactions identified.[170–175] The inhibitory effects on gastrointestinal motility may benefit patients with diarrhea and intestinal inflammation, because activation of cannabinoid receptors (CBRs) appears to reduce inflammation-associated hypermotility.[67,176,177] Comprehensive reviews of these mechanisms are available elsewhere.[41,173]

Epithelial cells, immune cells (B cells, natural killer cells, and mast cells),[178,179] and the enteric nervous system are all cellular targets of the endocannabinoid system.[169,180–182] Molecular targets include CBR type 1 (CB_1R) and CBR type 2 (CB_2R), as well as transient receptor potential vanilloid 1 receptors (TRPV1s, best known as the receptor for capsaicin), peroxisome proliferator-activated receptor alpha (PPARαs), and the orphan G-protein coupled receptors, GPR55 and GPR119.[169,183]

Endogenously derived bioactive lipids that activate CBRs include members of the N-acylethanolamine (NAE) family, namely 2-arachidonoylglycerol (2-AG), a promotor of gut barrier integrity, and N-arachidonoylethanolamine (AEA; also termed anandamide), a promotor of epithelial permeability,[184] as well as N-palmitoylethanolamine (PEA), N-oleoylethanolamine (OEA), N-stearoylethanolamine (SEA) and N-linoleylethanolamine (LEA).[185] These lipids can act as natural ligands for PPARα (OEA and PEA)[186,187] TRPV1 (AEA and OEA).[169,188,189] Other bioactive lipids belonging to the acylglycerol family, palmitoyl-glycerol (2-PG) and oleoylglycerol (2-OG), are also considered protective of barrier function.[190–193]

Mechanistic studies (both in vitro experiments and animal models) have suggested endocannabinoids, namely CB_1R and CB_2R, mediate gut barrier function, epithelial barrier permeability, and inflammatory processes, and thus may offer protective effects in IBD.[194–198] Conversely, intestinal biopsies of UC and CD patients revealed enhanced endocannabinoid or bioactive lipid levels, with or without increased CB receptor expression,[189,199–206] implying dysregulation of the endocannabinoid system plays a role in IBD pathogenesis. In addition, there is now evidence supporting a link between host intestinal microbiota and endocannabinoids in mediating intestinal integrity.[207]

Lactobacillus acidophilus was the first bacteria specifically shown to modulate the expression of CBRs and μ-opioid receptors in murine intestinal cells.[208] The effects of intestinal bacteria on CBR expression was well illustrated in an elaborate study implementing several models of gut microbiota modulation (HF diet, prebiotics, probiotics, or antibiotics), and mice bearing specific mutations involved in bacterial recognition (TLR, Myd88; myeloid differentiation primary response gene 88). Results indicated that gut microbiota modulation could activate colonic *Cnr1* expression, the gene encoding for CB_1R, which in turn influences gut permeability and plasma lipopolysaccharide levels.[207,209] Everard and colleagues[209] observed improvements in gut barrier function correlated with increased intestinal levels of 2-PG, 2-OG, and 2-AG in genetically susceptible obese and type 2 diabetic mice administered *A muciniphila* and fed an HF diet. More recently, the same group showed that intestinal epithelial Myd88 deletion in mice (IEC Myd99 KO) partially protected against inflammation and gut barrier disruption induced by an HF diet via mechanisms directly involving gut microbiota, and that in the absence of IEC Myd88, levels of AEA decreased, whereas both 2-AG and 2-OG increased. The investigators suggested that activation of GPR119 via 2-OG stimulates intestinal L-cell release of glucagon-like peptide-2, a peptide involved in barrier function.[210] Overall, cross-talk between the gut microbiota, endocannabinoid system, and metabolism of the host appears capable of inducing specific changes in the intestinal innate immune system and vice versa.

In a 2011 survey conducted in Mount Sinai Hospital, Toronto, Canada evaluating cannabis usage among IBD patients (N = 291), 50% of CD and 33% of UC patients reported having used cannabis as a CAM method to relieve IBD-related symptoms, such as pain, appetite loss, and diarrhea, at some point during their disease course.[211] One retrospective study (N = 30, CD)[212] and 2 prospective studies (N = 13, IBD; N = 21, CD)[213,214] have reported beneficial effects of cannabis usage for IBD symptom control, although study limitations included lack of standardization, dosing inconsistency, and diversity in cannabis plant strain. In addition, side effects ranged from addiction, dry mouth, drowsiness, increased appetite, to a sensation of "high." To this end, authorities now forbid motor vehicle use of for at least 3 to 4 hours after smoking, and 6 hours after oral ingestion.[215] Studies evaluating pharmacologic modulation of the endocannabinoid system are currently underway (experimental and clinical trials), but few of these account for the potential interaction between the gut microbiome and endogenous bioactive lipids.[216]

Nutrition-based modulation of the endocannabinoid system tone by reducing the ratio of *n*-6 to *n*-3 has proven effective in some obesity studies.[217–219] For example, docosahexaenoic acid (C22:0) administration was associated with decreased levels of AEA and 2-AG, and reductions in inflammation and fat mass in mice.[220] In obese individuals, daily supplementation with *n*-3 PUFAs from krill oil reduced plasma levels of 2-AG.[217] The implication of these findings in IBD is unclear considering the gastro-protective properties of 2-AG. Nutrition modulation of the endocannabinoid system, particularly in IBD, remains in the exploratory and discovery phase.

MIND-MICROBE BALANCE

Numerous studies advocate the neural, hormonal, and immune-related communication pathways that exist between the gut and brain of the host.[221–224] In IBD patients, various inflammatory mechanisms affecting epithelial integrity and proinflammatory cytokine production[225] have been proposed in explanation of the long-reported correlation between stress and increased relapse of disease.[226–230] However, it is possible that some of these proposed mechanisms are in fact consequences of altered gut bacteria, because stress has now been discovered to profoundly influence gut microbial communities.[231,232] Nevertheless, the converse is also true, with animal models showing that changes to intestinal microorganisms can indeed lead to alterations in behavior (for review, refer to Abautret-Daly and colleagues[226]).

Additional animal studies are required and should provide an invaluable first-line approach to understanding the physiologic changes that occur in the brain in response to intestinal microorganisms, in context to the internal and external milieu (host-specific) that constantly shapes both microbiome and brain. To this end, maintaining the host mind-microbe balance, via an ongoing consideration of this multifaceted communication pathway, could prove quintessential in attaining maximum efficacy of any treatment modality.

DIETETIC MANAGEMENT

Diet is recognized as one of the primary driving forces in shaping the composition of gut bacteria and metabolite production.[233–235] Notably, intestinal microbiota also play an important role in the synthesis of several vitamins (B vitamins, vitamin K, vitamin A)[236,237] and can affect the absorption of essential minerals such as iron,[238] magnesium, and calcium in the host.[239] Literature supports dietary intervention as a means of promoting beneficial host-bacteria interactions,[59,216,240] with new evidence revealing how single food ingredients (eg, turmeric) can interact with functional traits of intestinal microbiota to regulate host physiology.[241] However, the potential interactions between dietary compounds and host-specific microbial communities have not been investigated in most human diet intervention studies performed to date. A recent review of the known interactions between mucosal immunity, host genetics, gut microbiome, and diet is available.[242]

Macronutrients

Even small dietary changes have the potential to alter the composition of gut microbiota, in as little as a day.[243,244] Short-term dietary interventions, especially those devoid of carbohydrates, appear to have the most profound effect,[233] but taxonomic changes are not consistent among individuals,[235] perhaps a reflection of baseline microbiota composition. Fungal abundance has been linked to a carbohydrate-rich diet, with *Candida* abundance positively correlated with carbohydrate intake and negatively correlated with total saturated fatty acids.[245] Long-term dietary changes tend to impact ratios of *Bacteriodes*, *Prevotella*, and *Firmicutes*, with the most profound change in microbiota composition and bacterial metabolites resulting from diets high in red meat and fat, namely PUFAs.[235,246,247] Studies have suggested dietary fiber promotes *Prevotella*, whereas higher protein and fat intakes promote *Bacteroides* dominance.[235,246,247]

In IL-10$^{-/-}$ mice, significant blooms in the "pathobionts" *Bilophila wadsworthia* correlated with feeding an HF diet rich in saturated milk fat.[25] The sulfite-reducing properties of *B wadsworthia* led to an abundance of hydrogen sulfide production, a molecule disruptive to epithelial barrier function.[248,249] Other animal models have shown that an HF diet, in combination with high sugar, increases adherent invasive *E coli* (AIEC),[250] whereas others show that certain fibers (pectin, guar gum) can potentially mediate the proinflammatory effects of a dietary lipid.[251] Various IBD mouse models have suggested medium chain triglycerides (MCTs) can exert anti-inflammatory effects, thereby reducing intestinal inflammation.[252–254] In these studies, MCTs consisted of various saturated fatty acids sourced from coconut oil.

A predominantly meat-based diet was reported to decrease *Clostridiales*, a bacterium involved in plant-based fiber metabolism, while increasing abundance of bile-tolerant *Alistipes*.[233] In professional athletes, microbial diversity is markedly impacted by disproportionately high dietary intakes of protein, particularly within the genus *Akkermansia*.[255] Animal-based foods (ie, red meat) deliver L-carnitine to certain gut bacteria, producing trimethylamine N-oxide (TMAO),[256] a molecule identified to promote atherosclerosis in animal models[257] and humans.[258] In mice, potato resistant-starch appeared to attenuate detrimental effects of a meat-based diet, partly by promoting members the beneficial, *Lactobacillus* spp.[259,260]

Mediterranean diets, which are inherently low in red meat, has been suggested to beneficially impact gut microbiota,[261] whereas an energy-restricted diet, in combination with dietary fiber, was shown to increase microbial diversity in upwards of 25%, in individuals with low diversity.[262] Of interest, omnivores appear to produce more TMAO from dietary L-carnitine than that of vegans or vegetarians.[258] One plausible explanation could be archaeal lineages underlying the human gut microbiome. Certain strains of methanogens in the human gut, such as *Methanomassiliicoccus luminyensis* and *Methanosarcina barkeri*, strictly use methyl-based compounds, including trimethylamine (TMA), to enable their growth, thus could readily deplete TMA levels.[263] For instance, *M luminyensis* encodes a rare proteinogenetic amino acid pyrrolysine, a characteristic shared by few other bacteria.[264] The latter is a truly unique characteristic because methanogenesis of TMA (a methylated amine) is only possible in the presence of pyrrolysine in active catalytic site.[265] Notably, studies exploring the abundance and activity of archaeal taxa between human populations have identified significant differences in organism groups based on geographic location, as well as the consumption of specific food items such as salt-fermented seafood.[264,266–270]

B vitamins

The human gut microbiota supplies the host with B vitamins, including niacin (B3), riboflavin (B2), cobalamin (B12), biotin (B8), folate (B9), thiamin (B1), pantothenate (B5), and pyridoxine (B7). The host relies largely on microbiota-derived B vitamins as well as those obtained from dietary sources, because human cells alone do not produce sufficient quantities of B vitamins.[271] A comprehensive genome assessment of 256 common human gut bacteria revealed a diverse distribution in the presence and absence of B-vitamin biosynthesis pathways as well as that gut microbes actively exchange B vitamins among each other, and in doing so, enable organisms that are deficient in any of these vital biosynthesis pathways, to survive.[236] Three distinct genome patterns were identified, namely: (1) Actinobacteria are limited to niacin, pyridoxine, and thiamin pathways, (2) except for niacin, all pathways are lacking in 6 Firmicutes and 2 Actinobacteria genomes, and (3) 5 Firmicutes and 3 Proteobacteria genomes lack all pathways except for biotin and folate biosynthesis. Inverse patterns were also noted, implying complementary relationships between microbiota. For instance, the essential roles for folate metabolism were missing in all 4 *F prausnitzii* genomes. Findings indicate that perturbations to gut microbiota may impact not only individual B-vitamin requirements but also that deficiency in one or more B vitamin can lead to unfavorable blooms in proinflammatory organisms.[236] On the other hand, supplementation strategies using single or various combinations of B vitamins may provide a novel avenue for manipulating the gut microbiota.

Vitamin D
The vitamin D receptor (VDR) is abundantly expressed throughout the intestine and in all immune cells and is both directly and indirectly targeted by the bioactive forms of vitamin D, 1,25-dihydroxyvitamin D (1,25[OH]$_2$D and 1,25[OH]$_2$D$_3$).[272–274] There is evidence to support the interaction between vitamin D, the VDR, and gut microbial communities in immune-mediated disorders. For instance, compared with wild-type mice, VDR null mice have a depletion in *Alistipes* and *Odoribacter* with markedly increased levels of *Clostridium*, *Bacteroides*, and *Eggerthella* (cecum),[275] the latter bacterium implicated in UC and CD.[276] In a model of colitis-induced colorectal cancer, increased VDR expression following administration of VSL#3 was associated with lower colon damage and decreased richness and diversity of mucosally adherent bacteria.[277] Low vitamin D status is frequently observed in IBD, especially in CD patients.[278] One randomized controlled trial reported oral supplementation with *Lactobacillus reuteri* NCIMB 30242 increased circulating 25(OH)D concentrations.[279]

Elimination Diets
Elimination diets consist of an assortment of restrictive dietary regimens entailing the avoidance of specific foods or food groups that may, or may not, precede reintroduction of single food types for identification of those that initiate symptoms. Most elimination diets are not supported by gastroenterology organizations,[280–282] although approximately 70% of IBD patients report implementing some form of elimination diet while in remission.[283] Often, these self-imposed diets are based on nonmedical resources, such as the Internet or IBD support groups, with long-term avoidance of major food groups resulting in severe nutrient deficiencies and malnutrition.[125,284] Recent data show malnutrition can alter microbial composition and intraepithelial lymphocyte phenotype of the small intestine.[285]

FODMAP
A low-FODMAP (acronym of "Fermentable Oligo-, Di-, Mono-, and Polyols") diet encompasses the dietary restriction of fermentable oligosaccharides (many kinds of vegetables, including "onion family," legumes, wheat/rye), disaccharides (lactose-based dairy; milk, yogurt, cheeses), monosaccharides (many kinds of fruits, dried fruit, fruit juice), and polyols (honey, corn syrup, fructose, sweeteners ending in "-ol").[286] In principle, the diet may reduce symptoms of bloating and abdominal pain through the avoidance of short-chain carbohydrates (insoluble fibers), which undergo rapid fermentation by colonic bacteria.[286,287] In patients with existing disease or intestinal narrowing (strictures), avoidance of high-FODMAP foods (ie, insoluble fiber) thus may be appropriate.[283] However, most of the excluded FODMAP foods are indeed prebiotics, capable of beneficially modulating microbiota communities.[288,289] In IBS patients, one randomized controlled trial reported a low-FODMAP diet to significantly reduce *Bifidobacterium* spp,[289] with a second trial reporting greater bacterial diversity of butyrate-producing microbiota clusters in the high-FODMAP group

and reduced total bacterial abundance in the low-FODMAP group.[288] The high-FODMAP diet increased the relative abundance of anti-inflammatory *A muciniphila* and the butyrate-producing Clostridium cluster XIVa.[288] Oligosaccharides (soluble fiber) were reported to block adherence of pathogenic bacteria to epithelia in vitro, including mucosally associated AIEC, a bacterium frequently observed within the mucosa of CD patients.[290,291] Of the soluble plant fibers, soluble plantain fiber was reported the most consistently effective, inhibiting adherence of *Salmonella* spp, *Shigella* spp, Enterotoxigenic *E coli*, and *Clostridium difficile*.[292,293] Many of the oligosaccharide-containing cruciferous vegetables excluded from the FODMAP diet (eg, brussel sprouts, cabbage, collard greens, kale) are also rich in sulfur-containing compounds called glucosinolates, converted by gut microbiota to biologically active, anti-inflammatory compounds such as indoles, nitriles, and isothiocyanates.[242,294]

Specific carbohydrate diet

The specific carbohydrate diet (SCD) involves elimination of most dietary carbohydrates, primarily grains, starches, dairy, and sugars/sweeteners (except honey). Evidence to support effectiveness of SCD to induce or maintain remission in IBD is only available through small case series in CD and UC.[295–298] The proposed mechanisms underlying SCD beneficial effects include altered macronutrient ratio (protein, fat), reduced dietary gluten intake, or reduced intake of food additives (eg, emulsifiers), shown to influence gut microbiota and barrier function.[250,299,300] Animal models of gluten sensitivity support the modulatory role of gut microbiota in host responses to gluten,[301] with nonceliac, gluten-sensitive IBD patients reporting improvement in clinical symptoms following a gluten-free diet.[302]

Exclusive Elemental Nutrition

Exclusive enteral nutrition (EEN) is a formula-based therapy recommended as first-line therapy for induction of remission in pediatric CD, with an 85% efficacy rate.[303] Lower efficacy is noted in adult CD patients, possibly because of poor compliance or longer exposure to immunosuppressive treatments.[240] Some pediatric CD studies show EEN-induced alterations to *Bacteroides-Prevotella* correlate with therapeutic response,[304,305] whereas less impressive changes are observed in samples of adult CD patients posttreatment with enteral nutrition.[305] There is also literature suggesting that intestinal inflammation, relative to CD, may induce some changes in microbiota, such as reduced diversity and increased Proteobacteria.[290] Taken together, additional studies assessing the effects of EEN and enteral nutrition in adult CD patients are required.

MICROBIOME THERAPY

Microbiome therapy, such as additive (eg, probiotics), subtractive (eg, selective antibiotics, nutraceuticals with antimicrobial properties), or transformative (ie, FMT), is proving effective, although individual responsiveness varies substantially.

Subtractive Therapy

Subtractive therapy is the removal of specific bacterial species, or groups of species, from the gut to correct gut disease-associated dysbiosis, thereby restoring host microbial homeostasis. Elimination of host pathogenic gut bacteria, through conventional broad-spectrum antibiotics or nonconventional nutraceutical products with antimicrobial activity,[306] leads to a concomitant reduction in host commensals, possibly increasing host susceptibility to other infectious agents (eg, *C difficile*).

Next-generation subtractive therapies have overturned the concept of therapeutic probiotics, to that of therapeutic bacteriocins, a bacterially derived antimicrobial peptide with toxic activity.[307] Metagenomic and in vivo efforts demonstrate bacteriocin producers have a strong competitive/fitness advantage and increased protection against pathogens.[58,308–311] Subtractive therapy has also gone viral, via bacteriophage therapy, as a subset of viral species with the potential to bind and kill a narrow range of bacteria with impeccable specificity.[312–314] Bacteriophages, or phages, are highly abundant, naturally occurring organic entities. Viral genomes have been identified in both healthy and diseased individuals,[315–317] with healthy humans harboring an estimated 1200 viral genotypes.[318] Some IBD studies demonstrate reduced bacterial diversity with concomitant increase in bacteriophage richness, specifically in Caudovirales,[316] whereas others have reported decreased overall diversity.[319–321] Intestinal virome populations seem to be unique to each individual,[315,317] and phage community structure is highly susceptible to diet,[315] including other factors, such as geographic location.[316] Evidence indicates that viromes are also acquired via diet,[322] and it has been suggested that ingestion of viral communities occurs at a much higher rate than internal production.[323]

Current efforts to enhance or engineer bacteriophages, for host therapeutic benefit, have focused on enzymatic dispersal of bacteria in protective biofilms,[324] antibiotic resistance,[324,325] antimicrobial activity,[326] and modulation of gut microbial communities via cell death.[327–332] Therapeutic deployment of bacteriophage therapy in IBD has used naturally occurring or genetically engineered viral parasites.[327] Of interest, it is now proposed that phages could exert immunogenic effects,[333] with several studies demonstrating direct effects of intestinal phages on the immune system, including proinflammatory and anti-inflammatory responses.[318,334–343] Research exploring bacteriophage therapy remains in its early stages; however, the prospective that natural or engineered phages (ie, augmented antibacterial capability) can intimately control microbial population structure, while mediating mucosal immunity offers an intriguing prospect in the management of IBD patients.

Additive Therapy

Additive therapy entails supplementation of host microbiota with either individual or a combination of bacterial strains either natural (ie, probiotics) or genetically engineered in origin, such as probiotic strains with enhanced function.

Probiotics

Probiotics are live microorganisms that exert health benefits to the host when administered in sufficient quantity, with strains isolated from the human intestine suggested as preferential.[312] Animal and human investigations of various probiotic regimens in IBD have yielded controversial results, and animal data inconsistently reflect human IBD trials.[307] Two strains of probiotics, *E coli* Nissle 1917 and VSL#3, have shown some efficacy in UC and pouchitis[309,344–348]; however, no recommendations exist for probiotic administration in CD. Clinical intervention studies investigating their effects on the microbiota and human health have been limited by differences in probiotic formulation, timing of administration, and dosage as well as variability in patient diet and medication use (for reviews, see Refs.[125,226,349,350]). To date, no IBD-focused research has explored the potential therapeutic benefit of probiotics in alleviating anxiety or depression, although this has been explored in other disorders.[226]

Genetically Engineered Probiotics

Recent efforts are focusing on genetic modification of probiotic strains as an NG-CAM strategy. Advantages of enhanced bio-organisms can include stability of colonization (ie, bioavailability, longevity) and dynamic correction of disease-dysbiosis–related perturbations to prevent or resolve inflammation.[307] Application of cellular engineering in augmentation of prophylactic probiotics, such as E coli Nissle 1917 and Lactobacillus jensenii, has been successful in overcoming natural colonization resistance conferred by host resident gut microbiota.[351] Today, Lactococcus lactis is one of the most commonly applied bacterial chassis, a nonpathogenic, noncolonizing gram-positive bacterium used extensively throughout the dairy industry.[352] In mice, L lactis has been successfully engineered to secrete biologically active murine IL-10, a potent anti-inflammatory cytokine, relevant to IBD.[352,353] In addition, when synthesized in vivo, lower doses of IL-10 were required compared with systemic IL-10 administration.[353] Phase 1 clinical trials using IL-10–secreting L lactis have been well tolerated in CD patients, although efficacy was modest.[354] A nanobody-secreting modified strain of L lactis, delivering active anti-mTNF nanobodies locally to the colonic mucosa has proven highly efficacious in dextran sulfate sodium (DSS)-induced colitis and established enterocolitis IL-10 null mice.[355] Described for its anti-inflammatory properties, elafin is associated with restoring barrier function to damaged intestinal epithelia,[356–358] with reduced expression and subsequent defective elastolytic activity reported in patients with IBD.[359–361] Two strains of elafin-secreting bacteria, L lactis and L casei, were shown to decrease intestinal inflammation in mice, and to protect cultured human epithelial cells from increased epithelial permeability.[362] Other modifications of L lactis for treatment of diabetes and autoimmune disease[363,364] have been investigated, namely strains-producing auto-antigen proinsulin[365] and glutamic acid.[293] Administration of NAEs directly to the intestinal lumen to promote endocannabinoid function is also under investigation. Using a genetically modified strain of E coli Nissle 1917 to produce N-acylphosphatidylethanolamine (NAPE)-synthesizing enzymes, precursors to the NAE family of lipids, mice had lower food intake, insulin resistance, adiposity, and hepatosteatosis, with increases in hepatic NAE.[366] However, the effects on other bacterial members in the gut were not investigated.

To date, almost every type of known polyphenolic compound has been produced de novo or semi-de novo by genetically engineered strains of E coli or Saccharomyces cerevisiae.[367] Modified strains have also been used to produce alkaloids (amino acid–derived compounds),[285,368–372] polysaccharides,[373] and various forms of terpenoids (eg, lutein, lycopene, carotenes, and carotenoids), a group of phytochemicals typically present in green foods and soy plants.[374–378] Recently, tryptophan-derived indolyguco-sinolate was produced in a strain of S cerevisae after genome insertion with 8 plant genes.[379] This remarkable progress has also ensued development of novel or nonnatural polyphenolic compounds.[380,381]

One of the drawbacks to genetically engineered therapies is the very real concern of biosafety and environmental contamination.[353] The fact is, when administering a live genetically modified organism, that organism is also released into the environment. Once released, there is a possibility of unintentional colonization of individuals, or food industries (eg, dairy). Moreover, conditions in the human gastrointestinal tract favor natural horizontal gene transfer between bacterial members.[382,383] Engineered bacterium should thus inherently include a biological containment system, such as auxotrophy or other gene defect that necessitates supplementation with an essential metabolite or intact gene.[384] In addition, recombinant therapies designed on bacterial and probiotic strains currently listed by the US Food and Drug Administration as generally regarded as safe should be subject to strict reevaluation protocols via regulatory frameworks.[353]

To address the important issue of environmental safety, a modified strain of *Bacteriodes ovatus* (human commensal) was developed to deliver human transforming growth factor beta (TGF-β_1) but under the strict control dietary xylan (ie, sole energy source).[355,385,386] In a DSS model of colitis, xylan supplementation induced *B ovatus* secretion of human TGF-β_1 as well as significantly improved DSS-induced colitis, in some cases superior to that of steroid treatment.[386] Additional studies investigating specific dietary compounds and functional capacity as a means of controlling therapy delivery and biosafety of genetically modified bacteria are highly warranted.

Predicting Probiotic-Microbiota Interactions in the Host

In practice, a truly effective recombinant therapy would likely require long-term gastrointestinal colonization, and thus, should be capable of self-activation (or not) in response to specific environmental cues over time in the host. Development of effective therapies requires comprehensive understanding of the parameters governing competitive microbial colonization,[387] preferred areas of local microbial colonization (ie, small vs large bowel),[388] as well as how diet, environmental stimuli, and mucosal immunity influence microbial ecosystems, or possible latent effects of stimulated immune pathways on microbiota composition. For instance, *Bacteroides* spp appear to be resistant against antimicrobial peptides,[389] and their abilities for colonization and resilience are largely determined by the presence of carbohydrates.[390–392]

In order to predict the complex interactions between probiotic strains (natural or modified), mucosal immune systems, the gut microbiota (intestinal vs surface attached),[393–395] and host genetics, sophisticated in vitro systems, capable of dynamic, physiologically relevant environmental changes are essential.[307,396] At present, various in and ex vitro models, testing interbacterial interactions, have been applied, namely, single-[397] and multi-stage chemostat models,[396] synthetic 3-dimensional tissue scaffolds with villous features,[398] mouse ileal organoids,[399] and a human gut-on-a-chip microdevice.[218] Assessment of recombinant therapies in gene circuits allows for detection of disease biomarkers and sometimes drug production, but is shown to result in high cellular burden, and in turn, their condensed timeframes (ie, 24 hours) may not adequately gauge evolutionary stability of a recombinant therapy.[307] Stability of engineered therapies is a noted limitation as in vitro evolution experiments have shown bacteriophage functionality can reduce rapidly over time.[400,401] Moving forward, efforts to enhance both robustness and long-term durability of engineered therapies and their testing models should help in the realization of an environmentally autonomous "intelligent" engineered bio-organism as an NG-CAM strategy.

Transformative Therapy

Representing a somewhat more intrusive form of additive-type therapy, FMT focuses on changing intestinal microbiota communities as a whole. Procedures encompass infusion of fecal material sourced from a healthy donor, into the gut of an individual (ie, the recipient) for the treatment of disease-specific dysbiosis, with the aim of restoring microbial balance. Fecal microbiota inoculum is delivered either to the upper gastrointestinal tract via nasogastric/nasojejunal tube or upper endoscopy or to the lower intestinal area via enema or colonoscopy.[402] For treatment of recurrent *C difficile* infections, FMT boasts 90% clinical success, proving twice as effective as antibiotic therapy alone.[403] Mechanisms as to exactly why FMT is effective are not fully understood, although abundance of butyrate-producing species *Lachnospiraceae* in donor microbiota was recently proposed.[28,404]

Fecal Microbiota Transplantation

Cumulative evidence seems to indicate that FMT-induced remission is possible in a subset of both UC and CD patients,[405–407] although only 2 randomized controlled studies, bearing conflicting results, have evaluated FMT efficacy in UC patients, and no randomized controlled trial data are published for CD to date.[349,350,405,408] In a 2014 meta-analysis of 9 studies (included 79 UC and 39 CD patients), a remission rate of 36.2% in UC patients (pooled proportion) and 60.5% in CD patients (pooled estimate on subgroup analysis) was reported.[408,409] These effects, however, are not universal, nor are they sustained in either of the 2 IBD groups.

Failure of FMT in clinical studies may be attributed to various factors, including patient population (severe vs medically refractory), mechanism of action, stool donors, administration route and dosage, or other confounding factors, such as smoking, diet, and medication use.[406,408–411] A recent study comparing lyophilized FMT product with fresh or frozen products (using same donors) revealed lyophilized product had slightly lower efficacy (vs fresh), whereas no difference between fresh and frozen fecal product was identified.[412] The hygiene hypothesis, one of the longest standing theoretic frameworks associated with the pathogenesis of IBD,[4,413–416] also happens to underpin the single most unexplored aspects of FMT administration, namely optimum timing for microbiota modulation. It is plausible that remarkable efficacy may be observed if administered early in life, during certain key windows of plasticity in immune development. Equally, manipulation of microbial communities, perhaps early in diagnosis, could greatly improve long-term outcomes by attenuating disease progression.

One decidedly important issue concerning FMT therapy is the overall safety. The gut microbiome is a dynamic and living organism that constantly evolves over time, and a vast number of human-associated microbial and nonmicrobial (viruses, fungi) species remain undiscovered.[417] Although short-term infectious risks of FMT appear to be definable and quantifiable, the theoretic risk of introducing pathogenic organisms that could later exacerbate disease conditions[409,418] and the potential for unknown long-term consequences[410] are 2 caveats that continue to dampen enthusiasm in FMT clinical treatment. In an effort to mitigate these risks, several groups are currently investigating the use of an "artificial," synthetic stool mixture, designed to contain clinically active microbes.[419,420] The stool substitute appears capable of curing antibiotic-resistant *C difficile* colitis[419] and should be pursued as a feasible alternative. Overall, the concept of FMT holds strong potential within the repertoire of CAM and NG-CAM for management of IBD. In the future, the most effective FMT modalities will like encompass defined microbial communities[421] infused into precharacterized IBD recipients, pertaining to their gut microbiota community, diet, lifestyle, and medication intake.

SUMMARY

The human gastrointestinal tract is resident to a vastly diverse microbial consortium that coexists through strict rules of invasion, dominance, resilience, and succession. Although some members possess stronger capabilities for survival than others, each one retains a genome characteristic of their bacterial denomination that subsequently determines survival and ultimately the composition of a human gut microbiome. Collective evidence advocates the concept of gut microbiota modulation via dietary compounds, with or without nutraceutical supplementation. However, consistent reports of strong individuality in responsiveness suggest that initial composition of host microbiota mediates the effect of nutrition modulation. There is also a strong potential for the interaction between mind and microbe to influence responsiveness, although mechanistic understanding of these complex exchanges remains in its infancy at best. Synthetic stool for FMT is a next-generation microbiome therapy shown effective in treating *C difficile*,[419] which could provide a feasible alternative to current methods for patients with IBD. Nevertheless, studies investigating optimum timing for FMT administration are essential.

Animal and human studies are only starting to highlight the Pandora of interactions that endure between members of gut microbiome, their associated metabolites, dietary compounds, as well as host neurologic and immune systems, all of which are characteristic to each individual. Advanced research technologies have excelled in the scientific evidence in support of CAM and toward generating NG-CAM systems designed for the treatment of specific disease states, such as IBD. Although most envisioned NG-CAM strategies presently exist in their experimental and discovery phases, many show promise for future clinical application (**Fig. 1**).

REFERENCES

1. Bamias G, Pizarro TT, Cominelli F. Pathway-based approaches to the treatment of inflammatory bowel disease. Transl Res 2016;167(1):104–15.
2. Sartor RB. Microbial influences in inflammatory bowel diseases. Gastroenterology 2008;134(2):577–94.
3. Sartor RB, Wu GD. Roles for intestinal bacteria, viruses, and fungi in pathogenesis of inflammatory bowel diseases and therapeutic approaches. Gastroenterology 2017;152(2):327–39.e4.
4. Molodecky NA, Kaplan GG. Environmental risk factors for inflammatory bowel disease. Gastroenterol Hepatol (N Y) 2010;6(5):339–46.
5. Jimenez E, Fernández L, Marín ML, et al. Isolation of commensal bacteria from umbilical cord blood of healthy neonates born by cesarean section. Curr Microbiol 2005;51(4):270–4.
6. Veldhoen M, Ferreira C. Influence of nutrient-derived metabolites on lymphocyte immunity. Nat Med 2015;21(7):709–18.
7. Dominguez-Bello MG, Blaser MJ, Ley RE, et al. Development of the human gastrointestinal microbiota and insights from high-throughput sequencing. Gastroenterology 2011;140(6):1713–9.
8. Cultrone A, Tap J, Lapaque N, et al. Metagenomics of the human intestinal tract: from who is there to what is done there. Curr Opin Food Sci 2015;4:64–8.
9. Koenig JE, Spor A, Scalfone N, et al. Succession of microbial consortia in the developing infant gut microbiome. Proc Natl Acad Sci U S A 2011; 108(Suppl 1):4578–85.
10. Silverberg MS, Satsangi J, Ahmad T, et al. Toward an integrated clinical, molecular and serological classification of inflammatory bowel disease: report of a Working Party of the 2005 Montreal World Congress of Gastroenterology. Can J Gastroenterol 2005;19(Suppl A):5A–36A.
11. Kostic AD, Xavier RJ, Gevers D. The microbiome in inflammatory bowel disease: current status and the future ahead. Gastroenterology 2014;146(6):1489–99.
12. Ley RE, Hamady M, Lozupone C, et al. Evolution of mammals and their gut microbes. Science 2008;320(5883):1647–51.

13. Walker AW, Ince J, Duncan SH, et al. Dominant and diet-responsive groups of bacteria within the human colonic microbiota. ISME J 2011;5(2):220–30.
14. Tang J, Iliev ID, Brown J, et al. Mycobiome: approaches to analysis of intestinal fungi. J Immunol Methods 2015;421:112–21.
15. Kernbauer E, Ding Y, Cadwell K. An enteric virus can replace the beneficial function of commensal bacteria. Nature 2014;516(7529):94–8.
16. Iliev ID, Funari VA, Taylor KD, et al. Interactions between commensal fungi and the C-type lectin receptor Dectin-1 influence colitis. Science 2012;336(6086): 1314–7.
17. Richard ML, Lamas B, Liguori G, et al. Gut fungal microbiota: the Yin and Yang of inflammatory bowel disease. Inflamm Bowel Dis 2015;21(3):656–65.
18. Sokol H, Conway KL, Zhang M, et al. Card9 mediates intestinal epithelial cell restitution, T-helper 17 responses, and control of bacterial infection in mice. Gastroenterology 2013;145(3):591–601.e3.
19. Sokol H, Leducq V, Aschard H, et al. Fungal microbiota dysbiosis in IBD. Gut 2017;66(6):1039–48.
20. Odds FC. Candida and candidosis: a review and bibliography. Bailliere Tindall; 1988.
21. Chen X, Yang G, Song JH, et al. Probiotic yeast inhibits VEGFR signaling and angiogenesis in intestinal inflammation. PLoS One 2013;8(5):e64227.
22. Jawhara S, Poulain D. Saccharomyces boulardii decreases inflammation and intestinal colonization by Candida albicans in a mouse model of chemically-induced colitis. Med Mycol 2007;45(8):691–700.
23. Jawhara S, Thuru X, Standaert-Vitse A, et al. Colonization of mice by Candida albicans is promoted by chemically induced colitis and augments inflammatory responses through galectin-3. J Infect Dis 2008;197(7):972–80.
24. Zwolinska-Wcislo M, Brzozowski T, Budak A, et al. Effect of Candida colonization on human ulcerative colitis and the healing of inflammatory changes of the colon in the experimental model of colitis ulcerosa. J Physiol Pharmacol 2009;60(1):107–18.
25. Devkota S, Wang Y, Musch MW, et al. Dietary-fat-induced taurocholic acid promotes pathobiont expansion and colitis in Il10-/- mice. Nature 2012;487(7405): 104–8.
26. Gkouskou KK, Deligianni C, Tsatsanis C, et al. The gut microbiota in mouse models of inflammatory bowel disease. Front Cell Infect Microbiol 2014;4:28.
27. Hill DA, Hoffmann C, Abt MC, et al. Metagenomic analyses reveal antibiotic-induced temporal and spatial changes in intestinal microbiota with associated alterations in immune cell homeostasis. Mucosal Immunol 2010;3(2):148–58.
28. Natividad JM, Pinto-Sanchez MI, Galipeau HJ, et al. Ecobiotherapy rich in firmicutes decreases susceptibility to colitis in a humanized gnotobiotic mouse model. Inflamm Bowel Dis 2015;21(8):1883–93.
29. Thorburn AN, McKenzie CI, Shen S, et al. Evidence that asthma is a developmental origin disease influenced by maternal diet and bacterial metabolites. Nat Commun 2015;6:7320.
30. Sun M, He C, Cong Y, et al. Regulatory immune cells in regulation of intestinal inflammatory response to microbiota. Mucosal Immunol 2015;8(5):969–78.
31. Pabst O, Mowat AM. Oral tolerance to food protein. Mucosal Immunol 2012;5(3): 232–9.
32. Atarashi K, Tanoue T, Ando M, et al. Th17 cell induction by adhesion of microbes to intestinal epithelial cells. Cell 2015;163(2):367–80.

33. Atarashi K, Tanoue T, Oshima K, et al. Treg induction by a rationally selected mixture of Clostridia strains from the human microbiota. Nature 2013; 500(7461):232–6.
34. Kverka M, Zakostelska Z, Klimesova K, et al. Oral administration of Parabacteroides distasonis antigens attenuates experimental murine colitis through modulation of immunity and microbiota composition. Clin Exp Immunol 2011;163(2): 250–9.
35. Arpaia N, Campbell C, Fan X, et al. Metabolites produced by commensal bacteria promote peripheral regulatory T-cell generation. Nature 2013;504(7480): 451–5.
36. Furusawa Y, Obata Y, Fukuda S, et al. Commensal microbe-derived butyrate induces the differentiation of colonic regulatory T cells. Nature 2013;504(7480): 446–50.
37. Round JL, Mazmanian SK. The gut microbiota shapes intestinal immune responses during health and disease. Nat Rev Immunol 2009;9(5):313–23.
38. Sefik E, Geva-Zatorsky N, Oh S, et al. Mucosal immunology. Individual intestinal symbionts induce a distinct population of RORgamma(+) regulatory T cells. Science 2015;349(6251):993–7.
39. Ivanov II, Atarashi K, Manel N, et al. Induction of intestinal Th17 cells by segmented filamentous bacteria. Cell 2009;139(3):485–98.
40. Kanther M, Tomkovich S, Xiaolun S, et al. Commensal microbiota stimulate systemic neutrophil migration through induction of serum amyloid A. Cell Microbiol 2014;16(7):1053–67.
41. Yanai H, Salomon N, Lahat A. Complementary therapies in inflammatory bowel diseases. Curr Gastroenterol Rep 2016;18(12):62.
42. Koning M, Ailabouni R, Gearry RB, et al. Use and predictors of oral complementary and alternative medicine by patients with inflammatory bowel disease: a population-based, case-control study. Inflamm Bowel Dis 2013; 19(4):767–78.
43. Opheim R, Bernklev T, Fagermoen MS, et al. Use of complementary and alternative medicine in patients with inflammatory bowel disease: results of a cross-sectional study in Norway. Scand J Gastroenterol 2012;47(12):1436–47.
44. Opheim R, Hoivik ML, Solberg IC, et al. Complementary and alternative medicine in patients with inflammatory bowel disease: the results of a population-based inception cohort study (IBSEN). J Crohns Colitis 2012;6(3):345–53.
45. Sirois FM. Health-related self-perceptions over time and provider-based complementary and alternative medicine (CAM) use in people with inflammatory bowel disease or arthritis. Complement Ther Med 2014;22(4):701–9.
46. Canfora EE, Jocken JW, Blaak EE. Short-chain fatty acids in control of body weight and insulin sensitivity. Nat Rev Endocrinol 2015;11(10):577–91.
47. Dore J, Blottiere H. The influence of diet on the gut microbiota and its consequences for health. Curr Opin Biotechnol 2015;32:195–9.
48. Fischbach MA, Sonnenburg JL. Eating for two: how metabolism establishes interspecies interactions in the gut. Cell Host Microbe 2011;10(4):336–47.
49. Krishnan S, Alden N, Lee K. Pathways and functions of gut microbiota metabolism impacting host physiology. Curr Opin Biotechnol 2015;36:137–45.
50. Le Chatelier E, Nielsen T, Qin J, et al. Richness of human gut microbiome correlates with metabolic markers. Nature 2013;500(7464):541–6.
51. Dao MC, Everard A, Aron-Wisnewsky J, et al. Akkermansia muciniphila and improved metabolic health during a dietary intervention in obesity: relationship with gut microbiome richness and ecology. Gut 2016;65(3):426–36.

52. Biesalski HK, Aggett PJ, Anton R, et al. 26th Hohenheim Consensus Conference, September 11, 2010 Scientific substantiation of health claims: evidence-based nutrition. Nutrition 2011;27(10 Suppl):S1–20.
53. Sharma G, Prakash D. Phytochemicals of nutraceutical importance: do they defend against diseases. Phytochemicals of nutraceutical importance. Wallingford (CT): CAB International; 2014. p. 1–19.
54. Coppens P, Da Silva MF, Pettman S. European regulations on nutraceuticals, dietary supplements and functional foods: a framework based on safety. Toxicology 2006;221(1):59–74.
55. da Costa JoP. A current look at nutraceuticals – key concepts and future prospects. Trends in Food Science & Technology 2017;62:68–78.
56. Taylor CL. Regulatory frameworks for functional foods and dietary supplements. Nutr Rev 2004;62(2):55–9.
57. Scaldaferri F, Gerardi V, Lopetuso LR, et al. Gut microbial flora, prebiotics, and probiotics in IBD: their current usage and utility. Biomed Res Int 2013;2013: 435268.
58. Kommineni S, Bretl DJ, Lam V, et al. Bacteriocin production augments niche competition by enterococci in the mammalian gastrointestinal tract. Nature 2015;526(7575):719–22.
59. Thorburn AN, Macia L, Mackay CR. Diet, metabolites, and "western-lifestyle" inflammatory diseases. Immunity 2014;40(6):833–42.
60. Gibson GR, Roberfroid MB. Dietary modulation of the human colonic microbiota: introducing the concept of prebiotics. J Nutr 1995;125(6):1401–12.
61. Macfarlane S, Macfarlane GT, Cummings JH. Review article: prebiotics in the gastrointestinal tract. Aliment Pharmacol Ther 2006;24(5):701–14.
62. Cushing K, Alvarado DM, Ciorba MA. Butyrate and mucosal inflammation: new scientific evidence supports clinical observation. Clin Transl Gastroenterol 2015; 6:e108.
63. Kelly CJ, Zheng L, Campbell EL, et al. Crosstalk between microbiota-derived short-chain fatty acids and intestinal epithelial HIF augments tissue barrier function. Cell Host Microbe 2015;17(5):662–71.
64. Bordin M, D'Atri F, Guillemot L, et al. Histone deacetylase inhibitors up-regulate the expression of tight junction proteins. Mol Cancer Res 2004; 2(12):692–701.
65. Bindels LB, Walter J, Ramer-Tait AE. Resistant starches for the management of metabolic diseases. Curr Opin Clin Nutr Metab Care 2015;18(6):559–65.
66. Abrams SA, Griffin IJ, Hawthorne KM, et al. A combination of prebiotic short-and long-chain inulin-type fructans enhances calcium absorption and bone mineralization in young adolescents. Am J Clin Nutr 2005;82(2):471–6.
67. Kimball ES, Schneider CR, Wallace NH, et al. Agonists of cannabinoid receptor 1 and 2 inhibit experimental colitis induced by oil of mustard and by dextran sulfate sodium. Am J Physiol Gastrointest Liver Physiol 2006;291(2):G364–71.
68. Weaver CM, Martin BR, Nakatsu CH, et al. Galactooligosaccharides improve mineral absorption and bone properties in growing rats through gut fermentation. J Agric Food Chem 2011;59(12):6501–10.
69. Whisner CM, Martin BR, Schoterman MH, et al. Galacto-oligosaccharides increase calcium absorption and gut bifidobacteria in young girls: a double-blind cross-over trial. Br J Nutr 2013;110(07):1292–303.
70. Jakeman SA, Henry CN, Martin BR, et al. Soluble corn fiber increases bone calcium retention in postmenopausal women in a dose-dependent manner: a randomized crossover trial. Am J Clin Nutr 2016;104(3):837–43.

71. Guz-Mark A, Rinawi F, Egotubov O, et al. Pediatric-onset inflammatory bowel disease poses risk for low bone mineral density at early adulthood. Dig Liver Dis 2017;49(6):639–42.
72. Schüle S, Rossel JB, Frey D, et al. Prediction of low bone mineral density in patients with inflammatory bowel diseases. United Eur Gastroenterol J 2016;4(5): 669–76.
73. Zhao X, Zhou C, Chen H, et al. Efficacy and safety of medical therapy for low bone mineral density in patients with Crohn disease: a systematic review with network meta-analysis. Medicine (Baltimore) 2017;96(11):e6378.
74. Conlon MA, Kerr CA, McSweeney CS, et al. Resistant starches protect against colonic DNA damage and alter microbiota and gene expression in rats fed a Western diet. J Nutr 2012;142(5):832–40.
75. Kleessen B, Stoof G, Proll J, et al. Feeding resistant starch affects fecal and cecal microflora and short-chain fatty acids in rats. J Anim Sci 1997;75(9): 2453–62.
76. Wang X, Brown IL, Khaled D, et al. Manipulation of colonic bacteria and volatile fatty acid production by dietary high amylose maize (amylomaize) starch granules. J Appl Microbiol 2002;93(3):390–7.
77. Leitch EC, Walker AW, Duncan SH, et al. Selective colonization of insoluble substrates by human faecal bacteria. Environ Microbiol 2007;9(3):667–79.
78. Ze X, Duncan SH, Louis P, et al. Ruminococcus bromii is a keystone species for the degradation of resistant starch in the human colon. ISME J 2012;6(8): 1535–43.
79. Kanauchi O, Agata K, Fushiki T. Mechanism for the increased defecation and jejunum mucosal protein content in rats by feeding germinated barley foodstuff. Biosci Biotechnol Biochem 1997;61(3):443–8.
80. Kanauchi O, Suga T, Tochihara M, et al. Treatment of ulcerative colitis by feeding with germinated barley foodstuff: first report of a multicenter open control trial. J Gastroenterol 2002;37(Suppl 14):67–72.
81. Faghfoori Z, Navai L, Shakerhosseini R, et al. Effects of an oral supplementation of germinated barley foodstuff on serum tumour necrosis factor-alpha, interleukin-6 and -8 in patients with ulcerative colitis. Ann Clin Biochem 2011;48(Pt 3):233–7.
82. Hanai H, Kanauchi O, Mitsuyama K, et al. Germinated barley foodstuff prolongs remission in patients with ulcerative colitis. Int J Mol Med 2004;13(5):643–7.
83. Kanauchi O, Araki Y, Andoh A, et al. Effect of germinated barley foodstuff administration on mineral utilization in rodents. J Gastroenterol 2000;35(3): 188–94.
84. Mitsuyama K, Saiki T, Kanauchi O, et al. Treatment of ulcerative colitis with germinated barley foodstuff feeding: a pilot study. Aliment Pharmacol Ther 1998;12(12):1225–30.
85. Salminen S, Salminen E. Lactulose, lactic acid bacteria, intestinal microecology and mucosal protection. Scand J Gastroenterol Suppl 1997;222:45–8.
86. Hehemann J-H, Correc G, Barbeyron T, et al. Transfer of carbohydrate-active enzymes from marine bacteria to Japanese gut microbiota. Nature 2010; 464(7290):908–12.
87. Hehemann J-H, Kelly AG, Pudlo NA, et al. Bacteria of the human gut microbiome catabolize red seaweed glycans with carbohydrate-active enzyme updates from extrinsic microbes. Proc Natl Acad Sci U S A 2012;109(48): 19786–91.

88. Bindels LB, Delzenne NM, Cani PD, et al. Towards a more comprehensive concept for prebiotics. Nat Rev Gastroenterol Hepatol 2015;12(5):303–10.

89. Michel G, Nyval-Collen P, Barbeyron T, et al. Bioconversion of red seaweed galactans: a focus on bacterial agarases and carrageenases. Appl Microbiol Biotechnol 2006;71(1):23–33.

90. Thomas F, Hehemann JH, Rebuffet E, et al. Environmental and gut bacteroidetes: the food connection. Front Microbiol 2011;2:93.

91. Martens EC, Lowe EC, Chiang H, et al. Recognition and degradation of plant cell wall polysaccharides by two human gut symbionts. PLoS Biol 2011;9(12): e1001221.

92. He W, Fu L, Li G, et al. Production of chondroitin in metabolically engineered E. coli. Metab Eng 2015;27:92–100.

93. Zuo T, Cao L, Li X, et al. The squid ink polysaccharides protect tight junctions and adherens junctions from chemotherapeutic injury in the small intestinal epithelium of mice. Nutr Cancer 2015;67(2):364–71.

94. Zuo T, Cao L, Sun X, et al. Dietary squid ink polysaccharide could enhance SIgA secretion in chemotherapeutic mice. Food Funct 2014;5(12):3189–96.

95. Zuo T, Cao L, Xue C, et al. Dietary squid ink polysaccharide induces goblet cells to protect small intestine from chemotherapy induced injury. Food Funct 2015; 6(3):981–6.

96. Zuo T, He X, Cao L, et al. The dietary polysaccharide from Ommastrephes bartrami prevents chemotherapeutic mucositis by promoting the gene expression of antimicrobial peptides in Paneth cells. J Funct Foods 2015;12:530–9.

97. Lu S, Zuo T, Zhang N, et al. High throughput sequencing analysis reveals amelioration of intestinal dysbiosis by squid ink polysaccharide. J Funct Foods 2016;20:506–15.

98. Furlanetti AaM, Prata LF. Free and total GMP (glycomacropeptide) contents of milk during bovine lactation. Food Sci Technology (Campinas) 2003;23:121–5.

99. Barker HA. Amino acid degradation by anaerobic bacteria. Annu Rev Biochem 1981;50:23–40.

100. Mortensen PB, Holtug K, Bonnén H, et al. The degradation of amino acids, proteins, and blood to short-chain fatty acids in colon is prevented by lactulose. Gastroenterology 1990;98(2):353–60.

101. Neis EP, Dejong CH, Rensen SS. The role of microbial amino acid metabolism in host metabolism. Nutrients 2015;7(4):2930–46.

102. Nordgaard I, Mortensen PB, Langkilde AM. Small intestinal malabsorption and colonic fermentation of resistant starch and resistant peptides to short-chain fatty acids. Nutrition 1995;11(2):129–37.

103. Rasmussen HS, Holtug K, Mortensen PB. Degradation of amino acids to short-chain fatty acids in humans. An in vitro study. Scand J Gastroenterol 1988;23(2): 178–82.

104. Davila AM, Blachier F, Gotteland M, et al. Re-print of "Intestinal luminal nitrogen metabolism: role of the gut microbiota and consequences for the host". Pharmacol Res 2013;69(1):114–26.

105. Davila AM, Blachier F, Gotteland M, et al. Intestinal luminal nitrogen metabolism: role of the gut microbiota and consequences for the host. Pharmacol Res 2013; 68(1):95–107.

106. Requena P, Daddaoua A, Martínez-Plata E, et al. Bovine glycomacropeptide ameliorates experimental rat ileitis by mechanisms involving downregulation of interleukin 17. Br J Pharmacol 2008;154(4):825–32.

107. Brody EP. Biological activities of bovine glycomacropeptide. Br J Nutr 2000; 84(Suppl 1):S39–46.
108. Idota T, Kawakami H, Nakajima I. Growth-promoting effects of N-acetylneuraminic acid-containing substances on bifidobacteria. Biosci Biotechnol Biochem 1994;58(9):1720–2.
109. Yakabe T, Kawakami H, Idota T. Growth stimulation agent for bifidus and lactobacillus. Japanese patent. 1994;07–267866.
110. Sawin EA, De Wolfe TJ, Aktas B, et al. Glycomacropeptide is a prebiotic that reduces Desulfovibrio bacteria, increases cecal short-chain fatty acids, and is anti-inflammatory in mice. Am J Physiol Gastrointest Liver Physiol 2015; 309(7):G590–601.
111. Jimenez M, Cervantes-García D, Muñoz YH, et al. Novel mechanisms underlying the therapeutic effect of glycomacropeptide on allergy: change in gut microbiota, upregulation of TGF-β, and inhibition of mast cells. Int Arch Allergy Immunol 2016;171(3–4):217–26.
112. Hvas CL, Dige A, Bendix M, et al. Casein glycomacropeptide for active distal ulcerative colitis: a randomized pilot study. Eur J Clin Invest 2016;46(6):555–63.
113. Wernlund PG, Hvas CL, Christensen LA, et al. MON-PP058: randomised clinical trial: casein glycomacropeptide for active distal ulcerative colitis-a pilot study. Clin Nutr 34:S149.
114. Lull C, Wichers HJ, Savelkoul HF. Antiinflammatory and immunomodulating properties of fungal metabolites. Mediators Inflamm 2005;2005(2):63–80.
115. Valverde ME, Hernandez-Perez T, Paredes-Lopez O. Edible mushrooms: improving human health and promoting quality life. Int J Microbiol 2015;2015: 376387.
116. Wasser SP. Medicinal mushroom science: current perspectives, advances, evidences, and challenges. Biomed J 2014;37(6):345–56.
117. Cui J, Chisti Y. Polysaccharopeptides of coriolus versicolor: physiological activity, uses, and production. Biotechnol Adv 2003;21(2):109–22.
118. Ooi VE, Liu F. Immunomodulation and anti-cancer activity of polysaccharide-protein complexes. Curr Med Chem 2000;7(7):715–29.
119. Chang CJ, Lin CS, Lu CC, et al. Ganoderma lucidum reduces obesity in mice by modulating the composition of the gut microbiota. Nat Commun 2015;6:7489.
120. Jin M, Zhu Y, Shao D, et al. Effects of polysaccharide from mycelia of Ganoderma lucidum on intestinal barrier functions of rats. Int J Biol Macromol 2017;94:1–9.
121. Klupp NL, Chang D, Hawke F, et al. Ganoderma lucidum mushroom for the treatment of cardiovascular risk factors. Cochrane Database Syst Rev 2015;(2):CD007259.
122. Williamson G, Clifford MN. Role of the small intestine, colon and microbiota in determining the metabolic fate of polyphenols. Biochem Pharmacol 2017;139: 24–39.
123. TomÃ¡s-BarberÃ¡n FA, Selma MAV, EspÃ-n JC. Interactions of gut microbiota with dietary polyphenols and consequences to human health. Curr Opin Clin Nutr Metab Care 2016;19(6):471–6.
124. Dueñas M, Muñoz-González I, Cueva C, et al. A survey of modulation of gut microbiota by dietary polyphenols. Biomed Res Int 2015;2015:850902.
125. Uranga JA, López-Miranda V, Lombó F, et al. Food, nutrients and nutraceuticals affecting the course of inflammatory bowel disease. Pharmacol Rep 2016;68(4): 816–26.

126. Yang N, Sampathkumar K, Loo SC. Recent advances in complementary and replacement therapy with nutraceuticals in combating gastrointestinal illnesses. Clin Nutr 2017;36(4):968–79.

127. Cardona F, Andrés-Lacueva C, Tulipani S, et al. Benefits of polyphenols on gut microbiota and implications in human health. J Nutr Biochem 2013;24(8): 1415–22.

128. Ikarashi N, Ogawa S, Hirobe R, et al. Epigallocatechin gallate induces a hepatospecific decrease in the CYP3A expression level by altering intestinal flora. Eur J Pharm Sci 2017;100:211–8.

129. Oz HS, Chen T, de Villiers WJ. Green tea polyphenols and sulfasalazine have parallel anti-inflammatory properties in colitis models. Front Immunol 2013;4: 132.

130. Steinmann J, Buer J, Pietschmann T, et al. Anti-infective properties of epigallocatechin-3-gallate (EGCG), a component of green tea. Br J Pharmacol 2013;168(5):1059–73.

131. Unno T, Sakuma M, Mitsuhashi S. Effect of dietary supplementation of (-)-epigallocatechin gallate on gut microbiota and biomarkers of colonic fermentation in rats. J Nutr Sci Vitaminol (Tokyo) 2014;60(3):213–9.

132. Henning SM, Summanen PH, Lee RP, et al. Pomegranate ellagitannins stimulate the growth of Akkermansia muciniphila in vivo. Anaerobe 2017;43:56–60.

133. Landete JM, Arqués J, Medina M, et al. Bioactivation of phytoestrogens: intestinal bacteria and health. Crit Rev Food Sci Nutr 2016;56(11):1826–43.

134. Chen L, Tai WCS, Hsiao WLW. Dietary saponins from four popular herbal tea exert prebiotic-like effects on gut microbiota in C57BL/6 mice. J Funct Foods 2015;17:892–902.

135. Li Z, Henning SM, Lee RP, et al. Pomegranate extract induces ellagitannin metabolite formation and changes stool microbiota in healthy volunteers. Food Funct 2015;6(8):2487–95.

136. Barroso E, Muñoz-González I, Jiménez E, et al. Phylogenetic profile of gut microbiota in healthy adults after moderate intake of red wine. Mol Nutr Food Res 2017;61(3).

137. Cueva C, Gil-Sánchez I, Ayuda-Durán B, et al. An integrated view of the effects of wine polyphenols and their relevant metabolites on gut and host health. Molecules 2017;22(1) [pii:E99].

138. Ghouri YA, Richards DM, Rahimi EF, et al. Systematic review of randomized controlled trials of probiotics, prebiotics, and synbiotics in inflammatory bowel disease. Clin Exp Gastroenterol 2014;7:473–87.

139. Parkar SG, Stevenson DE, Skinner MA. The potential influence of fruit polyphenols on colonic microflora and human gut health. Int J Food Microbiol 2008; 124(3):295–8.

140. Remely M, Ferk F, Sterneder S, et al. EGCG prevents high fat diet-induced changes in gut microbiota, decreases of DNA strand breaks, and changes in expression and DNA methylation of Dnmt1 and MLH1 in C57BL/6J male mice. Oxidative Med Cell Longevity 2017;2017:3079148.

141. Sheflin AM, Melby CL, Carbonero F, et al. Linking dietary patterns with gut microbial composition and function. Gut Microbes 2017;8(2):113–29.

142. Smoliga JM, Blanchard O. Enhancing the delivery of resveratrol in humans: if low bioavailability is the problem, what is the solution? Molecules 2014;19(11): 17154–72.

143. Stevens JF, Maier CS. The chemistry of gut microbial metabolism of polyphenols. Phytochem Rev 2016;15(3):425–44.

144. Duda-Chodak A. The inhibitory effect of polyphenols on human gut microbiota. J Physiol Pharmacol 2012;63(5):497–503.
145. Duda-Chodak A, Tarko T, Satora P, et al. Interaction of dietary compounds, especially polyphenols, with the intestinal microbiota: a review. Eur J Nutr 2015;54(3):325–41.
146. Hervert-Hernandez D, Goñi I. Dietary polyphenols and human gut microbiota: a review. Food Rev Int 2011;27(2):154–69.
147. Laparra JMS, Sanz Y. Interactions of gut microbiota with functional food components and nutraceuticals. Pharmacol Res 2010;61(3):219–25.
148. Camuesco D, Comalada M, Concha A, et al. Intestinal anti-inflammatory activity of combined quercitrin and dietary olive oil supplemented with fish oil, rich in EPA and DHA (n-3) polyunsaturated fatty acids, in rats with DSS-induced colitis. Clin Nutr 2006;25(3):466–76.
149. Li W, Wang QL, Liu X, et al. Combined use of vitamin D3 and metformin exhibits synergistic chemopreventive effects on colorectal neoplasia in rats and mice. Cancer Prev Res (Phila) 2015;8(2):139–48.
150. Patten GS, Augustin MA, Sanguansri L, et al. Site specific delivery of microencapsulated fish oil to the gastrointestinal tract of the rat. Dig Dis Sci 2009;54(3): 511–21.
151. Zator ZA, Cantu SM, Konijeti GG, et al. Pretreatment 25-hydroxyvitamin D levels and durability of anti-tumor necrosis factor-alpha therapy in inflammatory bowel diseases. JPEN J Parenter Enteral Nutr 2014;38(3):385–91.
152. Goff JP, Koszewski NJ, Haynes JS, et al. Targeted delivery of vitamin D to the colon using beta-glucuronides of vitamin D: therapeutic effects in a murine model of inflammatory bowel disease. Am J Physiol Gastrointest Liver Physiol 2012;302(4):G460–9.
153. Woloszynska-Read A, Johnson CS, Trump DL. Vitamin D and cancer: clinical aspects. Best Pract Res Clin Endocrinol Metab 2011;25(4):605–15.
154. Dhaneshwar SS, Kandpal M, Vadnerkar G. L-glutamine conjugate of meselamine: a novel approach for targeted delivery to colon. J Drug Deliv Sci Technol 2009;19(1):67–72.
155. Teng Z, Luo Y, Wang Q. Carboxymethyl chitosan-soy protein complex nanoparticles for the encapsulation and controlled release of vitamin D(3). Food Chem 2013;141(1):524–32.
156. Das S, Ng KY. Colon-specific delivery of resveratrol: optimization of multiparticulate calcium-pectinate carrier. Int J Pharm 2010;385(1–2):20–8.
157. Almouazen E, Bourgeois S, Jordheim LP, et al. Nano-encapsulation of vitamin D3 active metabolites for application in chemotherapy: formulation study and in vitro evaluation. Pharm Res 2013;30(4):1137–46.
158. Beloqui A, Coco R, Memvanga PB, et al. pH-sensitive nanoparticles for colonic delivery of curcumin in inflammatory bowel disease. Int J Pharm 2014;473(1–2): 203–12.
159. Sareen R, Nath K, Jain N, et al. Curcumin loaded microsponges for colon targeting in inflammatory bowel disease: fabrication, optimization, and in vitro and pharmacodynamic evaluation. Biomed Res Int 2014;2014:340701.
160. Coradini K, Friedrich RB, Fonseca FN, et al. A novel approach to arthritis treatment based on resveratrol and curcumin co-encapsulated in lipid-core nanocapsules: in vivo studies. Eur J Pharm Sci 2015;78:163–70.
161. Aditya NP, Aditya S, Yang H, et al. Co-delivery of hydrophobic curcumin and hydrophilic catechin by a water-in-oil-in-water double emulsion. Food Chem 2015; 173:7–13.

162. Li Q, Zhai W, Jiang Q, et al. Curcumin-piperine mixtures in self-microemulsifying drug delivery system for ulcerative colitis therapy. Int J Pharm 2015;490(1–2): 22–31.

163. Tavano L, Muzzalupo R, Picci N, et al. Co-encapsulation of antioxidants into niosomal carriers: gastrointestinal release studies for nutraceutical applications. Colloids Surf B Biointerfaces 2014;114:82–8.

164. Ganta S, Amiji M. Coadministration of paclitaxel and curcumin in nanoemulsion formulations to overcome multidrug resistance in tumor cells. Mol Pharm 2009; 6(3):928–39.

165. Okuro PK, Thomazini M, Balieiro JCC, et al. Co-encapsulation of Lactobacillus acidophilus with inulin or polydextrose in solid lipid microparticles provides protection and improves stability. Food Res Int 2013;53(1):96–103.

166. Lee WL, Widjaja E, Loo SC. One-step fabrication of triple-layered polymeric microparticles with layer localization of drugs as a novel drug-delivery system. Small 2010;6(9):1003–11.

167. DiPatrizio NV, Piomelli D. Intestinal lipid-derived signals that sense dietary fat. J Clin Invest 2015;125(3):891–8.

168. DiPatrizio NV, Piomelli D. The thrifty lipids: endocannabinoids and the neural control of energy conservation. Trends Neurosci 2012;35(7):403–11.

169. Izzo AA, Sharkey KA. Cannabinoids and the gut: new developments and emerging concepts. Pharmacol Ther 2010;126(1):21–38.

170. Adami M, Frati P, Bertini S, et al. Gastric antisecretory role and immunohistochemical localization of cannabinoid receptors in the rat stomach. Br J Pharmacol 2002;135(7):1598–606.

171. Adami M, Zamfirova R, Sotirov E, et al. Gastric antisecretory effects of synthetic cannabinoids after central or peripheral administration in the rat. Brain Res Bull 2004;64(4):357–61.

172. Coruzzi G, Adami M, Guaita E, et al. Effects of cannabinoid receptor agonists on rat gastric acid secretion: discrepancy between in vitro and in vivo data. Dig Dis Sci 2006;51(2):310–7.

173. DiPatrizio NV. Endocannabinoids in the gut. Cannabis Cannabinoid Res 2016; 1(1):67–77.

174. Izzo AA, Mascolo N, Borrelli F, et al. Defaecation, intestinal fluid accumulation and motility in rodents: implications of cannabinoid CB1 receptors. Naunyn Schmiedebergs Arch Pharmacol 1999;359(1):65–70.

175. Izzo AA, Mascolo N, Pinto L, et al. The role of cannabinoid receptors in intestinal motility, defaecation and diarrhoea in rats. Eur J Pharmacol 1999;384(1):37–42.

176. Izzo AA, Fezza F, Capasso R, et al. Cannabinoid CB1-receptor mediated regulation of gastrointestinal motility in mice in a model of intestinal inflammation. Br J Pharmacol 2001;134(3):563–70.

177. Mathison R, Ho W, Pittman QJ, et al. Effects of cannabinoid receptor-2 activation on accelerated gastrointestinal transit in lipopolysaccharide-treated rats. Br J Pharmacol 2004;142(8):1247–54.

178. Klein TW, Newton C, Larsen K, et al. The cannabinoid system and immune modulation. J Leukoc Biol 2003;74(4):486–96.

179. Samson MT, Small-Howard A, Shimoda LM, et al. Differential roles of CB1 and CB2 cannabinoid receptors in mast cells. J Immunol 2003;170(10):4953–62.

180. Kulkarni-Narla A, Brown DR. Localization of CB1-cannabinoid receptor immunoreactivity in the porcine enteric nervous system. Cell Tissue Res 2000;302(1): 73–80.

181. Lynn AB, Herkenham M. Localization of cannabinoid receptors and nonsaturable high-density cannabinoid binding sites in peripheral tissues of the rat: implications for receptor-mediated immune modulation by cannabinoids. J Pharmacol Exp Ther 1994;268(3):1612–23.
182. Trautmann SM, Sharkey KA. The endocannabinoid system and its role in regulating the intrinsic neural circuitry of the gastrointestinal tract. Int Rev Neurobiol 2015;125:85–126.
183. Pertwee RG. Pharmacology of cannabinoid CB1 and CB2 receptors. Pharmacol Ther 1997;74(2):129–80.
184. Devane WA, Hanus L, Breuer A, et al. Isolation and structure of a brain constituent that binds to the cannabinoid receptor. Science 1992;258(5090):1946–9.
185. Cani PD, Plovier H, Van Hul M, et al. Endocannabinoids–at the crossroads between the gut microbiota and host metabolism. Nat Rev Endocrinol 2016;12(3):133–43.
186. De Petrocellis L, Di Marzo V. Non-CB1, non-CB2 receptors for endocannabinoids, plant cannabinoids, and synthetic cannabimimetics: focus on G-protein-coupled receptors and transient receptor potential channels. J Neuroimmune Pharmacol 2010;5(1):103–21.
187. Syed SK, Bui HH, Beavers LS, et al. Regulation of GPR119 receptor activity with endocannabinoid-like lipids. Am J Physiol Endocrinol Metab 2012;303(12):E1469–78.
188. Capasso R, Orlando P, Pagano E, et al. Palmitoylethanolamide normalizes intestinal motility in a model of post-inflammatory accelerated transit: involvement of CB(1) receptors and TRPV1 channels. Br J Pharmacol 2014;171(17):4026–37.
189. Izzo AA, Piscitelli F, Capasso R, et al. Peripheral endocannabinoid dysregulation in obesity: relation to intestinal motility and energy processing induced by food deprivation and re-feeding. Br J Pharmacol 2009;158(2):451–61.
190. Ben-Shabat S, Fride E, Sheskin T, et al. An entourage effect: inactive endogenous fatty acid glycerol esters enhance 2-arachidonoyl-glycerol cannabinoid activity. Eur J Pharmacol 1998;353(1):23–31.
191. Cani PD, Bibiloni R, Knauf C, et al. Changes in gut microbiota control metabolic endotoxemia-induced inflammation in high-fat diet-induced obesity and diabetes in mice. Diabetes 2008;57(6):1470–81.
192. Drucker DJ. Glucagon-like peptides. Diabetes 1998;47(2):159–69.
193. Lambert DM, Di Marzo V. The palmitoylethanolamide and oleamide enigmas: are these two fatty acid amides cannabimimetic? Curr Med Chem 1999;6(8):757–73.
194. Alhamoruni A, Wright KL, Larvin M, et al. Cannabinoids mediate opposing effects on inflammation-induced intestinal permeability. Br J Pharmacol 2012;165(8):2598–610.
195. Massa F, Marsicano G, Hermann H, et al. The endogenous cannabinoid system protects against colonic inflammation. J Clin Invest 2004;113(8):1202–9.
196. Storr MA, Keenan CM, Emmerdinger D, et al. Targeting endocannabinoid degradation protects against experimental colitis in mice: involvement of CB1 and CB2 receptors. J Mol Med (Berl) 2008;86(8):925–36.
197. Storr MA, Keenan CM, Zhang H, et al. Activation of the cannabinoid 2 receptor (CB2) protects against experimental colitis. Inflamm Bowel Dis 2009;15(11):1678–85.
198. Turcotte C, Chouinard F, Lefebvre JS, et al. Regulation of inflammation by cannabinoids, the endocannabinoids 2-arachidonoyl-glycerol and arachidonoyl-ethanolamide, and their metabolites. J Leukoc Biol 2015;97(6):1049–70.

199. Alhouayek M, Muccioli GG. Harnessing the anti-inflammatory potential of palmi-toylethanolamide. Drug Discov Today 2014;19(10):1632–9.
200. Borrelli F, Romano B, Petrosino S, et al. Palmitoylethanolamide, a naturally occurring lipid, is an orally effective intestinal anti-inflammatory agent. Br J Pharmacol 2015;172(1):142–58.
201. D'Argenio G, Petrosino S, Gianfrani C, et al. Overactivity of the intestinal endo-cannabinoid system in celiac disease and in methotrexate-treated rats. J Mol Med (Berl) 2007;85(5):523–30.
202. Di Marzo V, Izzo AA. Endocannabinoid overactivity and intestinal inflammation. Gut 2006;55(10):1373–6.
203. Esposito G, Capoccia E, Turco F, et al. Palmitoylethanolamide improves colon inflammation through an enteric glia/toll like receptor 4-dependent PPAR-alpha activation. Gut 2014;63(8):1300–12.
204. Guagnini F, Valenti M, Mukenge S, et al. Neural contractions in colonic strips from patients with diverticular disease: role of endocannabinoids and substance P. Gut 2006;55(7):946–53.
205. Ligresti A, Bisogno T, Matias I, et al. Possible endocannabinoid control of colo-rectal cancer growth. Gastroenterology 2003;125(3):677–87.
206. Smid SD. Gastrointestinal endocannabinoid system: multifaceted roles in the healthy and inflamed intestine. Clin Exp Pharmacol Physiol 2008;35(11):1383–7.
207. Muccioli GG, Naslain D, Bäckhed F, et al. The endocannabinoid system links gut microbiota to adipogenesis. Mol Syst Biol 2010;6:392.
208. Rousseaux C, Thuru X, Gelot A, et al. Lactobacillus acidophilus modulates intes-tinal pain and induces opioid and cannabinoid receptors. Nat Med 2007;13(1):35–7.
209. Everard A, Belzer C, Geurts L, et al. Cross-talk between Akkermansia mucini-phila and intestinal epithelium controls diet-induced obesity. Proc Natl Acad Sci U S A 2013;110(22):9066–71.
210. Everard A, Geurts L, Caesar R, et al. Intestinal epithelial MyD88 is a sensor switching host metabolism towards obesity according to nutritional status. Nat Commun 2014;5:5648.
211. Lal S, Prasad N, Ryan M, et al. Cannabis use amongst patients with inflamma-tory bowel disease. Eur J Gastroenterol Hepatol 2011;23(10):891–6.
212. Naftali T, Lev LB, Yablecovitch D, et al. Treatment of Crohn's disease with cannabis: an observational study. Isr Med Assoc J 2011;13(8):455–8.
213. Lahat A, Lang A, Ben-Horin S. Impact of cannabis treatment on the quality of life, weight and clinical disease activity in inflammatory bowel disease patients: a pilot prospective study. Digestion 2012;85(1):1–8.
214. Naftali T, Bar-Lev Schleider L, Dotan I, et al. Cannabis induces a clinical response in patients with Crohn's disease: a prospective placebo-controlled study. Clin Gastroenterol Hepatol 2013;11(10):1276–80.e1.
215. Kahan M, Srivastava A, Spithoff S, et al. Prescribing smoked cannabis for chronic noncancer pain: preliminary recommendations. Can Fam Physician 2014;60(12):1083–90.
216. Cani PD, Everard A. Talking microbes: when gut bacteria interact with diet and host organs. Mol Nutr Food Res 2016;60(1):58–66.
217. Banni S, Carta G, Murru E, et al. Krill oil significantly decreases 2-arachidonoyl-glycerol plasma levels in obese subjects. Nutr Metab (Lond) 2011;8(1):7.
218. Kim HJ, Li H, Collins JJ, et al. Contributions of microbiome and mechanical deformation to intestinal bacterial overgrowth and inflammation in a human gut-on-a-chip. Proc Natl Acad Sci U S A 2016;113(1):E7–15.

219. Kim J, Li Y, Watkins BA. Fat to treat fat: emerging relationship between dietary PUFA, endocannabinoids, and obesity. Prostaglandins Other Lipid Mediat 2013; 104-105:32–41.

220. Brown I, Cascio MG, Wahle KW, et al. Cannabinoid receptor-dependent and -independent anti-proliferative effects of omega-3 ethanolamides in androgen receptor-positive and -negative prostate cancer cell lines. Carcinogenesis 2010;31(9):1584–91.

221. Daniels GE. Psychiatric aspects of ulcerative colitis. N Engl J Med 1942;226(5): 178–84.

222. Murray CD. Psychogenic factors in the etiology of ulcerative colitis and bloody diarrhea. Am J Med Sci 1930;180(2):239–47.

223. Straker M. Ulcerative colitis: recovery of a patient with brief psychiatric treatment. Can Med Assoc J 1960;82:1224–7.

224. Sullivan AJ, Chandler CA. Ulcerative colitis of psychogenic origin: a report of six cases. Yale J Biol Med 1932;4(6):779–96.

225. Goldsmith DR, Rapaport MH, Miller BJ. A meta-analysis of blood cytokine network alterations in psychiatric patients: comparisons between schizophrenia, bipolar disorder and depression. Mol Psychiatry 2016;21(12):1696–709.

226. Abautret-Daly A, Dempsey E, Parra-Blanco A, et al. Gut-brain actions underlying comorbid anxiety and depression associated with inflammatory bowel disease. Acta Neuropsychiatr 2017;1–22 [Epub ahead of print].

227. Camilleri M, Madsen K, Spiller R, et al. Intestinal barrier function in health and gastrointestinal disease. Neurogastroenterol Motil 2012;24(6):503–12.

228. Matsunaga H, Hokari R, Ueda T, et al. Physiological stress exacerbates murine colitis by enhancing proinflammatory cytokine expression that is dependent on IL-18. Am J Physiol Gastrointest Liver Physiol 2011;301(3):G555–64.

229. Melgar S, Engström K, Jägervall A, et al. Psychological stress reactivates dextran sulfate sodium-induced chronic colitis in mice. Stress 2008;11(5): 348–62.

230. Singh S, Graff LA, Bernstein CN. Do NSAIDs, antibiotics, infections, or stress trigger flares in IBD? Am J Gastroenterol 2009;104(5):1298–313 [quiz: 1314].

231. Bangsgaard Bendtsen KM, Krych L, Sørensen DB, et al. Gut microbiota composition is correlated to grid floor induced stress and behavior in the BALB/c mouse. PLoS One 2012;7(10):e46231.

232. Lutgendorff F, Akkermans LM, Soderholm JD. The role of microbiota and probiotics in stress-induced gastro-intestinal damage. Curr Mol Med 2008;8(4): 282–98.

233. David LA, Maurice CF, Carmody RN, et al. Diet rapidly and reproducibly alters the human gut microbiome. Nature 2014;505(7484):559–63.

234. Sonnenburg ED, Smits SA, Tikhonov M, et al. Diet-induced extinctions in the gut microbiota compound over generations. Nature 2016;529(7585):212–5.

235. Wu GD, Chen J, Hoffmann C, et al. Linking long-term dietary patterns with gut microbial enterotypes. Science 2011;334(6052):105–8.

236. Magnusdottir S, Ravcheev D, de Crécy-Lagard V, et al. Systematic genome assessment of B-vitamin biosynthesis suggests co-operation among gut microbes. Front Genet 2015;6:148.

237. Rucker RB, Zempleni J, Suttie JW, et al. Handbook of vitamins. Boca Raton (FL): CRC Press; 2007.

238. Kau AL, Ahren PP, Goodman AL, et al. Human nutrition, the gut microbiome and the immune system. Nature 2011;474(7351):327–36.

239. Wallace TC, Marzorati M, Spence L, et al. New frontiers in fibers: innovative and emerging research on the gut microbiome and bone health. J Am Coll Nutr 2017;36(3):218–22.

240. Lee D, Albenberg L, Compher C, et al. Diet in the pathogenesis and treatment of inflammatory bowel diseases. Gastroenterology 2015;148(6):1087–106.

241. Dey N, Wagner VE, Blanton LV, et al. Regulators of gut motility revealed by a gnotobiotic model of diet-microbiome interactions related to travel. Cell 2015; 163(1):95–107.

242. Basson A, Trotter A, Rodriguez-Palacios A, et al. Mucosal interactions between genetics, diet, and microbiome in inflammatory bowel disease. Front Immunol 2016;7:290.

243. Donohoe DR, Garge N, Zhang X, et al. The microbiome and butyrate regulate energy metabolism and autophagy in the mammalian colon. Cell Metab 2011; 13(5):517–26.

244. Wanders D, Graff EC, Judd RL. Effects of high fat diet on GPR109A and GPR81 gene expression. Biochem Biophys Res Commun 2012;425(2):278–83.

245. Hoffmann C, Dollive S, Grunberg S, et al. Archaea and fungi of the human gut microbiome: correlations with diet and bacterial residents. PLoS One 2013;8(6):e66019.

246. De Filippo C, Cavalieri D, Di Paola M, et al. Impact of diet in shaping gut microbiota revealed by a comparative study in children from Europe and rural Africa. Proc Natl Acad Sci U S A 2010;107(33):14691–6.

247. Yatsunenko T, Rey FE, Manary MJ, et al. Human gut microbiome viewed across age and geography. Nature 2012;486(7402):222–7.

248. Attene-Ramos MS, Wagner ED, Plewa MJ, et al. Evidence that hydrogen sulfide is a genotoxic agent. Mol Cancer Res 2006;4(1):9–14.

249. Baron EJ, Summanen P, Downes J, et al. Bilophila wadsworthia, gen. nov. and sp. nov., a unique gram-negative anaerobic rod recovered from appendicitis specimens and human faeces. J Gen Microbiol 1989;135(12):3405–11.

250. Martinez-Medina M, Denizot J, Dreux N, et al. Western diet induces dysbiosis with increased E coli in CEABAC10 mice, alters host barrier function favouring AIEC colonisation. Gut 2014;63(1):116–24.

251. Jakobsdottir G, Xu J, Molin G, et al. High-fat diet reduces the formation of butyrate, but increases succinate, inflammation, liver fat and cholesterol in rats, while dietary fibre counteracts these effects. PLoS One 2013;8(11):e80476.

252. Mane J, Pedrosa E, Lorén V, et al. Partial replacement of dietary (n-6) fatty acids with medium-chain triglycerides decreases the incidence of spontaneous colitis in interleukin-10-deficient mice. J Nutr 2009;139(3):603–10.

253. Ohta N, Tsujikawa T, Nakamura T, et al. A comparison of the effects of medium- and long-chain triglycerides on neutrophil stimulation in experimental ileitis. J Gastroenterol 2003;38(2):127–33.

254. Tsujikawa T, Ohta N, Nakamura T, et al. Medium-chain triglycerides modulate ileitis induced by trinitrobenzene sulfonic acid. J Gastroenterol Hepatol 1999; 14(12):1166–72.

255. Clarke SF, Murphy EF, O'Sullivan O, et al. Exercise and associated dietary extremes impact on gut microbial diversity. Gut 2014;63(12):1913–20.

256. Wang Z, Klipfell E, Bennett BJ, et al. Gut flora metabolism of phosphatidylcholine promotes cardiovascular disease. Nature 2011;472(7341):57–63.

257. Lang DH, Yeung CK, Peter RM, et al. Isoform specificity of trimethylamine N-oxygenation by human flavin-containing monooxygenase (FMO) and P450 enzymes: selective catalysis by FMO3. Biochem Pharmacol 1998;56(8):1005–12.

258. Koeth RA, Wang Z, Levison BS, et al. Intestinal microbiota metabolism of L-carnitine, a nutrient in red meat, promotes atherosclerosis. Nat Med 2013; 19(5):576–85.

259. Paturi G, et al. Dietary combination of potato resistant starch and red meat up-regulates genes involved in colonic barrier function of rats. Int J Food Sci Technol 2013;48(11):2441–6.

260. Paturi G, Nyanhanda T, Butts CA, et al. Effects of potato fiber and potato-resistant starch on biomarkers of colonic health in rats fed diets containing red meat. J Food Sci 2012;77(10):H216–23.

261. De Filippis F, Pellegrini N, Vannini L, et al. High-level adherence to a Mediterranean diet beneficially impacts the gut microbiota and associated metabolome. Gut 2016;65(11):1812–21.

262. Cotillard A, Kennedy SP, Kong LC, et al. Dietary intervention impact on gut microbial gene richness. Nature 2013;500(7464):585–8.

263. Brugere JF, Borrel G, Gaci N, et al. Archaebiotics: proposed therapeutic use of archaea to prevent trimethylaminuria and cardiovascular disease. Gut Microbes 2014;5(1):5–10.

264. Horz HP. Archaeal lineages within the human microbiome: absent, rare or elusive? Life (Basel) 2015;5(2):1333–45.

265. Gaci N, Borrel G, Tottey W, et al. Archaea and the human gut: new beginning of an old story. World J Gastroenterol 2014;20(43):16062–78.

266. Le Marchand L, Wilkens LR, Harwood P, et al. Breath hydrogen and methane in populations at different risk for colon cancer. Int J Cancer 1993;55(6):887–90.

267. Nam YD, Chang HW, Kim KH, et al. Bacterial, archaeal, and eukaryal diversity in the intestines of Korean people. J Microbiol 2008;46(5):491–501.

268. Nava GM, Carbonero F, Ou J, et al. Hydrogenotrophic microbiota distinguish native Africans from African and European Americans. Environ Microbiol Rep 2012;4(3):307–15.

269. Segal I, Walker AR, Lord S, et al. Breath methane and large bowel cancer risk in contrasting African populations. Gut 1988;29(5):608–13.

270. Tyakht AV, Kostryukova ES, Popenko AS, et al. Human gut microbiota community structures in urban and rural populations in Russia. Nat Commun 2013;4: 2469.

271. Rucker RB, Steinberg FM, Johnston CS. Ascorbic acid, in handbook of vitamins. 4th edition. CRC Press; 2007.

272. Cantorna MT, Mahon BD. D-hormone and the immune system. J Rheumatol Suppl 2005;76:11–20.

273. Cantorna MT, Zhu Y, Froicu M, et al. Vitamin D status, 1,25-dihydroxyvitamin D3, and the immune system. Am J Clin Nutr 2004;80(6 Suppl):1717S–20S.

274. Lim WC, Hanauer SB, Li YC. Mechanisms of disease: vitamin D and inflammatory bowel disease. Nat Clin Pract Gastroenterol Hepatol 2005;2(7):308–15.

275. Jin D, Wu S, Zhang YG, et al. Lack of vitamin D receptor causes dysbiosis and changes the functions of the murine intestinal microbiome. Clin Ther 2015;37(5): 996–1009.e7.

276. Rehman A, Lepage P, Nolte A, et al. Transcriptional activity of the dominant gut mucosal microbiota in chronic inflammatory bowel disease patients. J Med Microbiol 2010;59(Pt 9):1114–22.

277. Appleyard CB, Cruz ML, Isidro AA, et al. Pretreatment with the probiotic VSL#3 delays transition from inflammation to dysplasia in a rat model of colitis-associated cancer. Am J Physiol Gastrointest Liver Physiol 2011;301(6): G1004–13.

278. Basson A. Vitamin D and Crohn's disease in the adult patient: a review. JPEN J Parenter Enteral Nutr 2014;38(4):438–58.
279. Jones ML, Martoni CJ, Prakash S. Oral supplementation with probiotic L. reuteri NCIMB 30242 increases mean circulating 25-hydroxyvitamin D: a post hoc analysis of a randomized controlled trial. J Clin Endocrinol Metab 2013;98(7): 2944–51.
280. Kornbluth A, Sachar DB. Ulcerative colitis practice guidelines in adults (update): American College of Gastroenterology, Practice Parameters Committee. Am J Gastroenterol 2004;99(7):1371–85.
281. Lichtenstein GR, Hanauer SB, Sandborn WJ. Management of Crohn's disease in adults. Am J Gastroenterol 2009;104(2):465–83 [quiz: 464, 484].
282. Turner D, Levine A, Escher JC, et al. Management of pediatric ulcerative colitis: joint ECCO and ESPGHAN evidence-based consensus guidelines. J Pediatr Gastroenterol Nutr 2012;55(3):340–61.
283. Owczarek D, Rodacki T, Domagała-Rodacka R, et al. Diet and nutritional factors in inflammatory bowel diseases. World J Gastroenterol 2016;22(3):895–905.
284. Hou JK, Lee D, Lewis J. Diet and inflammatory bowel disease: review of patient-targeted recommendations. Clin Gastroenterol Hepatol 2014;12(10):1592–600.
285. Brown S, Clastre M, Courdavault V, et al. De novo production of the plant-derived alkaloid strictosidine in yeast. Proc Natl Acad Sci U S A 2015; 112(11):3205–10.
286. Basson A. Nutrition management in the adult patient with Crohn's disease. South Afr J Clin Nutr 2016;25(4):164–72.
287. Donnellan CF, Yann LH, Lal S. Nutritional management of Crohn's disease. Therap Adv Gastroenterol 2013;6(3):231–42.
288. Halmos EP, Christophersen CT, Bird AR, et al. Diets that differ in their FODMAP content alter the colonic luminal microenvironment. Gut 2015;64(1):93–100.
289. Staudacher HM, Lomer MC, Anderson JL, et al. Fermentable carbohydrate restriction reduces luminal bifidobacteria and gastrointestinal symptoms in patients with irritable bowel syndrome. J Nutr 2012;142(8):1510–8.
290. Flanagan P, Campbell BJ, Rhodes JM. Bacteria in the pathogenesis of inflammatory bowel disease. Biochem Soc Trans 2011;39(4):1067–72.
291. Martin HM, Campbell BJ, Hart CA, et al. Enhanced Escherichia coli adherence and invasion in Crohn's disease and colon cancer. Gastroenterology 2004; 127(1):80–93.
292. Parsons BN, Wigley P, Simpson HL, et al. Dietary supplementation with soluble plantain non-starch polysaccharides inhibits intestinal invasion of Salmonella typhimurium in the chicken. PLoS One 2014;9(2):e87658.
293. Roberts CL, Keita AV, Parsons BN, et al. Soluble plantain fibre blocks adhesion and M-cell translocation of intestinal pathogens. J Nutr Biochem 2013;24(1): 97–103.
294. Zelante T, Iannitti RG, Cunha C, et al. Tryptophan catabolites from microbiota engage aryl hydrocarbon receptor and balance mucosal reactivity via interleukin-22. Immunity 2013;39(2):372–85.
295. Cohen SA, Gold BD, Oliva S, et al. Clinical and mucosal improvement with specific carbohydrate diet in pediatric Crohn disease. J Pediatr Gastroenterol Nutr 2014;59(4):516–21.
296. Kakodkar S, Farooqui AJ, Mikolaitis SL, et al. The specific carbohydrate diet for inflammatory bowel disease: a case series. J Acad Nutr Diet 2015;115(8): 1226–32.

297. Obih C, Wahbeh G, Lee D, et al. Specific carbohydrate diet for pediatric inflammatory bowel disease in clinical practice within an academic IBD center. Nutrition 2016;32(4):418–25.

298. Suskind DL, Wahbeh G, Gregory N, et al. Nutritional therapy in pediatric Crohn disease: the specific carbohydrate diet. J Pediatr Gastroenterol Nutr 2014; 58(1):87–91.

299. Chassaing B, Koren O, Goodrich JK, et al. Dietary emulsifiers impact the mouse gut microbiota promoting colitis and metabolic syndrome. Nature 2015; 519(7541):92–6.

300. Nickerson KP, Chanin R, McDonald C. Deregulation of intestinal anti-microbial defense by the dietary additive, maltodextrin. Gut Microbes 2015;6(1):78–83.

301. Galipeau HJ, McCarville JL, Huebener S, et al. Intestinal microbiota modulates gluten-induced immunopathology in humanized mice. Am J Pathol 2015; 185(11):2969–82.

302. Herfarth HH, Martin CF, Sandler RS, et al. Prevalence of a gluten-free diet and improvement of clinical symptoms in patients with inflammatory bowel diseases. Inflamm Bowel Dis 2014;20(7):1194–7.

303. Critch J, Day AS, Otley A, et al. Use of enteral nutrition for the control of intestinal inflammation in pediatric Crohn disease. J Pediatr Gastroenterol Nutr 2012; 54(2):298–305.

304. Lionetti P, Callegari ML, Ferrari S, et al. Enteral nutrition and microflora in pediatric Crohn's disease. JPEN J Parenter Enteral Nutr 2005;29(4 Suppl):S173–5 [discussion: S175–8, S184–8].

305. Shiga H, Kajiura T, Shinozaki J, et al. Changes of faecal microbiota in patients with Crohn's disease treated with an elemental diet and total parenteral nutrition. Dig Liver Dis 2012;44(9):736–42.

306. Ambrosio CMS, de Alancar SM, Moreno AM, et al. Antimicrobial activity of several essential oils on pathogenic and beneficial bacteria. Ind Crops Prod 2017;97:128–36.

307. Mimee M, Citorik RJ, Lu TK. Microbiome therapeutics - advances and challenges. Adv Drug Deliv Rev 2016;105(Pt A):44–54.

308. Corr SC, Li Y, Riedel CU, et al. Bacteriocin production as a mechanism for the antiinfective activity of Lactobacillus salivarius UCC118. Proc Natl Acad Sci U S A 2007;104(18):7617–21.

309. Millette M, Cornut G, Dupont C, et al. Capacity of human nisin- and pediocin-producing lactic Acid bacteria to reduce intestinal colonization by vancomycin-resistant enterococci. Appl Environ Microbiol 2008;74(7):1997–2003.

310. Walsh CJ, Guinane CM, Hill C, et al. In silico identification of bacteriocin gene clusters in the gastrointestinal tract, based on the Human Microbiome Project's reference genome database. BMC Microbiol 2015;15:183.

311. Zheng J, Gänzle MG, Lin XB, et al. Diversity and dynamics of bacteriocins from human microbiome. Environ Microbiol 2015;17(6):2133–43.

312. McCarville JL, Caminero A, Verdu EF. Novel perspectives on therapeutic modulation of the gut microbiota. Therap Adv Gastroenterol 2016;9(4):580–93.

313. Reyes A, Wu M, McNulty NP, et al. Gnotobiotic mouse model of phage-bacterial host dynamics in the human gut. Proc Natl Acad Sci U S A 2013;110(50): 20236–41.

314. Rodriguez-Valera F, Martin-Cuadrado AB, Rodriguez-Brito B, et al. Explaining microbial population genomics through phage predation. Nat Rev Microbiol 2009;7(11):828–36.

315. Minot S, Sinha R, Chen J, et al. The human gut virome: inter-individual variation and dynamic response to diet. Genome Res 2011;21(10):1616–25.
316. Norman JM, Handley SA, Baldridge MT, et al. Disease-specific alterations in the enteric virome in inflammatory bowel disease. Cell 2015;160(3):447–60.
317. Reyes A, Haynes M, Hanson N, et al. Viruses in the faecal microbiota of monozygotic twins and their mothers. Nature 2010;466(7304):334–8.
318. Mills S, Shanahan F, Stanton C, et al. Movers and shakers: influence of bacteriophages in shaping the mammalian gut microbiota. Gut Microbes 2013;4(1): 4–16.
319. Lepage P, Colombet J, Marteau P, et al. Dysbiosis in inflammatory bowel disease: a role for bacteriophages? Gut 2008;57(3):424–5.
320. Perez-Brocal V, García-López R, Vázquez-Castellanos JF, et al. Study of the viral and microbial communities associated with Crohn's disease: a metagenomic approach. Clin Transl Gastroenterol 2013;4:e36.
321. Wagner J, Maksimovic J, Farries G, et al. Bacteriophages in gut samples from pediatric Crohn's disease patients: metagenomic analysis using 454 pyrosequencing. Inflamm Bowel Dis 2013;19(8):1598–608.
322. Zhang T, Breitbart M, Lee WH, et al. RNA viral community in human feces: prevalence of plant pathogenic viruses. PLoS Biol 2006;4(1):e3.
323. Letarov A, Kulikov E. The bacteriophages in human- and animal body-associated microbial communities. J Appl Microbiol 2009;107(1):1–13.
324. Lu TK, Collins JJ. Engineered bacteriophage targeting gene networks as adjuvants for antibiotic therapy. Proc Natl Acad Sci U S A 2009;106(12):4629–34.
325. Edgar R, Friedman N, Molshanski-Mor S, et al. Reversing bacterial resistance to antibiotics by phage-mediated delivery of dominant sensitive genes. Appl Environ Microbiol 2012;78(3):744–51.
326. Westwater C, Kasman LM, Schofield DA, et al. Use of genetically engineered phage to deliver antimicrobial agents to bacteria: an alternative therapy for treatment of bacterial infections. Antimicrob Agents Chemother 2003;47(4): 1301–7.
327. Ando H, Lemire S, Pires DP, et al. Engineering modular viral scaffolds for targeted bacterial population editing. Cell Syst 2015;1(3):187–96.
328. Bikard D, Euler CW, Jiang W, et al. Exploiting CRISPR-Cas nucleases to produce sequence-specific antimicrobials. Nat Biotechnol 2014;32(11):1146–50.
329. Citorik RJ, Mimee M, Lu TK. Sequence-specific antimicrobials using efficiently delivered RNA-guided nucleases. Nat Biotechnol 2014;32(11):1141–5.
330. Gibson DG, Young L, Chuang RY, et al. Enzymatic assembly of DNA molecules up to several hundred kilobases. Nat Methods 2009;6(5):343–5.
331. Hagens S, Habel A, von Ahsen U, et al. Therapy of experimental pseudomonas infections with a nonreplicating genetically modified phage. Antimicrob Agents Chemother 2004;48(10):3817–22.
332. Kiro R, Shitrit D, Qimron U. Efficient engineering of a bacteriophage genome using the type I-E CRISPR-Cas system. RNA Biol 2014;11(1):42–4.
333. Riley PA. Bacteriophages in autoimmune disease and other inflammatory conditions. Med Hypotheses 2004;62(4):493–8.
334. Dabrowska K, Switała-Jeleń K, Opolski A, et al. Possible association between phages, Hoc protein, and the immune system. Arch Virol 2006;151(2):209–15.
335. Dabrowska K, Zembala M, Boratynski J, et al. Hoc protein regulates the biological effects of T4 phage in mammals. Arch Microbiol 2007;187(6):489–98.
336. Gorski A, Kniotek M, Perkowska-Ptasińska A, et al. Bacteriophages and transplantation tolerance. Transplant Proc 2006;38(1):331–3.

337. Gorski A, Nowaczyk M, Weber-Dabrowska B, et al. New insights into the possible role of bacteriophages in transplantation. Transplant Proc 2003; 35(6):2372–3.
338. Gorski A, Wazna E, Dabrowska BW, et al. Bacteriophage translocation. FEMS Immunol Med Microbiol 2006;46(3):313–9.
339. Gorski A, Weber-Dabrowska B. The potential role of endogenous bacterio-phages in controlling invading pathogens. Cell Mol Life Sci 2005;62(5):511–9.
340. Kniotek M, et al. Phages as immunomodulators of antibody production. Immu-nology 2004;33–7.
341. Miedzybrodzki R, Switala-Jelen K, Fortuna W, et al. Bacteriophage preparation inhibition of reactive oxygen species generation by endotoxin-stimulated poly-morphonuclear leukocytes. Virus Res 2008;131(2):233–42.
342. Pajtasz-Piasecka E, Rossowska J, Duś D, et al. Bacteriophages support anti-tumor response initiated by DC-based vaccine against murine transplantable colon carcinoma. Immunol Lett 2008;116(1):24–32.
343. Przerwa A, Zimecki M, Switała-Jeleń K, et al. Effects of bacteriophages on free radical production and phagocytic functions. Med Microbiol Immunol 2006; 195(3):143–50.
344. Gionchetti P, Rizzello F, Venturi A, et al. Oral bacteriotherapy as maintenance treatment in patients with chronic pouchitis: a double-blind, placebo-controlled trial. Gastroenterology 2000;119(2):305–9.
345. Henker J, Müller S, Laass MW, et al. Probiotic Escherichia coli Nissle 1917 (EcN) for successful remission maintenance of ulcerative colitis in children and adoles-cents: an open-label pilot study. Z Gastroenterol 2008;46(9):874–5.
346. Kruis W, Fric P, Pokrotnieks J, et al. Maintaining remission of ulcerative colitis with the probiotic Escherichia coli Nissle 1917 is as effective as with standard mesalazine. Gut 2004;53(11):1617–23.
347. Mimura T, Rizzello F, Helwig U, et al. Once daily high dose probiotic therapy (VSL#3) for maintaining remission in recurrent or refractory pouchitis. Gut 2004;53(1):108–14.
348. Sood A, Midha V, Makharia GK, et al. The probiotic preparation, VSL#3 induces remission in patients with mild-to-moderately active ulcerative colitis. Clin Gas-troenterol Hepatol 2009;7(11):1202–9, 1209.e1.
349. Vindigni SM, Zisman TL, Suskind DL, et al. The intestinal microbiome, barrier function, and immune system in inflammatory bowel disease: a tripartite patho-physiological circuit with implications for new therapeutic directions. Therap Adv Gastroenterol 2016;9(4):606–25.
350. Yadav V, Varum F, Bravo R, et al. Inflammatory bowel disease: exploring gut pathophysiology for novel therapeutic targets. Transl Res 2016;176:38–68.
351. Duan F, March JC. Engineered bacterial communication prevents Vibrio chol-erae virulence in an infant mouse model. Proc Natl Acad Sci U S A 2010; 107(25):11260–4.
352. Lagenaur LA, Sanders-Beer BE, Brichacek B, et al. Prevention of vaginal SHIV transmission in macaques by a live recombinant Lactobacillus. Mucosal Immu-nol 2011;4(6):648–57.
353. Steidler L, Hans W, Schotte L, et al. Treatment of murine colitis by Lactococcus lactis secreting interleukin-10. Science 2000;289(5483):1352–5.
354. Braat H, Rottiers P, Hommes DW, et al. A phase I trial with transgenic bacteria expressing interleukin-10 in Crohn's disease. Clin Gastroenterol Hepatol 2006; 4(6):754–9.

355. Vandenbroucke K, de Haard H, Beirnaert E, et al. Orally administered L. lactis secreting an anti-TNF nanobody demonstrate efficacy in chronic colitis. Mucosal Immunol 2010;3(1):49–56.
356. Bergstrom A, Skov TH, Bahl MI, et al. Establishment of intestinal microbiota during early life: a longitudinal, explorative study of a large cohort of Danish infants. Appl Environ Microbiol 2014;80(9):2889–900.
357. Maurice CF, Haiser HJ, Turnbaugh PJ. Xenobiotics shape the physiology and gene expression of the active human gut microbiome. Cell 2013;152(1–2): 39–50.
358. Morgan XC, Tickle TL, Sokol H, et al. Dysfunction of the intestinal microbiome in inflammatory bowel disease and treatment. Genome Biol 2012;13(9):R79.
359. Carmody RN, Gerber GK, Luevano JM Jr, et al. Diet dominates host genotype in shaping the murine gut microbiota. Cell Host Microbe 2015;17(1):72–84.
360. Voreades N, Kozil A, Weir TL. Diet and the development of the human intestinal microbiome. Front Microbiol 2014;5:494.
361. Zhang C, Zhang M, Pang X, et al. Structural resilience of the gut microbiota in adult mice under high-fat dietary perturbations. ISME J 2012;6(10):1848–57.
362. Motta JP, Bermúdez-Humarán LG, Deraison C, et al. Food-grade bacteria expressing elafin protect against inflammation and restore colon homeostasis. Sci Transl Med 2012;4(158):158ra144.
363. Bermudez-Humaran LG, Cortes-Perez NG, Lefèvre F, et al. A novel mucosal vaccine based on live Lactococci expressing E7 antigen and IL-12 induces systemic and mucosal immune responses and protects mice against human papillomavirus type 16-induced tumors. J Immunol 2005;175(11):7297–302.
364. Daniel C, Roussel Y, Kleerebezem M, et al. Recombinant lactic acid bacteria as mucosal biotherapeutic agents. Trends Biotechnol 2011;29(10):499–508.
365. Takiishi T, Korf H, Van Belle TL, et al. Reversal of autoimmune diabetes by restoration of antigen-specific tolerance using genetically modified Lactococcus lactis in mice. J Clin Invest 2012;122(5):1717–25.
366. Chen Z, Guo L, Zhang Y, et al. Incorporation of therapeutically modified bacteria into gut microbiota inhibits obesity. J Clin Invest 2014;124(8):3391–406.
367. Wang J, Guleria S, Koffas MA, et al. Microbial production of value-added nutraceuticals. Curr Opin Biotechnol 2016;37:97–104.
368. Fossati E, Ekins A, Narcross L, et al. Reconstitution of a 10-gene pathway for synthesis of the plant alkaloid dihydrosanguinarine in Saccharomyces cerevisiae. Nat Commun 2014;5:3283.
369. Hawkins KM, Smolke CD. Production of benzylisoquinoline alkaloids in Saccharomyces cerevisiae. Nat Chem Biol 2008;4(9):564–73.
370. Minami H, Kim JS, Ikezawa N, et al. Microbial production of plant benzylisoquinoline alkaloids. Proc Natl Acad Sci U S A 2008;105(21):7393–8.
371. Nakagawa A, Matsuzaki C, Matsumura E, et al. (R,S)-tetrahydropapaveroline production by stepwise fermentation using engineered Escherichia coli. Sci Rep 2014;4:6695.
372. Nakagawa A, Minami H, Kim JS, et al. A bacterial platform for fermentative production of plant alkaloids. Nat Commun 2011;2:326.
373. Zhang C, Liu L, Teng L, et al. Metabolic engineering of Escherichia coli BL21 for biosynthesis of heparosan, a bioengineered heparin precursor. Metab Eng 2012;14(5):521–7.
374. Jain N, Ramawat KG. Nutraceuticals and antioxidants in prevention of diseases. In: Natural products. Springer Berlin Heidelberg 2013; p. 2559–80.

375. Li X-R, Tian GQ, Shen HJ, et al. Metabolic engineering of Escherichia coli to produce zeaxanthin. J Ind Microbiol Biotechnol 2015;42(4):627–36.
376. Marienhagen J, Bott M. Metabolic engineering of microorganisms for the synthesis of plant natural products. J Biotechnol 2013;163(2):166–78.
377. Mora-Pale M, Sanchez-Rodriguez SP, Linhardt RJ, et al. Metabolic engineering and in vitro biosynthesis of phytochemicals and non-natural analogues. Plant Sci 2013;210:10–24.
378. Zhao J, Li Q, Sun T, et al. Engineering central metabolic modules of Escherichia coli for improving β-carotene production. Metab Eng 2013;17:42–50.
379. Mikkelsen MD, Buron LD, Salomonsen B, et al. Microbial production of indolyl-glucosinolate through engineering of a multi-gene pathway in a versatile yeast expression platform. Metab Eng 2012;14(2):104–11.
380. Bhan N, Cress BF, Linhardt RJ, et al. Expanding the chemical space of polyketides through structure-guided mutagenesis of Vitis vinifera stilbene synthase. Biochimie 2015;115:136–43.
381. Bhan N, Li L, Cai C, et al. Enzymatic formation of a resorcylic acid by creating a structure-guided single-point mutation in stilbene synthase. Protein Sci 2015; 24(2):167–73.
382. Juhas M. Horizontal gene transfer in human pathogens. Crit Rev Microbiol 2015; 41(1):101–8.
383. Soucy SM, Huang J, Gogarten JP. Horizontal gene transfer: building the web of life. Nat Rev Genet 2015;16(8):472–82.
384. Sola-Oladokun B, Culligan EP, Sleator RD. Engineered probiotics: applications and biological containment. Annu Rev Food Sci Technol 2017;8:353–70.
385. Hamady ZZ, Scott N, Farrar MD, et al. Xylan-regulated delivery of human keratinocyte growth factor-2 to the inflamed colon by the human anaerobic commensal bacterium Bacteroides ovatus. Gut 2010;59(4):461–9.
386. Hamady ZZ, Scott N, Farrar MD, et al. Treatment of colitis with a commensal gut bacterium engineered to secrete human TGF-beta1 under the control of dietary xylan 1. Inflamm Bowel Dis 2011;17(9):1925–35.
387. Seedorf H, Griffin NW, Ridaura VK, et al. Bacteria from diverse habitats colonize and compete in the mouse gut. Cell 2014;159(2):253–66.
388. Donaldson GP, Lee SM, Mazmanian SK. Gut biogeography of the bacterial microbiota. Nat Rev Microbiol 2016;14(1):20–32.
389. Cullen TW, Schofield WB, Barry NA, et al. Gut microbiota. Antimicrobial peptide resistance mediates resilience of prominent gut commensals during inflammation. Science 2015;347(6218):170–5.
390. Lee SM, Donaldson GP, Mikulski Z, et al. Bacterial colonization factors control specificity and stability of the gut microbiota. Nature 2013;501(7467):426–9.
391. Sonnenburg ED, Zheng H, Joglekar P, et al. Specificity of polysaccharide use in intestinal bacteroides species determines diet-induced microbiota alterations. Cell 2010;141(7):1241–52.
392. Wu M, McNulty NP, Rodionov DA, et al. Genetic determinants of in vivo fitness and diet responsiveness in multiple human gut Bacteroides. Science 2015; 350(6256):aac5992.
393. Earle KA, Billings G, Sigal M, et al. Quantitative imaging of gut microbiota spatial organization. Cell Host Microbe 2015;18(4):478–88.
394. Li H, Limenitakis JP, Fuhrer T, et al. The outer mucus layer hosts a distinct intestinal microbial niche. Nat Commun 2015;6:8292.
395. Nava GM, Friedrichsen HJ, Stappenbeck TS. Spatial organization of intestinal microbiota in the mouse ascending colon. ISME J 2011;5(4):627–38.

396. Van den Abbeele P, Belzer C, Goossens M, et al. Butyrate-producing Clostridium cluster XIVa species specifically colonize mucins in an in vitro gut model. ISME J 2013;7(5):949–61.
397. Auchtung JM, Robinson CD, Britton RA. Cultivation of stable, reproducible microbial communities from different fecal donors using minibioreactor arrays (MBRAs). Microbiome 2015;3:42.
398. Costello CM, Sorna RM, Goh YL, et al. 3-D intestinal scaffolds for evaluating the therapeutic potential of probiotics. Mol Pharm 2014;11(7):2030.
399. Lukovac S, Belzer C, Pellis L, et al. Differential modulation by Akkermansia muciniphila and Faecalibacterium prausnitzii of host peripheral lipid metabolism and histone acetylation in mouse gut organoids. MBio 2014;5(4) [pii:e01438-14].
400. Gladstone EG, Molineux IJ, Bull JJ. Evolutionary principles and synthetic biology: avoiding a molecular tragedy of the commons with an engineered phage. J Biol Eng 2012;6(1):13.
401. Springman R, Molineux IJ, Duong C, et al. Evolutionary stability of a refactored phage genome. ACS Synth Biol 2012;1(9):425–30.
402. Borody TJ, Campbell J. Fecal microbiota transplantation: techniques, applications, and issues. Gastroenterol Clin North Am 2012;41(4):781–803.
403. van Nood E, Vrieze A, Nieuwdorp M, et al. Duodenal infusion of donor feces for recurrent Clostridium difficile. N Engl J Med 2013;368(5):407–15.
404. Moayyedi P, Surette MG, Kim PT, et al. Fecal microbiota transplantation induces remission in patients with active ulcerative colitis in a randomized controlled trial. Gastroenterology 2015;149(1):102–9.e6.
405. Cammarota G, Ianiro G, Cianci R, et al. The involvement of gut microbiota in inflammatory bowel disease pathogenesis: potential for therapy. Pharmacol Ther 2015;149:191–212.
406. Pigneur B, Sokol H. Fecal microbiota transplantation in inflammatory bowel disease: the quest for the Holy Grail. Mucosal Immunol 2016;9(6):1360–5.
407. Reinisch W. Fecal microbiota transplantation in inflammatory bowel disease. Dig Dis 2017;35(1–2):123–6.
408. Colman RJ, Rubin DT. Fecal microbiota transplantation as therapy for inflammatory bowel disease: a systematic review and meta-analysis. J Crohns Colitis 2014;8(12):1569–81.
409. Rubin DT. Curbing our enthusiasm for fecal transplantation in ulcerative colitis. Am J Gastroenterol 2013;108(10):1631–3.
410. Angelberger S, Reinisch W, Makristathis A, et al. Temporal bacterial community dynamics vary among ulcerative colitis patients after fecal microbiota transplantation. Am J Gastroenterol 2013;108(10):1620–30.
411. Kump PK, Gröchenig HP, Lackner S, et al. Alteration of intestinal dysbiosis by fecal microbiota transplantation does not induce remission in patients with chronic active ulcerative colitis. Inflamm Bowel Dis 2013;19(10):2155–65.
412. Jiang ZD, Ajami NJ, Petrosino JF, et al. Randomised clinical trial: faecal microbiota transplantation for recurrent Clostridium difficile infection - fresh, or frozen, or lyophilised microbiota from a small pool of healthy donors delivered by colonoscopy. Aliment Pharmacol Ther 2017;45(7):899–908.
413. Cholapranee A, Ananthakrishnan AN. Environmental hygiene and risk of inflammatory bowel diseases: a systematic review and meta-analysis. Inflamm Bowel Dis 2016;22(9):2191–9.
414. Gent AE, Hellier MD, Grace RH, et al. Inflammatory bowel disease and domestic hygiene in infancy. Lancet 1994;343(8900):766–7.

415. Guarner F. Hygiene, microbial diversity and immune regulation. Curr Opin Gastroenterol 2007;23(6):667–72.
416. Koloski NA, Bret L, Radford-Smith G. Hygiene hypothesis in inflammatory bowel disease: a critical review of the literature. World J Gastroenterol 2008;14(2): 165–73.
417. Lloyd-Price J, Abu-Ali G, Huttenhower C. The healthy human microbiome. Genome Med 2016;8(1):51.
418. Robert S, Gysemans C, Takiishi T, et al. Oral delivery of glutamic acid decarboxylase (GAD)-65 and IL10 by Lactococcus lactis reverses diabetes in recent-onset NOD mice. Diabetes 2014;63(8):2876–87.
419. Petrof EO, Gloor GB, Vanner SJ, et al. Stool substitute transplant therapy for the eradication of Clostridium difficile infection: 'RePOOPulating' the gut. Microbiome 2013;1(1):3.
420. Petrof EO, Khoruts A. From stool transplants to next-generation microbiota therapeutics. Gastroenterology 2014;146(6):1573–82.
421. Ianiro G, Bibbò S, Scaldaferri F, et al. Fecal microbiota transplantation in inflammatory bowel disease: beyond the excitement. Medicine (Baltimore) 2014; 93(19):e97.

Dietary Therapies in Pediatric Inflammatory Bowel Disease
An Evolving Inflammatory Bowel Disease Paradigm

Erin R. Lane, MD, Dale Lee, MD, David L. Suskind, MD*

KEYWORDS

- Pediatrics • Inflammatory bowel disease • Ulcerative colitis • Crohn disease
- Enteral nutrition • Prebiotics • Dietary therapy

KEY POINTS

- Western diets, typically high in fat and sugar and low in fiber, have been associated with increased risk of developing inflammatory bowel disease (IBD).
- Exclusive enteral nutrition is the most robustly evaluated exclusion diet and has been shown to be effective for induction of clinical remission and mucosal healing.
- Whole foods exclusion diets, such as the specific carbohydrate diet, are promising dietary interventions for the treatment of pediatric IBD.
- Repeated nutritional assessments and targeted interventions are critical to promote adequate growth in children with IBD.

INTRODUCTION

Inflammatory bowel disease (IBD) is a heterogeneous group of immune-mediated chronic inflammatory diseases affecting the gastrointestinal tract. Ulcerative colitis (UC) and Crohn disease (CD) are the 2 primary phenotypes of IBD. UC is characterized by contiguous, circumferential, isolated colonic mucosal inflammation extending proximally from the rectum, whereas the stereotypical inflammation seen in CD is patchy, transmural, and may affect the gastrointestinal tract at any location.

Globally, the incidence of IBD has been rapidly increasing, supporting the hypothesis that environmental factors play a critical role in the pathogenesis of IBD.[1,2] Evidence of the strong environmental impact on disease development is supported

None of the authors have a conflict of interest in regard to this article except for D.L. Suskind who has written a patient handbook on nutrition in IBD, *Nutrition in Immune Balance*.
Department of Pediatrics, Division of Gastroenterology, Seattle Children's Hospital, University of Washington, 4800 Sandpoint Way Northeast, Seattle, WA 98105, USA
* Corresponding author.
E-mail address: David.Suskind@seattlechildrens.org

Gastroenterol Clin N Am 46 (2017) 731–744
http://dx.doi.org/10.1016/j.gtc.2017.08.012
0889-8553/17/© 2017 Elsevier Inc. All rights reserved.

by the observation of discordant incidence of IBD in industrialized compared with nonindustrialized countries, as well as the rising incidence of IBD in countries as they undergo demographic and economic development.[3,4] Similarly, children emigrating from countries of low IBD-prevalence to countries of high-IBD prevalence develop the same risk of developing IBD as their peers who have resided in high-IBD prevalence areas for many generations.[5] Among the potential environmental factors associated with the development of IBD, diet and its modulation of the intestinal microbiome are important areas of ongoing research that, because they are modifiable, make attractive targets for novel therapies.[6]

The etiologic factors of IBD are incompletely understood but recent data support the hypotheses that IBD results from a complex interplay of genetics, immune dysregulation, and environmental triggers. Current theories postulate that, in genetically predisposed individuals, pathologic alterations in the intestinal microbiome trigger an aberrant mucosal immune response, leading to the development of chronic intestinal inflammation. Such perturbations in the gut microbiome, often referred to as dysbiosis, are an essential factor in driving inflammation in IBD rather than merely a consequence of the chronic inflammation.[7] Abundant evidence supports the integral role the intestinal microbiome plays in the pathogenesis of IBD.[8–26] However, it is important to be aware of association versus causation in the study of these relationships.

Although advances in bioinformatics, genomics, and experimental models of IBD have identified how environmental factors, such as dietary exposures, contribute to the development of IBD, many questions remain. This article reviews the data supporting diet as a potential contributing factor in the pathogenesis of IBD and explores current knowledge on diet as a primary and adjunctive therapy for pediatric IBD.

ROLE OF DIET IN PATHOGENESIS OF INFLAMMATORY BOWEL DISEASE

Diet and nutrition play a critical role at many time points along the complex course of pediatric IBD, ranging from influencing the risk of developing disease to induction and maintenance of remission. In both retrospective and prospective cohort studies, specific dietary factors have been shown to either protect against or serve as risk factors for the development of IBD.[4,27–30] Although such studies inherently introduce some element of bias because they are based on dietary recalls, additional studies have supported these findings and proposed potential biological mechanisms.

Throughout different stages of life, diet seems to have a major influence on microbial composition and function, as well as influence the risk of developing IBD.[31] Early-life dietary exposures may play an important role in development of the intestinal microbiome and influence the risk of IBD. Infant diet has been shown to affect the composition of the intestinal microbiome and there seems to be an associated risk-reduction in development of IBD among infants who were breastfed.[32,33] A potential biological mechanism has been sought by evaluating the intestinal microbial alterations in breastfed versus formula-fed infants. Exclusively breastfed infants have been found to have increased numbers of Actinobacteria, whereas formula-fed infants have higher levels of γ-Proteobacteria.[34,35] Interestingly, intestinal microbiota of breastfed infants are significantly less diverse than formula-fed infants; however, their microbial genes demonstrated a more robust interaction with the host immune system, metabolism, and biosynthesis.[36] The cessation of breastfeeding and associated reduction in passage of maternal immunoglobulin (Ig)-A induces changes in the microbiome characteristic of an adult microbiome, including increased prominence of Firmicutes and Bacteroidetes; however, peak microbial diversity and microbiome stability is often not reached until adulthood.[37–39]

Dietary exposures in childhood and later in life also have a significant effect on the development of IBD. Several large longitudinal studies have demonstrated an association between reduced risk of IBD and a diet high in fruits and vegetables, and an elevated risk of IBD in those who consumed diets rich in animal fats and refined sugars.[4,27,28] In addition, western diets high in fat have been demonstrated to increase risk of IBD; specifically, consumption of a high ratio of omega-6 fatty acids (proinflammatory) to omega-3 fatty acids (anti-inflammatory) has been associated with an increased incidence of UC.[27,40] A controlled study examining the effects of diet on the microbiome demonstrated that the composition of gut microbiota is changed dramatically by increases in dietary fat and decreases in dietary fiber compared with low-fat and high-fiber diets.[41] African children on traditional high-fiber diets demonstrate different gut microbiomes than their European peers, whose diets are typified by high-sugar, fat, and animal-protein.[42]

In an experimental model of colitis using interleukin (IL)-10 knock-out mice, diets rich in milk-derived saturated fat demonstrated increased incidence and severity of spontaneous colitis, suggesting a potential mechanistic link between the observed association between the proliferation of westernized diets and increased incidence of IBD globally.[43] Additionally, murine models of colitis (IL-10 knockout mice) fed common commercial food emulsifiers, carboxymethylcellulose and polysorbate-80, demonstrated thinning of the colonic mucosal layer, invasion of bacteria into the lamina propria, an altered microbiome, and worsening colitis.[44] Nickerson and colleagues[45] suggest a link between the increasing dietary prevalence of maltodextrin (MDX), a common starch-based food additive, and the rising incidence of CD. A series of experiments to uncover potential mechanisms demonstrated that exposure to MDX enhances mucosal adhesion and biofilm formation by *Escherichia coli*, including adherent-invasive *E coli*, and increases viability of intracellular Salmonella in mucosal macrophages and epithelial cells. Using this evidence, the investigators hypothesize that MDX may contribute to the development of IBD by priming the intestinal mucosal to be more sensitive to epithelial damage due to a reduction in epithelial antimicrobial defense mechanisms.[45]

Although abundant data support nutritional factors as having either proinflammatory or anti-inflammatory effect on the intestinal microbiome, further research is required to delineate the specific mechanism by which dietary alterations are useful in the treatment of IBD.

DIETARY INTERVENTIONS AS PRIMARY THERAPY FOR INFLAMMATORY BOWEL DISEASE
Exclusive Enteral Nutrition

Diet has been well-studied as a therapy for IBD. Perhaps the largest body of literature on use of diet as a specific therapy for IBD centers on the use of exclusive enteral nutrition (EEN). EEN is a formula-based, complete exclusion diet in which patients receive 100% of their daily calorie intake through either intact protein or semielemental or elemental formulas rather than from table foods. EEN has been shown to improve clinical symptoms, mucosal healing, and nutritional status in children with CD, with clinical remission rates equivalent to systemic corticosteroids.[46] A meta-analysis evaluating the efficacy of EEN versus corticosteroids for induction of remission in children with active CD identified 4 randomized controlled trials (RCTs). Although there was significant heterogeneity of duration of EEN (range 3–10 weeks) and type of formula (elemental, semielemental, or polymeric) used in EEN groups, a pooled analysis of RCTs suggested no difference in the percentage of children achieving remission (measured by disease activity scores) between those treated with EEN versus those treated with corticosteroids (risk ratio 0.96, 95% CI 0.6–1.14).[47] Although EEN may be equivalent to EEN corticosteroids in so far as induction of clinical remission, mucosal healing seems to be more robust with EEN than with corticosteroids.[46] Although the importance of achieving complete mucosal healing is well-documented in adults with CD, the significance in the pediatric population may be heightened given the timing of growth and development, as well as the future duration of disease.[48] Similar clinical results comparing the efficacy of EEN versus corticosteroids have not been reproduced in adults, although some investigators suggest that this finding may be a question of compliance versus efficacy.[49]

Given the many benefits of EEN for the treatment of pediatric CD, including improved adverse-effect profile over corticosteroids and beneficial effect on linear growth, recent expert consensus guidelines put forth by the North American Society for Pediatric Gastroenterology, Hepatology, and Nutrition (NASPGHAN) strongly recommend that EEN be considered as an effective induction therapy in newly diagnosed and active CD.[50] These guidelines also recommend use of EEN for a period of at least 8 weeks for induction of remission but acknowledge the benefits of EEN for longer durations (up to 12 weeks), especially for those children with growth failure or pubertal delay.[50–54]

Studies using metagenomics have demonstrated alterations in the intestinal microbiome before and after treatment with EEN as soon as 1 week after initiation.[55] Similarly, in a prospective, case-control study evaluating changes in fecal microbial diversity and metabolic activity of 15 children with CD treated with EEN, fecal microbiota diversity decreased, as did concentrations of previously identified commensal microbes.[56] These observations correlated with an improvement in clinical disease activity and reduction in inflammatory markers. Interestingly, these differences in the microbiome were more pronounced in study subjects who responded to EEN versus those who did not, potentially identifying biomarkers of disease phenotype and aiding future selection of individual patients who are more likely to respond to particular therapies. Noting that patients demonstrate variable responses to nutritional therapy, Frivolt and colleagues,[57] in a retrospective cohort analysis of children with CD treated with EEN for induction of remission, evaluated patient-specific genetic polymorphisms associated with a more robust response to EEN. Specifically, NOD2 genotypes associated with a poorer sustained response to EEN, measured by higher relapse rates at 1-year post-EEN, included 92% R702 W or G908 R versus 50% 1007 fs versus 60% wild-type ($P<.01$).[57]

Partial Enteral Nutrition

Although EEN for induction of remission is clearly beneficial for children with CD, it is often less feasible for long-term maintenance of remission. When combined with a regular diet, the addition of partial nutrition provided by formula, partial enteral nutrition (PEN), reduces the rate of CD relapse by 50%.[58] However, the efficacy in achieving clinical remission and mucosal healing is greatest when 100% EEN is used, rather than PEN.[59,60] In an RCT of children with active CD, those randomized to receive EEN versus PEN (defined as 50% of calories provided by formula), clinical remission rate with PEN was lower than that with EEN (15% vs 42%; $P = .035$).[61] Although clinical measures of disease activity, measured by the pediatric CD disease activity index (PCDAI) improved in both groups, the reduction in PCDAI with PEN was due to symptomatic and nutritional benefits. Only the group treated with EEN demonstrated a significant reduction in serologic measures of disease activity, including improvement in serum albumin and hemoglobin, and reduction in serum erythrocyte sedimentation rate.[61] Interestingly, changes to the composition of the intestinal micro-biome have not been demonstrated in children on PEN, suggesting that the changes to the microbiome seen with EEN may stem from exclusion of table foods rather than the addition of formula.[49]

Specific Carbohydrate Diet

Because patients find EEN prohibitively restrictive and difficult to maintain, there have been efforts to identify whole foods diets that may confer similar therapeutic benefit. One of the most studied whole foods exclusion diets for treatment of IBD is the specific carbohydrate diet (SCD). The SCD diet was developed by Dr Sydney Haas, a pediatrician in the 1930s who developed the diet as a treatment of celiac disease. This diet removes all grains, sweeteners except for honey, most processed foods, and all milk products except for hard cheeses and yogurt fermented longer than 24 hours, and was the primary treatment of celiac disease before the discovery of gluten as the offending antigen. The SCD diet was popularized by Elaine Gottschall as a treatment of IBD after her daughter's UC was successfully treated with the diet. In a survey of 417 subjects with IBD (47% CD, 43% UC) who used the SCD as a treatment, 33% self-reported clinical remission at 2 months after initiation of the SCD, and 42% at 6 and 12 months on the diet. For individuals who reported reaching remission, 47% of individuals reported associated improvement in abnormal laboratory values.[62] Suskind and colleagues[63] reported clinical remission in 7 children with active CD after initiation of the SCD diet without use of concomitant treatment. In addition to clinical remission, these children demonstrated significant improvement and normalization of inflammatory markers, including stool calprotectin. Cohen and colleagues[64] reported both clinical and mucosal improvements, documented with capsule endoscopy in 7 children with CD who used the SCD for 52 weeks. Additionally, a case series including more than 75 subjects with CD and UC, demonstrated clinical and laboratory improvement on SCD.[65]

In a recent prospective multicenter study of the SCD in pediatric subjects with mild to moderate CD or UC, 8 out of 12 subjects (aged 10–17 years) followed for 12 weeks demonstrated clinical remission, 2 out of 12 subjects did not improve, whereas 2 out of 12 individuals were unable to maintain the diet. Mean C-reactive protein decreased from 24.1 plus or minus 22.3 mg/L to 7.1 plus or minus 0.4 mg/L at 12 weeks in the Seattle cohort (nl<8.0 mg/L) and decreased from 20.7 plus or minus 10.9 mg/L to 4.8 plus or minus 4.5 mg/L at 12 weeks in the Atlanta cohort (nl<4.9 mg/L). Concomitant with clinical and laboratory improvements, significant changes in microbial composition occurred with the dietary change.[66]

Crohn Disease Exclusion Diet

Given the successes in clinical remission seen with the SCD diet, other exclusion diets have been used for reduction of inflammation and symptom improvement in IBD. The CD exclusion diet (CDED), designed and evaluated by a group in Israel led by Dr Arie Levine, is based on the hypothesis that the efficacy of EEN depends on exclusion of components of western diets that may promote a proinflammatory microbiome and potentiate intestinal permeability. The CDED focuses primarily on excluding processed foods, specifically excluding gluten, dairy, gluten-free baked goods, animal fat, processed meats, products containing emulsifiers, and all canned or processed foods. In a prospective cohort of pediatric and adult subjects with mild to moderate CD treated with 50% PEN and the CDED, Sigall-Boneh and colleagues[67] showed this exclusion diet was successful in achieving induction of clinical remission, including a reduction in inflammatory markers. Additionally, a small subgroup of

7 subjects treated with 100% of total daily calories from the CDED alone also achieved clinical remission.[67]

Inflammatory Bowel Disease–Anti-inflammatory Diet

The IBD–anti-inflammatory diet (IBD-AID) was developed by a group at University of Massachusetts Medical School, and is derived from the SCD. It is a whole foods–based diet that generally restricts the intake of complex carbohydrates, such as refined sugar, gluten-based grains, and certain starches from the diet, but also incorporates ingestion of prebiotics and probiotics. It also incorporates 4 phases of food textures, beginning with softened or pureed foods for patients with active inflammation or structuring phenotypes.[68] In a small, retrospective case-series of 11 adult subjects with CD and UC adherent to the IBD-AID diet for at least 4 weeks, all demonstrated improvement in reported clinical symptoms and reportedly all subjects were able to discontinue at least 1 prior IBD medication.[68] To date, however, there is a paucity of prospective data or application of IBD-AID in the pediatric population.

Other Exclusion Diets

It is well-known that individuals with both inflammatory and functional gastrointestinal disorders often report specific foods or elements of a standard western diet that trigger clinical symptoms. Many exclusion diets that have been less rigorously evaluated use this concept in promoting clinical remission or improvement in symptoms. Foods most frequently excluded due to intolerances included cereals, dairy products, and yeast. In a small cohort of adults with active CD, after induction with an elemental diet, those who excluded trigger foods had prolonged clinical remission and improvement in serum inflammatory markers compared with those who consumed a regular diet.[69] Similarly, an RCT found that, whereas IgG4-targeted exclusion diets for adults with active CD resulted in symptomatic improvement, no significant reduction in objective measures of inflammation, such as serum inflammatory markers, was observed.[70–72] In a small, prospective controlled study of adults with CD in clinical remission, Chiba and colleagues[73] demonstrated that a lacto-ovo-vegetarian diet resulted in reduction in relapse and prolongation of time to relapse versus a standard omnivorous diet. Although these exclusion diets hold promise for induction or maintenance of remission in CD, further research is necessary to characterize their effects on mucosal healing and alterations in the intestinal microbiome.

Other diets have shown clinical improvement in IBD patients but have been less rigorously evaluated with regard to reduction in inflammatory burden in IBD. Specifically, low-lactose diets have been shown to reduce clinical symptoms of IBD. Similarly, patients with IBD report symptom improvement on a low fermentable oligosaccharide, disaccharide, monosaccharide, and polyol (FODMAP) diet but there is a paucity of data that supports a reduction in intestinal mucosal inflammation.[74,75] Low-FODMAP diets have been found to reduce potentially favorable bacterial species within the colon, particularly *Faecalibacterium prausnitzii*, and reduced production of butyrate.[76] However, these alterations in the microbiome have unclear clinical consequences. Other restriction diets, such as the vegan and vegetarian diets, are popular among some patient populations. Zimmer and colleagues[77] demonstrated alterations in the ratios of *Bacteroides* spp, *Bifidobacterium* spp, and *Enterobacteriaceae* in patients adherent to vegan and vegetarian diets. Further studies are required before these restriction diets can be recommended in the treatment of IBD.

The mechanism by which exclusion diets reduce clinical symptoms and intestinal inflammation remains unclear; however, the growing numbers of animal and human studies have helped elucidate potential mechanisms by which alteration of dietary components helps or hinders treatment of intestinal inflammation. In general, studies evaluating the effects of diet in intestinal inflammation can be categorized into 2 broad categories: (1) exclusion of proinflammatory mediators and (2) inclusion of anti-inflammatory mediators. For example, it may be that restriction diets act through exclusion or inclusion of certain nutritional substrates that modulate the composition or function of the intestinal microbiome or mucosal immune system.[6,49]

Probiotics and Prebiotics

Several studies have evaluated the role of probiotics and prebiotics in induction and maintenance of remission in IBD. Probiotics, in general, have not shown clinical efficacy in the treatment of CD; however, there may be some role for the use of specific probiotics in the management of mild to moderate active UC or recurrent pouchitis after ileoanal anastomosis.[78] VSL#3 is 1 such probiotic formulation that contains a highly concentrated probiotic preparation of 8 different types of bacteria within the *Lactobacillus*, *Streptococcus*, and *Bifidobacterium* spp. In placebo-controlled trials, treatment with VSL#3 prevented recurrence of pouchitis.[79,80] Although data exist to support the limited utility of certain probiotics in the treatment of IBD, further studies are required to delineate the anti-inflammatory mechanism of probiotics in IBD.[81]

Prebiotics are dietary compounds that change the structure or metabolome of the intestinal microbiota. Inulin and oligofructose are 2 prebiotics that have been shown to promote the growth of beneficial *Bifidobacterium* and *lactobacillus* spp in humans and in rats.[82,83] Additionally, cellobiose and rice fiber are dietary-fiber sourced prebiotics that have been shown to reduce proinflammatory cytokines in experimental models of colitis; however, few studies examine the beneficial clinical effects of prebiotics in active IBD.[84] In a randomized, placebo-controlled study of adults with active CD, Benjamin and colleagues[85] evaluated changes in disease activity after administration of fructo-oligosaccharides (FOS). Despite some changes to immunoregulation of dendritic cells observed in those receiving FOS, no significant clinical improvements were seen nor were there significant changes to the fecal microbiome between the groups at baseline or after the 4-week intervention. Fermentable fiber, another form of prebiotic, is metabolized by colonic bacteria to short-chain fatty acids (SCFAs; ie, acetate, propionate, and butyrate), which are known to modulate cell proliferation, histone acetylation, gene expression, and immune response.[86] In adults with IBD, fecal samples demonstrated reduced concentrations of butyrate and acetate compared with healthy controls, suggesting that SCFA may play some protective role in the prevention of intestinal inflammation.[87] In animal models of IBD, supplementation with soluble fiber has been shown to reduce intestinal inflammation by increasing the production of SCFA and altering the intestinal microbiome.[88,89] Proposed mechanisms have stemmed from studies that have evaluated the immunomodulatory effects of SCFA in vivo as well as in animal models of colitis. SCFA-producing bacterial strains in Clostridia clusters IV, XIVa, and XVII from healthy individuals induce colonic CD4+ regulatory T cells (Tregs) differentiation, expansion, and function.[90] SCFA produced by *Clostridia* spp have been found to induce Tregs and reduce colitis in mouse models.[91,92] In humans, dietary fiber may reduce the risk of flare in patients with CD, although additional studies are required to recommend fiber supplementation as an anti-inflammatory therapy in IBD.[93]

DIETARY INTERVENTIONS AS ADJUNCTIVE THERAPY FOR INFLAMMATORY BOWEL DISEASE

IBD poses unique challenges in the pediatric age group because chronic inflammation places children at risk of growth failure, weight loss, pubertal delay, and impaired bone mineral density.[29] Growth failure is relatively common among children with CD and has been reported to affect 25% to 88% of children with CD at initial diagnosis and at follow-up during the course of the disease.[94] The development of malnutrition in children with IBD is often complex and may be secondary to several factors, including (1) reduced caloric intake, (2) malabsorption, and (3) increased metabolic demands due to chronic inflammation and altered metabolism.[95] Multiple studies suggest that energy needs of children with active CD may be increased above recommended dietary intakes by as little as 5% and as much as 35%, depending on nutritional status and degree of systemic inflammatory burden.[94] Additionally, linear growth and nutritional status may be influenced by the pharmacologic therapies used to treat IBD, corticosteroids being the most notable for their negative influence on linear growth velocity.[96] Early recognition of evolving poor nutritional status and aggressive intervention are critical to avoid irreversible consequences later in life.

In an effort to underscore the importance of early and frequent nutritional interventions in the treatment of pediatric IBD, the European Society for Pediatric Gastroenterology, Hepatology and Nutrition and NASPGHAN have established consensus clinical guidelines recommending frequent screening of nutritional status.[94,97] The recommended screening should occur at all clinical visits, and should include measurements of body weight, height, can calculation of body mass index. These data should be plotted on appropriate standardized growth charts and followed longitudinally.[94] Weight loss, poor weight gain, or deceleration of linear growth velocity should alert providers that aggressive nutritional intervention, or change in medical therapy should be considered.

For restoration of nutritional status in patients without contraindications to enteral intake, enteral nutrition is preferred over parenteral nutrition. As previously discussed, enteral nutrition is associated with multiple markers of remission, including improved clinical disease activity scores, mucosal healing, and downregulation of proinflammatory cytokines, as well as improved weight gain, linear growth, and overall nutritional status.[94,97–100] However, total parenteral nutrition (TPN) may be used as nutritional support in children with IBD when the enteral route either cannot be used or has been incompletely effective in supporting adequate nutritional status.[94] Additionally, TPN may be used as a primary nutritional therapy in pediatric patients with IBD to reduce postoperative complications in malnourished patients who are not candidates for enteral nutrition support.[94]

SUMMARY

The relationship between diet, nutrition, and pediatric IBD is complex. Dietary exposures may be responsible, in part, for promoting intestinal inflammation and establishment of disease, largely through alteration of the intestinal microbiome and mucosal immunity. As such, the manipulation of diet provides an intriguing mechanism for treatment of IBD. Strong evidence exists to support the use of EEN for both induction and maintenance of remission in pediatric IBD. EEN is the most well-studied, has been shown to be at least as efficacious as corticosteroids in inducing remission in pediatric CD, and remains an attractive therapy given its many benefits, including minimal side effects, advantages in terms of mucosal healing, restoration of nutritional status, improved bone health, and linear growth in children. Whole foods exclusion diets, such as the SCD diet, are gaining in popularity as the evidence grows to support their use in the treatment of pediatric IBD; however, further research is required.

REFERENCES

1. Miyoshi J, Chang EB. The gut microbiota and inflammatory bowel diseases. Transl Res 2017;179:38–48.
2. Loftus EV Jr. Clinical epidemiology of inflammatory bowel disease: incidence, prevalence, and environmental influences. Gastroenterology 2004;126: 1504–17.
3. Molodecky NA, Soon IS, Rabi DM, et al. Increasing incidence and prevalence of the inflammatory bowel diseases with time, based on systematic review. Gastroenterology 2012;142:46–54.e42 [quiz: e30].
4. Ananthakrishnan AN, Khalili H, Konijeti GG, et al. A prospective study of long-term intake of dietary fiber and risk of Crohn's disease and ulcerative colitis. Gastroenterology 2013;145:970–7.
5. Ponder A, Long MD. A clinical review of recent findings in the epidemiology of inflammatory bowel disease. Clin Epidemiol 2013;5:237–47.
6. Lee D, Albenberg L, Compher C, et al. Diet in the pathogenesis and treatment of inflammatory bowel diseases. Gastroenterology 2015;148:1087–106.
7. Hansen JJ, Sartor RB. Therapeutic manipulation of the microbiome in ibd: current results and future approaches. Curr Treat Options Gastroenterol 2015;13: 105–20.
8. Frank DN, Robertson CE, Hamm CM, et al. Disease phenotype and genotype are associated with shifts in intestinal-associated microbiota in inflammatory bowel diseases. Inflamm Bowel Dis 2011;17:179–84.
9. Morgan XC, Tickle TL, Sokol H, et al. Dysfunction of the intestinal microbiome in inflammatory bowel disease and treatment. Genome Biol 2012;13:R79.
10. Li J, Butcher J, Mack D, et al. Functional impacts of the intestinal microbiome in the pathogenesis of inflammatory bowel disease. Inflamm Bowel Dis 2015;21: 139–53.
11. Gevers D, Kugathasan S, Denson LA, et al. The treatment-naive microbiome in new-onset Crohn's disease. Cell Host Microbe 2014;15:382–92.
12. Frank DN, St Amand AL, Feldman RA, et al. Molecular-phylogenetic characterization of microbial community imbalances in human inflammatory bowel diseases. Proc Natl Acad Sci U S A 2007;104:13780–5.
13. Ott SJ, Musfeldt M, Wenderoth DF, et al. Reduction in diversity of the colonic mucosa associated bacterial microflora in patients with active inflammatory bowel disease. Gut 2004;53:685–93.
14. Manichanh C, Rigottier-Gois L, Bonnaud E, et al. Reduced diversity of faecal microbiota in Crohn's disease revealed by a metagenomic approach. Gut 2006;55: 205–11.
15. Fichera A, McCormack R, Rubin MA, et al. Long-term outcome of surgically treated Crohn's colitis: a prospective study. Dis Colon Rectum 2005;48:963–9.
16. Lee YK, Mazmanian SK. Has the microbiota played a critical role in the evolution of the adaptive immune system? Science 2010;330:1768–73.
17. Jostins L, Ripke S, Weersma RK, et al. Host-microbe interactions have shaped the genetic architecture of inflammatory bowel disease. Nature 2012;491: 119–24.

18. McGovern DP, Jones MR, Taylor KD, et al. Fucosyltransferase 2 (FUT2) non-secretor status is associated with Crohn's disease. Hum Mol Genet 2010; 19:3468–76.
19. Rausch P, Rehman A, Kunzel S, et al. Colonic mucosa-associated microbiota is influenced by an interaction of Crohn disease and FUT2 (Secretor) genotype. Proc Natl Acad Sci U S A 2011;108:19030–5.
20. Elinav E, Strowig T, Kau AL, et al. NLRP6 inflammasome regulates colonic microbial ecology and risk for colitis. Cell 2011;145:745–57.
21. Dheer R, Santaolalla R, Davies JM, et al. Intestinal epithelial toll-like receptor 4 signaling affects epithelial function and colonic microbiota and promotes a risk for transmissible colitis. Infect Immun 2016;84:798–810.
22. Sartor RB. Therapeutic manipulation of the enteric microflora in inflammatory bowel diseases: antibiotics, probiotics, and prebiotics. Gastroenterology 2004;126:1620–33.
23. Rietdijk ST, D'Haens GR. Recent developments in the treatment of inflammatory bowel disease. J Dig Dis 2013;14:282–7.
24. Perencevich M, Burakoff R. Use of antibiotics in the treatment of inflammatory bowel disease. Inflamm Bowel Dis 2006;12:651–64.
25. Saleh M, Trinchieri G. Innate immune mechanisms of colitis and colitis-associated colorectal cancer. Nat Rev Immunol 2011;11:9–20.
26. Kennedy RJ, Hoper M, Deodhar K, et al. Interleukin 10-deficient colitis: new similarities to human inflammatory bowel disease. Br J Surg 2000;87:1346–51.
27. Ananthakrishnan AN, Khalili H, Konijeti GG, et al. Long-term intake of dietary fat and risk of ulcerative colitis and Crohn's disease. Gut 2014;63:776–84.
28. Jantchou P, Morois S, Clavel-Chapelon F, et al. Animal protein intake and risk of inflammatory bowel disease: the E3N prospective study. Am J Gastroenterol 2010;105:2195–201.
29. Penagini F, Dilillo D, Borsani B, et al. Nutrition in pediatric inflammatory bowel disease: from etiology to treatment. A systematic review. Nutrients 2016;8:1–27.
30. Hou JK, Abraham B, El-Serag H. Dietary intake and risk of developing inflammatory bowel disease: a systematic review of the literature. Am J Gastroenterol 2011;106:563–73.
31. David LA, Maurice CF, Carmody RN, et al. Diet rapidly and reproducibly alters the human gut microbiome. Nature 2014;505:559–63.
32. Barclay AR, Russell RK, Wilson ML, et al. Systematic review: the role of breastfeeding in the development of pediatric inflammatory bowel disease. J Pediatr 2009;155:421–6.
33. Azad MB, Konya T, Maughan H, et al. Gut microbiota of healthy Canadian infants: profiles by mode of delivery and infant diet at 4 months. CMAJ 2013; 185:385–94.
34. Bezirtzoglou E, Tsiotsias A, Welling GW. Microbiota profile in feces of breast- and formula-fed newborns by using fluorescence in situ hybridization (FISH). Anaerobe 2011;17:478–82.
35. Penders J, Thijs C, Vink C, et al. Factors influencing the composition of the intestinal microbiota in early infancy. Pediatrics 2006;118:511–21.
36. Praveen P, Jordan F, Priami C, et al. The role of breast-feeding in infant immune system: a systems perspective on the intestinal microbiome. Microbiome 2015;3:41.
37. Backhed F, Roswall J, Peng Y, et al. Dynamics and stabilization of the human gut microbiome during the first year of life. Cell Host Microbe 2015;17:852.

38. Planer JD, Peng Y, Kau AL, et al. Development of the gut microbiota and mucosal IgA responses in twins and gnotobiotic mice. Nature 2016;534:263–6.
39. Lozupone CA, Stombaugh JI, Gordon JI, et al. Diversity, stability and resilience of the human gut microbiota. Nature 2012;489:220–30.
40. IBD in EPIC Study Investigators, Tjonneland A, Overvad K, Bergmann MM, et al. Linoleic acid, a dietary n-6 polyunsaturated fatty acid, and the aetiology of ulcerative colitis: a nested case-control study within a European prospective cohort study. Gut 2009;58:1606–11.
41. Wu GD, Chen J, Hoffmann C, et al. Linking long-term dietary patterns with gut microbial enterotypes. Science 2011;334:105–8.
42. De Filippo C, Cavalieri D, Di Paola M, et al. Impact of diet in shaping gut microbiota revealed by a comparative study in children from Europe and rural Africa. Proc Natl Acad Sci U S A 2010;107:14691–6.
43. Devkota S, Wang Y, Musch MW, et al. Dietary-fat-induced taurocholic acid promotes pathobiont expansion and colitis in Il10-/- mice. Nature 2012;487:104–8.
44. Chassaing B, Koren O, Goodrich JK, et al. Dietary emulsifiers impact the mouse gut microbiota promoting colitis and metabolic syndrome. Nature 2015;519:92–6.
45. Nickerson KP, Chanin R, McDonald C. Deregulation of intestinal anti-microbial defense by the dietary additive, maltodextrin. Gut Microbes 2015;6:78–83.
46. Borrelli O, Cordischi L, Cirulli M, et al. Polymeric diet alone versus corticosteroids in the treatment of active pediatric Crohn's disease: a randomized controlled open-label trial. Clin Gastroenterol Hepatol 2006;4:744–53.
47. Dziechciarz P, Horvath A, Shamir R, et al. Meta-analysis: enteral nutrition in active Crohn's disease in children. Aliment Pharmacol Ther 2007;26:795–806.
48. Baert F, Moortgat L, Van Assche G, et al. Mucosal healing predicts sustained clinical remission in patients with early-stage Crohn's disease. Gastroenterology 2010;138:463–8 [quiz: e10–11].
49. Lewis JD, Abreu MT. Diet as a trigger or therapy for inflammatory bowel diseases. Gastroenterology 2017;152:398–414.e6.
50. Critch J, Day AS, Otley A, et al. Use of enteral nutrition for the control of intestinal inflammation in pediatric Crohn disease. J Pediatr Gastroenterol Nutr 2012;54:298–305.
51. Newby EA, Sawczenko A, Thomas AG, et al. Interventions for growth failure in childhood Crohn's disease. Cochrane Database Syst Rev 2005;(3):CD003873.
52. Thomas AG, Taylor F, Miller V. Dietary intake and nutritional treatment in childhood Crohn's disease. J Pediatr Gastroenterol Nutr 1993;17:75–81.
53. Hannon TS, Dimeglio LA, Pfefferkorn MD, et al. Acute effects of enteral nutrition on protein turnover in adolescents with Crohn disease. Pediatr Res 2007;61:356–60.
54. Shamir R, Phillip M, Levine A. Growth retardation in pediatric Crohn's disease: pathogenesis and interventions. Inflamm Bowel Dis 2007;13:620–8.
55. Lewis JD, Chen EZ, Baldassano RN, et al. Inflammation, antibiotics, and diet as environmental stressors of the gut microbiome in pediatric Crohn's disease. Cell Host Microbe 2015;18:489–500.
56. Gerasimidis K, Bertz M, Hanske L, et al. Decline in presumptively protective gut bacterial species and metabolites are paradoxically associated with disease improvement in pediatric Crohn's disease during enteral nutrition. Inflamm Bowel Dis 2014;20:861–71.

57. Frivolt K, Schwerd T, Werkstetter KJ, et al. Repeated exclusive enteral nutrition in the treatment of paediatric Crohn's disease: predictors of efficacy and outcome. Aliment Pharmacol Ther 2014;39:1398–407.

58. Takagi S, Utsunomiya K, Kuriyama S, et al. Effectiveness of an 'half elemental diet' as maintenance therapy for Crohn's disease: a randomized-controlled trial. Aliment Pharmacol Ther 2006;24:1333–40.

59. Grover Z, Muir R, Lewindon P. Exclusive enteral nutrition induces early clinical, mucosal and transmural remission in paediatric Crohn's disease. J Gastroenterol 2014;49:638–45.

60. Lee D, Baldassano RN, Otley AR, et al. Comparative effectiveness of nutritional and biological therapy in north American children with active Crohn's disease. Inflamm Bowel Dis 2015;21:1786–93.

61. Johnson T, Macdonald S, Hill SM, et al. Treatment of active Crohn's disease in children using partial enteral nutrition with liquid formula: a randomised controlled trial. Gut 2006;55:356–61.

62. Suskind DL, Wahbeh G, Cohen SA, et al. Patients perceive clinical benefit with the specific carbohydrate diet for inflammatory bowel disease. Dig Dis Sci 2016; 61:3255–60.

63. Suskind DL, Wahbeh G, Gregory N, et al. Nutritional therapy in pediatric Crohn disease: the specific carbohydrate diet. J Pediatr Gastroenterol Nutr 2014;58: 87–91.

64. Cohen SA, Gold BD, Oliva S, et al. Clinical and mucosal improvement with specific carbohydrate diet in pediatric Crohn disease. J Pediatr Gastroenterol Nutr 2014;59:516–21.

65. Kakodkar S, Farooqui AJ, Mikolaitis SL, et al. The specific carbohydrate diet for inflammatory bowel disease: a case series. J Acad Nutr Diet 2015;115:1226–32.

66. Suskind DL, Cohen SA, Brittnacher MJ, et al. Clinical and fecal microbial changes with diet therapy in active inflammatory bowel disease. J Clin Gastroenterol 2016. [Epub ahead of print].

67. Sigall-Boneh R, Pfeffer-Gik T, Segal I, et al. Partial enteral nutrition with a Crohn's disease exclusion diet is effective for induction of remission in children and young adults with Crohn's disease. Inflamm Bowel Dis 2014;20:1353–60.

68. Olendzki BC, Silverstein TD, Persuitte GM, et al. An anti-inflammatory diet as treatment for inflammatory bowel disease: a case series report. Nutr J 2014; 13:5.

69. Riordan AM, Hunter JO, Cowan RE, et al. Treatment of active Crohn's disease by exclusion diet: East Anglian multicentre controlled trial. Lancet 1993;342: 1131–4.

70. Rajendran N, Kumar D. Food-specific IgG4-guided exclusion diets improve symptoms in Crohn's disease: a pilot study. Colorectal Dis 2011;13:1009–13.

71. Lee D, Suskind D. Individualized food-based dietary therapy for Crohn's disease: are we making progress? Dig Dis Sci 2016;61:958–60.

72. Gunasekeera V, Mendall MA, Chan D, et al. Treatment of Crohn's disease with an IgG4-guided exclusion diet: a randomized controlled trial. Dig Dis Sci 2016;61: 1148–57.

73. Chiba M, Abe T, Tsuda H, et al. Lifestyle-related disease in Crohn's disease: relapse prevention by a semi-vegetarian diet. World J Gastroenterol 2010;16: 2484–95.

74. Gearry RB, Irving PM, Barrett JS, et al. Reduction of dietary poorly absorbed short-chain carbohydrates (FODMAPs) improves abdominal symptoms in

patients with inflammatory bowel disease-a pilot study. J Crohns Colitis 2009;3: 8–14.

75. Prince AC, Myers CE, Joyce T, et al. Fermentable carbohydrate restriction (Low FODMAP Diet) in clinical practice improves functional gastrointestinal symptoms in patients with inflammatory bowel disease. Inflamm Bowel Dis 2016;22:1129–36.

76. Halmos EP, Christophersen CT, Bird AR, et al. Consistent prebiotic effect on gut microbiota with altered FODMAP intake in patients with Crohn's Disease: a randomised, controlled cross-over trial of well-defined diets. Clin Transl Gastroenterol 2016;7:e164.

77. Zimmer J, Lange B, Frick JS, et al. A vegan or vegetarian diet substantially alters the human colonic faecal microbiota. Eur J Clin Nutr 2012;66:53–60.

78. Mack DR. Probiotics in inflammatory bowel diseases and associated conditions. Nutrients 2011;3:245–64.

79. Gionchetti P, Rizzello F, Venturi A, et al. Oral bacteriotherapy as maintenance treatment in patients with chronic pouchitis: a double-blind, placebo-controlled trial. Gastroenterology 2000;119:305–9.

80. Mimura T, Rizzello F, Helwig U, et al. Once daily high dose probiotic therapy (VSL#3) for maintaining remission in recurrent or refractory pouchitis. Gut 2004;53:108–14.

81. Matsuoka K, Kanai T. The gut microbiota and inflammatory bowel disease. Semin Immunopathol 2015;37:47–55.

82. Guarner F. Prebiotics in inflammatory bowel diseases. Br J Nutr 2007;98(Suppl 1): S85–9.

83. Arribas B, Suarez-Pereira E, Ortiz Mellet C, et al. Di-D-fructose dianhydride-enriched caramels: effect on colon microbiota, inflammation, and tissue damage in trinitrobenzenesulfonic acid-induced colitic rats. J Agric Food Chem 2010;58:6476–84.

84. Nishimura T, Andoh A, Hashimoto T, et al. Cellobiose prevents the development of Dextran Sulfate Sodium (DSS)-Induced experimental colitis. J Clin Biochem Nutr 2010;46:105–10.

85. Benjamin JL, Hedin CR, Koutsoumpas A, et al. Randomised, double-blind, placebo-controlled trial of fructo-oligosaccharides in active Crohn's disease. Gut 2011;60:923–9.

86. Kim S, Kim JH, Park BO, et al. Perspectives on the therapeutic potential of short-chain fatty acid receptors. BMB Rep 2014;47:173–8.

87. Huda-Faujan N, Abdulamir AS, Fatimah AB, et al. The impact of the level of the intestinal short chain fatty acids in inflammatory bowel disease patients versus healthy subjects. Open Biochem J 2010;4:53–8.

88. Koleva PT, Valcheva RS, Sun X, et al. Inulin and fructo-oligosaccharides have divergent effects on colitis and commensal microbiota in HLA-B27 transgenic rats. Br J Nutr 2012;108:1633–43.

89. Joo E, Yamane S, Hamasaki A, et al. Enteral supplement enriched with glutamine, fiber, and oligosaccharide attenuates experimental colitis in mice. Nutrition 2013;29:549–55.

90. Atarashi K, Tanoue T, Shima T, et al. Induction of colonic regulatory T cells by indigenous clostridium species. Science 2011;331:337–41.

91. Xavier RJ. Microbiota as therapeutic targets. Dig Dis 2016;34:558–65.

92. Smith PM, Howitt MR, Panikov N, et al. The microbial metabolites, short-chain fatty acids, regulate colonic Treg cell homeostasis. Science 2013;341:569–73.

93. Brotherton CS, Martin CA, Long MD, et al. Avoidance of fiber is associated with greater risk of Crohn's disease flare in a 6-month period. Clin Gastroenterol Hepatol 2016;14:1130–6.

94. Kleinman RE, Baldassano RN, Caplan A, et al. Nutrition support for pediatric patients with inflammatory bowel disease: a clinical report of the North American Society for Pediatric Gastroenterology, Hepatology And Nutrition. J Pediatr Gastroenterol Nutr 2004;39:15–27.

95. Azcue M, Rashid M, Griffiths A, et al. Energy expenditure and body composition in children with Crohn's disease: effect of enteral nutrition and treatment with prednisolone. Gut 1997;41:203–8.

96. Gerasimidis K, McGrogan P, Edwards CA. The aetiology and impact of malnutrition in paediatric inflammatory bowel disease. J Hum Nutr Diet 2011;24:313–26.

97. Ruemmele FM, Veres G, Kolho KL, et al. Consensus guidelines of ECCO/ESPGHAN on the medical management of pediatric Crohn's disease. J Crohns Colitis 2014;8:1179–207.

98. Belli DC, Seidman E, Bouthillier L, et al. Chronic intermittent elemental diet improves growth failure in children with Crohn's disease. Gastroenterology 1988;94:603–10.

99. Sanderson IR, Udeen S, Davies PS, et al. Remission induced by an elemental diet in small bowel Crohn's disease. Arch Dis Child 1987;62:123–7.

100. Polk DB, Hattner JA, Kerner JA Jr. Improved growth and disease activity after intermittent administration of a defined formula diet in children with Crohn's disease. JPEN J Parenter Enteral Nutr 1992;16:499–504.

Diet as a Therapeutic Option for Adult Inflammatory Bowel Disease

 CrossMark

Samir Kakodkar, MD[a], Ece A. Mutlu, MD, MS, MBA[b],*

KEYWORDS

- Diet • Inflammatory bowel disease • Ulcerative colitis • Crohn's disease
- Specific carbohydrate diet • Low FODMAP diet • Exclusive enteral nutrition

KEY POINTS

- Diet can have an impact on inflammatory bowel disease (IBD) through multiple mechanisms.
- Exclusive enteral nutrition can be used to induce remission in adult Crohn's disease patients when corticosteroids are contraindicated.
- There is preliminary evidence to suggest efficacy of the Specific Carbohydrate Diet and the low FODMAP diet in IBD.

INTRODUCTION

There is suspicion that the pathogenesis of inflammatory bowel disease (IBD) may involve the Western diet which is known to be low in fruits and vegetables and high in fat, n-6 polyunsaturated fatty acids (PUFA) and red/processed foods.[1] Westernization has become a global phenomenon, this may explain why there is an increasing incidence of IBD in countries where it was previously rare.[2] Diet has not traditionally been part of the gastroenterologist's armamentarium against IBD that affects adults. In fact, many patients are informed that diet likely does not play any part in the development or perpetuation of inflammation, and there is no one particular diet that has been shown to be effective in treating IBD. Patients are often told, "Eat what you can tolerate." Despite this refrain, approximately 40% of patients with Crohn's disease (CD) believe that diet can control symptoms and approximately 80% believe diet is important in the overall management of disease.[3] In addition, 40% of patients with IBD have attempted various diets, often without the assistance of a physician or dietician.[4] There are now mechanisms posited to explain how foods can be both

---

[a] Divison of Gastroenterology and Hepatology, Northwestern University Feinberg School of Medicine, 420 East Superior Street, Chicago, IL 60611, USA; [b] Division of Digestive Diseases & Nutrition, Rush University Medical Center, 1725 West Harrison Street, Suite 206, Chicago, IL 60612, USA
* Corresponding author.
E-mail address: Ece_Mutlu@rush.edu

Gastroenterol Clin N Am 46 (2017) 745–767
http://dx.doi.org/10.1016/j.gtc.2017.08.016
0889-8553/17/© 2017 Elsevier Inc. All rights reserved.

proinflammatory and antiinflammatory. The resistance to adopting diet amongst gastroenterologists is multifactorial. It partly stems from lack of data demonstrating mucosal healing, which does not correlate well with perceived improvement in symptoms, particularly in CD. There is fear of causing more weight loss in a patient population that may already be malnourished, and implementing a dietary protocol may be too time consuming in a clinic setting. The belief that patients will jettison evidence-based medical therapy and instead adopt an unproven dietary intervention is particularly pervasive. These assumptions may be unsubstantiated. Diet deserves further consideration given the evidence assessed in this review.

It is not possible to fit all preclinical data and its potential implications into a single short article. It should be noted that current clinical data in dietary therapy for IBD is in its infancy, and randomized, clinical trials are largely lacking. In the absence of such data, we also present what we do in our clinics to generate a starting point or guide for clinicians who seek such information for their patients and for researchers coming into the field who are looking into new areas of investigation. Macronutrient associations with IBD are reviewed with an emphasis on the mechanistic basis behind how food contributes to intestinal inflammation. There are many diets described in the medical literature and lay press for IBD: the IgG-4 guided exclusion diet, the semivegetarian diet, the low-fat, fiber-limited exclusion diet, the paleolithic diet, the maker's diet, the vegan diet, and the low-carbohydrate diet.[5–11] This review predominantly focuses on exclusive enteral nutrition (EEN), which has the most robust evidence to support its use for inducing remission in CD, and the Specific Carbohydrate Diet (SCD), which perhaps already has the largest following among patients with IBD, and has some preliminary evidence published to support its efficacy. The Low FODMAP diet is also discussed because of its current widespread use in the IBS patient population and similar mechanism to the SCD.

MACRONUTRIENT ASSOCIATIONS WITH INFLAMMATORY BOWEL DISEASE

The association of carbohydrates, protein, fats, and fiber with IBD has been investigated. The evidence primarily comes from epidemiologic studies looking at dietary associations before the onset of IBD with only a few studies looking at flares in existing patients with IBD. Several general and systematic reviews have been published summarizing these epidemiologic associations of diet and IBD development.[1,12–15] Many of the studies suffer from recall and selection bias, small sample size, and short follow-up periods. The data is often conflicting and inconclusive. The current body of literature tends to consider only the macronutrient in question and does not attempt to control for confounders, which understandably would be a difficult undertaking. It is also premature to dismiss diet as a therapeutic tool just because there is not a consistent association among macronutrients with development of IBD; it does not necessarily mean limiting a macronutrient cannot help to alleviate symptoms or inflammation once the disease process has begun.

The Western diet, high in carbohydrates and refined sugars, has been shown to induce dysbiosis in mouse models. Furthermore, a diet composed of highly processed sugars and carbohydrates can lead to obesity, which is associated with a proinflammatory state and increased bowel permeability. There have been several studies published from the 1970s through the 1990s investigating the association between various classifications of carbohydrates and CD, and the results have been conflicting.[16] Unfortunately, almost all of these were retrospective, case-control studies subject to recall and selection bias. Patients were often asked to remember diets eaten years before diagnosis, and the accuracy of this data has been called into question. Most studies also did not subdivide carbohydrates into monosaccharides, disaccharides, oligosaccharides, and polysaccharides. There have been many studies investigating the association of sugar, that is, disaccharides and monosaccharides, with IBD with a trend toward showing a positive association, more so with CD, but also with ulcerative colitis (UC) to a lesser extent.[17–19] A much larger study by Chan and colleagues[20] addressed prior design weaknesses in a large prospective fashion using the EPIC-IBD study (Emerging Practice in IBD Collaborative) cohort from 8 European countries. The cohort of initially healthy subjects was given a validated food frequency questionnaire at recruitment to measure intake of carbohydrate, sugar, and starch during the previous year. Cases were identified as those subjects who subsequently developed IBD. Each case was compared with 4 controls who did not develop IBD. There was no association in univariate or multivariate analyses for carbohydrates or any dietary pattern with IBD risk when adjusted for total energy intake, body mass index, and cigarette smoking. However, in a subgroup analysis, there was a positive association between a "high sugar and soft drinks" pattern and UC when comparing the highest and lowest consumers, and the risk was present only if they also had low vegetable intakes.

Protein derived from meat, cheese, milk, fish, nuts, and eggs provides colonic bacteria with sulfate and sulfite, which are fermented to form hydrogen sulfide. This combination may have a negative effect on colonocytes by inhibiting butyrate oxidation. The association between protein intake and development of IBD has been studied. Reif and colleagues[21] used a preillness dietary questionnaire in newly diagnosed patients with IBD in Israel to show there was no statistically significant association with total protein intake. Consumption of eggs did show a positive association with UC but not CD, and there was no association with fish and both types of IBD. Another epidemiologic analysis of CD incidence in Japan showed a positive correlation with animal and milk protein intake, but there was no correlation with fish protein. There was a negative correlation with vegetable protein.[22] A prospective cohort study of middle-aged French women showed an association between risk of IBD and total protein intake, specifically with meat and fish but not eggs or dairy.[23]

Dietary fat has a substantial theoretic basis for playing a role in both driving and ameliorating inflammation in the intestine depending on the subtype. n-6 PUFAs such as linoleic acid are precursors for arachidonic acid (which itself is a precursor of prostaglandins and leukotrienes), and dietary omega-3 PUFA is a competitive substrate for n-6 PUFA metabolism.[24] Docosahexaenoic acid (DHA) can alter expression of cyclooxygenase-2 in the gastrointestinal (GI) tract and thus inhibit LTB4/PGE2 release and inhibit angiogenesis.[25,26] Lipoxins derived from n-6 PUFA and resolvins derived from omega-3 PUFA are antiinflammatory and can inhibit dendritic cell function and LTB4 production.[27,28] The omega-3 PUFA can inhibit T-cell proliferation and decrease antigen presentation,[29,30] and can modulate chemotaxis of immune cells by inhibiting IL-8 and ICAM-1 expression[25,31]; reduce inflammation via the nuclear factor-κB and peroxisome proliferator activated receptor alpha pathways[32,33]; and can bind to receptors such as GPR20 (G-protein–coupled receptor) causing antiinflammatory effects in macrophages.[34] Long-chain triglycerides can produce increased lymphocytes fluxes and enhanced proliferative response in intestinal lymph,[35] whereas medium chain triglycerides can suppress IL-8, a neutrophil chemottractant expressed in high levels in actively inflamed mucosa of both CD and UC.[36,37] Fats can also alter the microbiome,[38–40] which can lead to upregulation of Toll-like receptor and NOD-mediated inflammation,[41–43] as well as increased intestinal permeability from altered tight junction proteins.[44,45] Milk-derived saturated fats can alter the bile acid composition and allow for growth of sulfate-reducing bacteria such as *Bilophila wadsworthia*, which produce toxic hydrogen sulfide and can aggravate colitis in IL-10 knockout mouse models.[46,47] Dietary fat can activate mast cells, which can indirectly affect gut permeability via regulation of transcellular and paracellular transport.[48,49]

Studies of the association of fat with IBD have similar methodologic shortcomings. Most studies have been retrospective case control, are subject to bias in determining pre-illness diet and fail to account for confounders.[1,50–54] Although some studies have shown an association of CD with total fat, monounsaturated fatty acids, total PUFA, total omega-3 fatty acid, and omega-6 fatty acids, there are also other studies that show no such association.[23,55–59] For UC, there have been associations with total fat, MUFAs, total PUFA, and omega-6 fatty acids[21,23,52,56,60]; however, there are studies that show no such association.[59,61] Negative and positive associations with omega-3 fatty acids have been reported.[52,53,56] Two studies have shown a statistically significant decrease in the risk of UC with high intake of DHA.[52,53] One of the only prospective studies published used the Nurses' Health Study cohort and found that there was no association of total fat, saturated fat, total monounsaturated fatty acids, or total PUFA with risk of IBD.[62] There was an association with high intake of transunsaturated fatty acids and UC but not CD. There was an inverse association between long-term intake of omega-3 PUFA, particularly DHA and EPA, and risk of UC but not CD. Unfortunately, randomized, controlled trials have shown that using fish oil or omega-3 PUFA in those already diagnosed with IBD is not a very effective strategy.[63,64]

A lower intake of fiber may change the microbiome and lead to diminished production of short-chain fatty acids (SCFA),thereby reducing their expected immunoregulatory effects.[65] SCFAs, particularly acetate and propionate, are the only known ligands for a G-protein–coupled receptor GPR43 expressed on neutrophils, eosinophils, and activated macrophages. Another SCFA butyrate is the main energy source for colonocytes and helps to maintain the epithelium. SCFAs also inhibit histone deacetylases and can inhibit nuclear factor-κB. Certain soluble plant fibers have also been shown to inhibit translocation of *Escherichia coli* across M-cells in Peyer's patches.[66] The retrospective study published by Reif and colleagues[21] showed that fiber had a negative association with IBD, although this did not reach statistical significance. The prospective Nurses' Health Study cohort study showed an association between the highest quintile of cumulative dietary fiber intake and reduced risk of developing CD but not UC. Fiber from fruits and vegetables reduced risk of CD, but this was not true for fiber from whole grains or legumes.[67] Li and colleagues[68] published a metaanalysis of case-controlled studies that showed an inverse relationship between vegetable consumption and UC but not CD. A subgroup analysis did show an inverse relationship between vegetable consumption and CD only in European studies, but not Asian studies. There was an inverse relationship between fruit consumption for both UC and CD. Although the overall negative association between fiber intake and IBD is relatively consistent, these conclusions have been questioned in CD; it is possible that patients could have intentionally limited fiber during a prolonged, symptomatic period preceding the official diagnosis of CD.[69]

VITAMINS AND MICRONUTRIENTS

The reader is referred in Fayez K. Ghishan and Pawel R. Kiela's article, "Vitamins and Minerals in IBD," for a discussion of vitamins and trace elements in this issue. Briefly, vitamin D is a fat-soluble vitamin that, in addition to regulating bone, calcium, and phosphorus metabolism, can regulate the adaptive and innate immune systems.[70,71] Polymorphisms of the vitamin D receptor have been identified as a genetic factor in patients with IBD. Patients with IBD, particularly CD, are more likely to be vitamin D deficient. A higher serum level is associated with improved outcomes.[72–77] However, vitamin D deficiency can be a cause or consequence of IBD, and therapeutic trials in CD have yielded only modest results.[78–80] A low vitamin D level may also be a proxy for northern latitude, reduced ultraviolet light exposure, and a disrupted circadian rhythm, which may be associated with dysbiosis and increased IBD-related hospitalizations.[81,82] Abnormalities in vitamin D absorption have also been identified, especially when IBD is active, suggesting that simple megadose supplementation strategies may not be adequate or appropriate in active disease, especially in those who are not calcium replete.

Zinc is an essential micronutrient and deficiency has been associated with excessive loss of GI secretions from chronic diarrhea or fistula drainage. It is an enzyme cofactor involved in wound healing, cellular immunity, and growth.[83] The prevalence of zinc deficiency in IBD ranges from 15% to 40%.[84–87] A low serum zinc level has also been associated with hospitalization, operation, or other complications in patients with CD.[88] Patients with UC with low serum zinc levels also have increased hospitalizations and a trend toward increased complications. The accuracy of serum zinc levels has been called into question because acute illness can diminish plasma levels and shift zinc stores into the liver.[83] Despite this limitation, serum zinc levels may still have clinical value; normalization those in patients with IBD who are deficient has been associated with improved outcomes.

Other common deficiencies in IBD, more notably in CD than UC, include vitamin B_1, B_6, B_{12}, D, K, folic acid, selenium, and iron.[89] There is some evidence to suggest that oral iron may modify the microbiome, and enable adherent invasive *E coli* penetration and survival in macrophages, and is associated with increased intestinal inflammation,[90,91] though such effects have not been associated with intravenous iron formulations.

Taking into account this evidence, we currently recommend a multivitamin with trace elements to our patients with IBD, especially those on dietary therapy and following restricted diets. We do measure vitamin levels once a year and additionally replace the deficient trace element or vitamin as necessary based on the results.

FOOD ADDITIVES

A significant variety of food additives that have a GRAS (Generally Regarded As Safe) status by the US Food and Drug Administration are being used in common foods and could potentially have an impact on IBD. Although few clinical studies have been conducted, we generally recommend avoidance of food additives in patients with IBD because substances that have been shown to be safe in a healthy individual may not be so in those individuals who are genetically and/or environmentally susceptible to GI inflammation. Additionally, most food additives do not enhance the nutrient content of food and are not essential components of a healthy diet. Excluding them is not expected to bring about any physical harm and has the potential advantage of replacing processed foods with whole and naturally occurring foods that have higher nutritional value.

One such food additive is carrageenan, which usually is used as a thickening, stabilizing, texturizing, or emulsifying agent in a variety of foods, even those that are regarded as "healthy" by the public. For example, dairy products such as chocolate milk; nondairy milks that are derived from soy, rice, and nuts like almonds; cottage cheese, mayonnaise, sour cream, cooking cream, whipping cream, ice cream; lunch meats and rotisserie chicken; and even infant formula can have added carrageenan. Estimates of intake can vary from 20 mg to several grams per day with an estimated mean of 250 mg/d.[92,93] Because carrageenan is derived from seaweed, it is considered "natural". Evidently the label "natural" on food packaging does not guarantee a lack of food additives. Preclinical evidence clearly demonstrates that carrageenan can cause colitis when given to animals in sufficient quantities in multiple models (eg, guinea pigs, rats, mice), which share similarities with human IBD[92,93]. This inflammation can be ameliorated by antibiotics and is partially driven by the gut microbiota,[94,95] but inflammatory signals can also occur in the absence of gut microbiota.[95] Multiple in vitro studies using human colonic tissues also attribute inflammatory effects to carrageenan.[92] In a pilot, randomized, placebo-controlled clinical trial, 12 patients with UC were maintained on a carrageenan-free diet and were administered either placebo or carrageenan-containing capsules at a low dose (200 mg/d, which is less than the estimated intake in the US diet). There were no relapses in those patients with UC who were carrageenan free and taking placebo capsules three patients taking carrageenan capsules had earlier relapse associated with elevated fecal calprotectin levels and elevated inflammatory cytokines such as IL-6.[93]

Another ubiquitous additive is maltodextrin which is used as a thickener. It is derived from corn starch and other starches and therefore is considered natural. Its use over the past few years seems to have increased and is correlated with the increase in the incidence of CD.[96] It is found in many packaged foods (about 60% of all items), sugars, candy, beer, baby formula, cereal and health bars, nearly all flavored chips, and similar snacks. Maltodextrin has been shown to promote colonic inflammation in the form of necrotizing enterocolitis in young piglets and promotes growth of E coli in the ileum.[96] In humans, patients with IBD seem to have a microbiome enriched in the metabolism of maltodextrin. E coli, including adherent invasive E coli strains from patients with CD, form thicker biofilms and enhanced adhesion in the presence of maltodextrin. This suggests that this compound may be increasing the colonization of pathogenic bacteria in IBD.[96,97] Furthermore, recent studies suggest that maltodextrin may be deregulating cellular and mucosal barrier–related host antibacterial defenses.[96]

Sodium caprate is a medium-chain fatty acid constituent of milk fat that has been shown to increase paracellular permeability of the ileum in CD via dilation of tight junctions and disassembly of perijunctional filamentous actin.[98] Polysorbate 80 and carboxymethyl cellulose have been shown to induce colitis in IBD mouse models.[99,100] Polysorbate 80 is an emulsifier found in processed foods that enhances E coli translocation across M cells and human Peyer's patches in CD.[66] Carboxymethyl cellulose is found in industrialized milk products, breads, sauces, and sausages, and has been shown to enhance bacterial adherence to the epithelium and distend spaces between villi, leading to bacterial infiltration in IL-10 gene-deficient mice.[94,100]

DIETS FOR THE TREATMENT OF INFLAMMATORY BOWEL DISEASE
Exclusive Enteral Nutrition

EEN is as effective as steroids in inducing remission in children with CD.[101] Enteral feeds are also effective in the adult CD population, but a meta-analysis showed that they were inferior to corticosteroids for inducing remission.[102] EEN has not been shown to be effective for UC.[103] EEN is the first-line therapy for CD in Asian countries. Its mechanism of action is not clear, but it may restore the epithelial barrier and correct dysbiosis. Other studies have shown that EEN paradoxically decreases Faecalibacterium prausnitzii (a beneficial bacterium) and bacterial microbiota diversity (which are well-recognized changes that characterize the dysbiotic microbiome in IBD). EEN-associated fecal microbiota seems to be farther away from that of a healthy individual in compositional studies; therefore, it is plausible that EEN-related micro-biota improvements are only in depleting the gut microbiome of potentially harmful bacteria rather than restoring a totally healthy microbiome. EEN may also work by excluding certain dietary components known to increase intestinal permeability and adherence of adherent invasive *E coli*.[104,105] Open-label trials have demonstrated endoscopic healing, decreased mucosal cytokine production, and improved quality of life in patients with CD.[106–108]

Enteral feeds are classified based on their nitrogen content.[102] There are 3 types: elemental (amino acid based), semielemental (oligopeptide based), and polymeric (whole protein based). Elemental and semielemental formulas are hypoallergenic; the amino acids or chains of amino acids are not long enough for antigen recognition or presentation. The nitrogen source likely is not relevant to therapeutic efficacy; there has not been a statistically significant difference in efficacy between different formulations.[102,109] A nonsignificant trend favoring very low fat and/or very low long chain triglyceride content has been noted.[102] The main criticism regarding the use of enteral nutrition is its lack of palatability; however, this mainly applies to elemental formula, which has a bitter aftertaste. Polymeric formulas, which again are noninferior, may be more palatable and could be used as an alternative to steroids for inducing remission in adults. There remains the concern regarding insufficient caloric intake when a patient drinks EEN by mouth versus using a nasogastric or gastrostomy tube. EEN may additionally have insufficient vitamins and minerals such as vitamin D and zinc for patients with IBD on steroids and with diarrhea, respectively.[110] EEN has successfully been used sequentially and also in combination with various exclusion diets to induce and maintain remission, but this method requires more research before it can be recommended routinely.[111–113] Yamamoto and colleagues[114] published a study demonstrating partial enteral nutrition with a low fat diet was associated with decreased postoperative recurrence of CD. There are also data to suggest that partial enteral nutrition supplementation can decrease loss of response to infliximab.[115,116]

There are probably multiple mechanisms through which dietary substances work to help IBD and these can vary from antigenicity of the foods to nutrient repletion. Paradoxically, the changes to the microbiome induced by EEN are not toward enriching bacterial diversity; nevertheless, this treatment can be effective in patients.

The Specific Carbohydrate Diet

The SCD is one of the most popular diets for IBD available in the lay press. It was initially developed by gastroenterologist Dr Sidney Haas in 1951 and later popularized by biochemist Elaine Gottschall in the book *Breaking the Vicious Cycle: Intestinal Health through Diet*.[117,118] Gottschall's theory is based on the assumption that carbohydrates have the most influence on the microbiota's maintenance and growth. She states that patients with IBD have small bowel mucosal injury, which may be due to bacterial overgrowth leading to excessive fermentation of undigested carbohydrates. This leads to the formation of lactic, acetic, or other organic acids, which also may cause further injury to the small bowel mucosa. As a defense mechanism, the small intestine produces mucus that prevents the brush border intestinal enzymes from making contact with disaccharides and amylopectin, causing more maldigestion. Gottschall states, "The diet is based on the principle that specifically selected carbohydrates, requiring minimal digestive processes are absorbed and leave virtually none to be used for furthering microbial growth in the intestine." It is worth noting that, despite Gottschall's claim, there is no small bowel injury known to commonly occur with UC besides that of backwash ileitis and rarely panenteritis following colectomy. Gottschall likens the mechanism of action of the SCD to exclusive elemental nutrition because the principal carbohydrates in both are monosaccharides. However, as noted, the classification of elemental formula is based on nitrogen content and not carbohydrate content. Vivonex Plus Essential and Peptamen, both manufactured by Nestle (Vevey, Switzerland) as elemental formulas, have maltodextrin and cornstarch listed as ingredients, which are not monosaccharides. Additionally, elemental and polymeric formulas are effective for only CD when the SCD claims to be effective for both UC and CD.

Essential features of the SCD are as follows. It is primarily a modified carbohydrate diet, which allows consumption of monosaccharides and excludes disaccharides, and most polysaccharides (such as linear or branch-chained multiple sugars or starches). The diet is supplemented with homemade yogurt, fermented for 24 hours to free it of lactose. Recommended cultures include *Lactobacillus bulgaricus*, *Lactobacillus acidophilus*, and *Streptococcus thermophile*. The SCD allows almost all fruits, vegetables containing more amylose (a linear-chain polysaccharide, rather than amylopectin, which is a branch-chained polysaccharide), nuts, nut-derived flours, low lactose dairy such as dry curd cottage cheese, meats, eggs, butters, and oils. It excludes sucrose, maltose, isomaltose, lactose, all true and pseudograins and grain-derived flours, potatoes, okra, corn, fluid milk, soy, and cheeses containing high amounts of lactose, as well as some food additives and preservatives. The SCD may be one of the most difficult diets available because it is several degrees more restrictive than the gluten-free diet and the author advises "fanatical adherence." Food labels for prepared foods are not to be trusted unless the company offers a letter in writing stating the ingredients are SCD legal. Juices from concentrate or with "natural flavors" are not allowed because Gottschall asserted these could still have illegal sugars added that are not listed on the label. Even small amounts of lactose, sucrose, or starch that can be fillers in medications or supplements are typically considered illegal. If a medication is essential, however, it is still allowed even with illegal ingredients. An online survey showed that 56% of patients continued to take medications along with the SCD.[119]

Several studies have been published that suggest that SCD may be effective in IBD and most clinical observations have been in pediatric disease. These studies are reviewed in Erin R. Lane and colleagues' article, "Dietary Therapies in Pediatric Inflammatory Bowel Disease: An Evolving IBD Paradigm," elsewhere in this issue. In adults, our group demonstrated that the fecal microbiome of patients with IBD following the SCD may be different and more biodiverse than patients with IBD following a Western diet based on 16srRNA analysis of fecal microbiota composition.[120,121] We also published a case series of 50 patients with IBD on the SCD and showed that SCD followers had decreased symptom scores and a high quality of life.[122] The majority of these patients had colonic CD and some were able to maintain clinical remission using diet without maintenance medications. There is also evidence that following the diet is associated with improvements in the erythrocyte sedimentation rate, C-reactive protein, calprotectin, and Lewis score on capsule endoscopy; nevertheless, concomitant medication use in some of these patients is a potential confounder.[123–125] Results of an online survey of patients with IBD following the SCD hints at the possibility of the diet helping to prevent IBD complications and hospitalizations, although this is only patient reported and needs further study prospectively.[119]

Although Gottschall recommends strict adherence to the SCD, there are some data to suggest some liberalization may be possible with continued maintenance of remission,[124] and patients in our published case series and in our clinical observations have tolerated and done well with some of the "illegal" food items on an individual basis. This suggests that SCD is a starting point for patients with IBD to explore their individual diet–disease relationship, especially in the maintenance phase. Patients could potentially conduct trial and error experiments on themselves with the aid of a health provider who can follow how they respond with objective assessments. Unfortunately, the appropriate time from diet initiation to liberalization is not clearly defined. Gottschall recommends staying on the SCD for at least 1 year after the last symptom has disappeared, but there are no formal recommendations regarding how to liberalize from there. In our clinics, we suggest that an attempt at liberalization should occur preferably after the disease is well-controlled and is in the inactive phase. This allows the patient and the clinician to be able to better delineate clinical food–symptom correlations. We also recommend that during liberalization foods be introduced one at a time in small quantities over weeks rather than a few days.

The Anti-Inflammatory Diet for IBD is based on the SCD, encourages the use of omega-3 fatty acids, utilizes food-based prebiotics and probiotics, and uses a graded approach of food introduction based on food textures. The Anti-Inflammatory Diet for IBD does include otherwise SCD "illegal" foods such as oatmeal, soy milk, flax and chia seeds, fenugreek, and hummus, although it still has been successful in reducing Harvey Bradshaw Index in CD and the Modified Truelove and Witts Severity Index in UC symptomatically.[126] Currently there is an ongoing trial that is looking at the effectiveness of the SCD versus a Mediterranean-style diet in active CD funded by the Patient-Centered Outcomes Research Institute.[127]

There are also some practical considerations when implementing the SCD. The SCD is not simply a list of "legal" and "illegal" foods. There are many other rules regarding which foods to eat depending on presence of symptoms and duration of the SCD. For example, it would be incorrect for a patient with active cramping and diarrhea to start the SCD eating a salad, even if the ingredients of a salad were all technically "legal." With active diarrhea, fruits, raw vegetables, eggs, and large amounts of honey should be avoided. A patient is supposed to start off the SCD with the introductory diet consisting of dry curd cottage cheese, yogurt, eggs, apple cider or other juice, homemade gelatin, chicken soup, and broiled fish or beef patty for 2 to 5 days. From there, the allowed foods are slowly liberalized. The efficacy of the SCD should be judged at the earliest after 1 month of adherence. We recommend a formal assessment of symptoms using appropriate symptom scores and also markers of inflammation including C-reactive protein, fecal calprotectin, and possibly colonoscopy if clinically appropriate. If there are no improvements in symptoms and/or inflammation, it may be reasonable to discontinue the SCD. Hwang and colleagues[110] discussed the nutritional deficiencies that can possibly occur with the SCD including folate, thiamine, vitamin B_6, vitamin D, vitamin C, vitamin A, calcium, and potassium deficiencies, although this is purely speculative. It is reasonable for the patient's diet to be monitored by a dietician to assess for such potential deficiencies.

The SCD is not an approach suited for every patient with IBD. It may not be practical for a CD patient with a significant amount of small bowel strictures because it can tend to be higher in fiber and may lead to an obstruction (although some of our patients have been able to juice to get part of the nutritional contents of fruits and vegetables rather than directly consuming them raw). Because most of the food consumed on SCD is prepared from scratch, ready access to fresh produce is necessary, and it may not be possible to follow the SCD if a patient lives in a "food desert" without access to transportation to a grocery or produce store that has reasonable pricing. At least a high school education is likely necessary to be able to read the *Breaking the Vicious Cycle* book, implement the protocol, and trouble shoot the diet using online message boards. If eating out is an integral part of a patient's social life and/or happiness, the SCD may be too onerous, especially if disease activity is absent or mild, and other medical therapy is efficacious. In our experience, patients who have failed multiple medical therapies are more likely to find the restrictions of the SCD acceptable and worth the sacrifice, even though this patient population may not necessarily be the most likely to respond. We believe most patients with IBD should be notified that this and other exclusion diets exist so that they can make a personal decision if diet is the right strategy according to their circumstances. We also believe that all exclusion diets, including the SCD, should be adjunctive to clinically appropriate medical therapy.

Unfortunately, the nature of the SCD protocol makes some degree of orthorexia nervosa unavoidable. This syndrome is characterized by obsessive focus on food choice, planning, purchase, preparation, and consumption of food with the belief that this can control or reverse disease. The SCD's improvement in symptoms can increase quality of life and the restrictions can also decrease it. The gastroenterologist and patient should be vigilant in monitoring the net effect of this to determine if the SCD is helping and worth continuing. Cooking and preparing meals can be difficult for a patient who has significant disease activity, so family support is an important factor associated with success in implementing SCD in our experience. Websites do exist that offer ready-made food products that are SCD legal for purchase. If a patient has the financial means to pay for these foods, these websites can help to significantly reduce the time burden of cooking.

The Low FODMAP Diet

Many patients in the active phase of IBD and also those in remission can have functional symptoms similar to those seen in IBS patients for whom the low FODMAP diet has been promoted. The theory behind the low FODMAP diet is partially similar to that of the SCD in that it tries to exclude poorly absorbed short-chain carbohydrates that can be fermented by intestinal bacteria resulting in gas, bloating, abdominal pain, and change in bowel habits. FODMAPs are osmotically active and can lead to more fluid delivery to the colon. The low FODMAP diet specifically limits fructose, lactose, fructans, galactans, and polyols, and has been shown to be effective in improving IBS symptoms.[128] IBS is prevalent in the IBD population; one study showed that 57% of patients with CD and 33% of patients with UC experienced IBS symptoms in the preceding week.[129] There is limited evidence that the low FODMAP diet may improve IBS symptoms in patients with IBD. Gearry and colleagues[130] published an uncontrolled study of 52 patients with CD and 20 patients with UC with inactive disease and showed approximately one-half had some response to the low FODMAP diet. The diet was effective in alleviating abdominal pain, diarrhea, bloating, and gas. There was a trend toward more constipation in patients with UC, but this difference was not significant. There is a theoretic concern that the low FODMAP diet excludes inulin, fructooligossacharides, and fructose, which are known prebiotics. This exclusion could potentially exacerbate the dysbiosis that is known to already exist in the IBD population; however, at this time there is no evidence that this does indeed occur.

Differing from the SCD, the low FODMAP diet limits certain sources of fructose (honey apples, dates, watermelon, and other fruits), fructans (onions, garlic), and galactans (beans, lentils, and legumes) that are otherwise allowed on the SCD. Another notable difference is that the low FODMAP diet allows use of sucrose, which is one of the main exclusions of the SCD. Overall, the low FODMAP diet is less restrictive because it is also not as exclusionary of additives and preservatives, which makes eating at restaurants and eating processed foods easier. The dietary exclusions also tend to be more temporary, because reintroduction of FODMAPS after several weeks of strict adherence is encouraged.

Our Own Recommendations for an Inflammatory Bowel Disease Diet

We have previously developed and tested an "anti-IBD" diet that restricts disaccharides; wheat and other grains except white rice; PUFAs and most saturated fats; processed meats and large amounts of red meats; and is devoid of all additives and preservatives. Additionally, foods that are rich in protease inhibitors (raw foods, nuts and seeds, uncooked root vegetables, etc) were reduced or avoided, and foods were advised to be cooked (with all methods except rapid high-heat such as charring), because cooking with heat exposure reduces the protease inhibitor content of foods. Protease inhibitors naturally occur in plants to neutralize digestive proteases in the intestinal lumen of the consuming person as well as those released by pests of the plant, and are a survival/defense mechanism of the plant. However, in the GI tract, neutralization of digestive proteases by large amounts of protease inhibitors within the food allows for bacterial toxins to survive small bowel transit and potentially create inflammation in the distal parts of the GI tract. One such example is a disease called pigbel, which is a clostridial bacterial toxin related to acute or chronic necrotizing enteritis initially noted in the Papua New Guinea Highlanders who consume large amounts of foods that contain trypsin inhibitors.[131]

In this diet, we encourage the consumption of all vegetables and fruits, replacement of red meat with fish high in omega 3 fatty acid content and chicken, and encouraged cooking with monounsaturated fats such as olive oil, which have been reported to be antiinflammatory. Coconut oil, which has been shown to have some antiinflammatory and anticarcinogenic properties, was the saturated fat alternative for the patients (especially for baking), and other fats were discouraged. Contrary to other diets limiting all grains, white rice was allowed, because very little of it is expected to be remaining in the distal small bowel or colon.

We evaluated this diet as a maintenance treatment in adult patients with CD in a randomized, placebo-controlled, double-blind pilot study. We enrolled 54 subjects with quiescent CD, with medical induction of remission. Patients were randomized into 3 groups: (1) a prebiotic fructooligosaccharides intervention (receiving active fructooligosaccharides supplement + a placebo diet); (2) placebo (receiving placebo supplement + the placebo diet); and (3) diet intervention (receiving placebo supplement + the anti-IBD diet). The subjects were followed until either they had a flare (defined as the need for a new medication for treatment or a rise in the Crohn's Disease Activity Index) or up to 12 months. Flares, quality of life, compliance with treatments, and 16s DNA-based microbiome composition in colonic biopsy samples before and after the interventions were assessed. The results demonstrated that this anti-IBD diet resulted in a reduction of the flares compared with placebo and a fructooligosaccharides supplement with a moderate effect size (in fact, none of the subjects flared in the diet intervention group during the study); quality of life did not decline with the interventions; and beneficial bacteria such as *Roseburia* (which produce short chain fatty acids and are noted to be lower in patients with IBD compared with healthy individuals in multiple microbiome studies) increased at the end of treatment.[132]

Other Diets for Inflammatory Bowel Disease

Several other diets have been described both in the medical literature and lay press for the treatment of IBD. A summary list of food exclusions is noted in **Table 1** for each of

Table 1
Food exclusions for diets

Food Restrictions	Grains	Meat	Dairy	Fats and Oils	Vegetables	Fruits	Beans and Legumes	Nuts and Seeds	Beverages	Sweeteners	Miscellaneous
SCD	All excluded	Processed meats	Lactose-containing dairy (ie, milk from animals, soft cheeses)	Margarine, but all other permitted	Potatoes, yams, parsnips, okra, corn, none in cans or jars	No additional sweeteners except honey	Chick peas, bean sprouts, soy, mung, fava, garbanzo beans; other beans need to be soaked and drained	Shelled peanuts, nuts in salted mixtures	Juice from concentrate, juices packed in boxes, lactose-free milk or with lactase enzyme, fortified wines	Refined sugar, molasses, corn or maple syrup, agave	Cornstarch, arrowroot, tapioca, sago starch, chocolate, carob, agar agar, carrageenan, guar gum, pectin, soy sauce
ªLow FODMAP diet	Chicory root, inulin, with HFCS, wheat, flour tortillas, rye	No high FODMAP sauces or with HFCS	Buttermilk, cottage cheese, ice cream, sweetened condensed or evaporated milk, soft cheeses, sour cream, whipped cream, and yogurt	None	Artichokes, asparagus, beets, leeks, broccoli, Brussel sprouts, cabbage, cauliflower, fennel, mushrooms, okra, summer squash, garlic, onion	Avocado, apples, applesauce, apricots, dates, canned fruit, cherries, dried fruits, figs, guava, lychee, mango, nectarines, pears, papaya, peaches, plums, prunes, persimmon, watermelon	Green beans, snow peas, blackeye peas, split peas, haricot verts, kidney beans, mung beans, soy beans	Pistachios, cashews, coconut milk	Any with HFCS, high FODMAP fruit/vegetable juices, fortified wines	HFCS, agave, honey, molasses, sorbitol, mannitol, isomalt, xylitol	Soy products, carob powder
IgG-4 guided exclusion	Wheat, rice	Shrimp, egg, pork, beef, cod fish, lamb, chicken	Milk, cheddar cheese	None	Potato	Tomato	None	Peanuts	None	None	Yeast, soya

Semivegetarian diet	Bread, white rice (brown allowed)	Minced or processed meat, fish allowed once a week, meat once every 2 wk	Cheese	Margarine, butter	None	None	None	None	Carbonated beverages, juices, moderate or no alcohol	Desserts	Fast food, no eating between meals
[a]LOFFLEX Diet	Wheat, oats, rye, barley	Pork, ham, bacon, eggs, processed meats	Cow, goat, sheep milk products, ice cream	Corn oil, vegetable, oil, nut oil, margarine, butter	Corn, onions, sweet corn, tomato	Citrus fruit, apples, bananas, dried fruit, and marmalade	Peas, beans, and lentils	Nuts and seeds	Tea, coffee, fruit squash, carbonated drinks, citrus juice, apple juice, tomato juice, alcohol		Pies, pâté, yeast, salad cream/ dressings, mustard, soy sauce
Paleolithic diet	All grains	Processed meats	Milk from animals, cheese, ice cream	Butter	Corn, starchy tubers, manioc, potatoes, sweet potatoes, tapioca pudding, yams		All beans, peas, lentils	Peanuts	Soda, colas, fruit drinks, candy	Sucrose	Miso, tofu
[a]Maker's diet	All grains	Pork (including sausage), bacon, ham, ostrich, emu, imitation meat, shellfish, eel, catfish, squid, fried or breaded fish or chicken, lunch meat, imitation eggs	Soy milk, rice milk, almond milk, cow's milk	Safflower, sunflower, cottonseed, soy, canola, corn oils; margarine, lard, hydrogenated oils	Corn, sweet and white potatoes	Apples, bananas, apricots, grapes, melon, peaches, oranges, pears dried fruit, canned fruit	Soy, black, navy, garbanzo, kidney, white, and lima beans	Honey-roasted nuts, macadamia nuts, hazelnuts, peanuts, cashews, walnuts, pecans brazil nuts, peanut butter, nuts or seeds dry roasted in oil	Alcoholic beverages, fruits juice, soda, chlorinated tap water, preground commercial coffee	Sugar, heated honey, artificial sweeteners, sorbitol, xylitol	Tofu, protein powder from rice, soy, whey or cow's milk

(continued on next page)

Table 1
(continued)

Food Restrictions	Grains	Meat	Dairy	Fats and Oils	Vegetables	Fruits	Beans and Legumes	Nuts and Seeds	Beverages	Sweeteners	Miscellaneous
[a]Vegan diet	All grains	All meat	All dairy	Heated and fried oils	Raw vegetables (except juiced), onion, radish, mustard green, garlic, chili pepper	Citrus fruits, pineapples, peaches, nectarines, berries (except blueberries), tomatoes, tomatillos, avocado	All legumes, soybeans	All nuts and seeds	Coffee, caffeinated teas, pasteurized drinks, soft drinks, sports drinks	Sucrose	Salt, spices, fermented products, chemical additives and preservatives
Low-carbohydrate diet	Limit bread, pastries, cereals, grains, pasta	N/A	N/A	N/A	Limit potatoes	Limit sweet fruits	N/A	N/A	N/A	Limit sweetened foods	Limit total carbohydrates to <72 g in 24 h

Abbreviations: HFCS, high-fructose corn syrup; LOFFLEX, low-fat, fiber-limited exclusion; N/A, not applicable; SCD, Specific Carbohydrate Diet.

[a] These diets have foods listed that are initially excluded but later on there is some liberalization.

the exclusion diets; however, the many subtleties of their respective protocols are beyond the scope of this review.

The IGG4 exclusion diet

Gunasekeera and colleagues[5] published a randomized, controlled trial of an IgG4-guided exclusion diet for CD. IgG4 titers were drawn for the foods noted in **Table 1**. The foods corresponding with the 4 highest IgG4 titers were eliminated for 4 weeks, and beef, pork, and egg were most commonly excluded, although exclusions varied for each person. There were significant improvements in the Short Inflammatory Bowel Disease Questionnaire and Crohn's Disease Activity Index. Fecal calprotectin only improved in those with severe disease, that is, a Crohn's Disease Activity Index of greater than 150. A major lesson from the observations with this diet is that food can and perhaps should be personalized and customized for each IBD patient.

Semivegetarian (flexitarian) diet

Chiba and associates[6] described a semivegetarian diet for CD as a departure from the Western diet known to be associated with the development of IBD. The diet includes brown rice, miso soup, pickled and other vegetables, fruit, green tea, eggs, yogurt, potatoes, and milk. Meat and fish are limited but not completely excluded. Fast food, sweets, carbonated beverages, cola, juices, alcohol, margarine, butter, cheese, and bread are discouraged. An uncontrolled, prospective trial of patients with CD in medically or surgically induced remission showed that the semivegetarian diet may be effective for maintaining remission for up to 2 years of follow-up.

Others

The low-fat, fiber-limited exclusion diet dietary protocol uses elemental formula to induce remission in CD and followed by a preliminary diet with exclusions noted in **Table 1**.[7] There is then a structured protocol for food reintroduction as the patient keeps a food diary to monitor for reactions. The Paleolithic diet (as described in *The Paleo Diet* by Cordain[8]), Maker's Diet (as described in *The Maker's Diet* by Rubin[9]), a vegan diet (as described in *Self Healing Colitis & Crohn's* by Klein[10]), and a low carbohydrate diet (as described in *Life without Bread* by Allan and Lutz[10]) are described only in the lay press with some associated anecdotal success, but no clinical trials or case reports have been published in peer-reviewed medical journals.[8–11]

SUMMARY

Diet remains a controversial but very promising treatment modality for adult patients with IBD. Data on diet and IBD is full of contradictions and is sparse in terms of good quality clinical trials. Although numerous mechanisms have been put forth to explain how dietary carbohydrates, fat, protein, and other components can cause or reduce inflammation, many of these mechanisms pertain to mouse models, which are tools to enhance our understanding of diet–disease relationships, but cannot reproduce the full set of responses to inflammatory stresses in humans.[133] Current data suggest limiting omega-6 PUFAs, saturated fats, animal protein, and food additives may be helpful in IBD. The SCD, one of the most popular diets already being used by patients with IBD, instead restricts certain carbohydrates and pays little attention to the types of fat or protein consumed. Despite these contradictions, there is preliminary evidence that the SCD helps to improve symptoms, decrease inflammation, and may lead to increased biodiversity of the microbiome so should remain an option for the appropriate IBD patient in conjunction with appropriate medical therapy. Similarly, the low FODMAP diet focuses on excluding particular carbohydrates, is less restrictive, and may be appropriate in patients with IBD without active disease to decrease IBS-like symptoms. EEN seems to paradoxically reduce the biodiversity of the microbiome, but can induce remission, which may be helpful when corticosteroids are contraindicated. Clinical trials are needed to answer the many questions generated by patients and guide dietary therapies that have the potential to reduce flares in patients with IBD.

REFERENCES

1. Hou JK, Abraham B, El-Serag H. Dietary intake and risk of developing inflammatory bowel disease: a systematic review of the literature. Am J Gastroenterol 2011;106:563–73.
2. Thia KT, Loftus EV Jr, Sandborn WJ, et al. An update on the epidemiology of inflammatory bowel disease in Asia. Am J Gastroenterol 2008;103:3167–82.
3. McDonald PJ, Fazio VW. What can Crohn's patients eat? Eur J Clin Nutr 1988; 42(8):703–8.
4. Moser G, Tillinger W, Sachs G, et al. Relationship between the use of unconventional therapies and disease-related concerns: a study of patients with inflammatory bowel disease. J Psychosom Res 1996;40(5):503–9.
5. Gunasekeera V, Mendall M, Chan D, et al. Treatment of Crohn's disease with an IgG4-guided exclusion diet: a randomized controlled trial. Dig Dis Sci 2016; 61(4):1148–57.
6. Chiba M, Abe T, Tsuda H, et al. Lifestyle-related disease in Crohn's disease: relapse prevention by a semi-vegetarian diet. World J Gastroenterol 2010; 16(20):2484–95.
7. Hunter J. Inflammatory bowel disease. Vermillion (United Kingdom): Random House UK; 2011.
8. Cordain L. The paleo diet: lose weight and get healthy by eating the foods you were designed to eat. New York (NY): John Wiley & Sons; 2010.
9. Rubin JS. The Maker's diet. Shippensburg (PA): Destiny Image; 2013.
10. Klein D. Self healing colitis & Crohn's. Maui (HI): Colitis & Crohn's Health Recovery Center; 2011.
11. Allan CB, Lutz W. Life without bread: how a low-carbohydrate diet can save your life. Los Angeles (CA): Keats; 2000.
12. Sporen CEGM, Peirik MJ, Zeegers MP, et al. Review article: the association of diet with onset and relapse in patient with inflammatory bowel disease. Aliment Pharmacol Ther 2013;38:1172–87.
13. Lewis JD, Abreu MT. Diet as a trigger or therapy for inflammatory bowel disease. Gastroenterology 2017;152:398–414.
14. Dixon LJ, Kabi A, Nickerson KP, et al. Combinatorial effects of diet and genetics on inflammatory bowel disease pathogenesis. Inflamm Bowel Dis 2015;21(4): 912–22.
15. Wedrychowicz A, Zajac A, Tomasik P. Advances in nutritional therapy in inflammatory bowel diseases: review. World J Gastroenterol 2016;22(3):1045–66.
16. Riordan AM, Ruxton CH, Hunter JO. A review of associations between Crohn's disease and consumption of sugars. Eur J Clin Nutr 1998;52(4):229–38.
17. Mayberry JF, Rhodes J, Allan R, et al. Diet in Crohn's disease. Dig Dis Sci 1981; 26:444–8.
18. Panza E, Franceschi S, La Vecchia C, et al. Dietary factors in aetiology of inflammatory bowel disease. Ital J Gastroenterol 1987;19:205–9.

19. Persson PG, Ahlbom A, Hellers G. Diet and inflammatory bowel disease: a case control study. Epidemiology 1992;3:47–52.
20. Chan SS, Luben R, van Schaik F, et al. Carbohydrate intake in the etiology of Crohn's disease and ulcerative colitis. Inflamm Bowel Dis 2014;20(11):2013–21.
21. Reif S, Klein I, Lubin F, et al. Pre-illness dietary factors in inflammatory bowel disease. Gut 1997;40(6):754–60.
22. Shoda R, Matsueda K, Yamato S, et al. Epidemiologic analysis of Crohn disease in Japan: increased dietary intake of n-6 polyunsaturated fatty acids and animal protein relates to the increased incidence of Crohn disease in Japan. Am J Clin Nutr 1996;63(5):741–5.
23. Jantchou P, Morois S, Clavel-Chapelon F, et al. Animal protein intake and risk of inflammatory bowel disease: the E3N Prospective Study. Am J Gastroenterol 2010;105:2195–201.
24. Schmitz G, Ecker J. The opposing effects of n-3 and n-6 fatty acids. Prog Lipid Res 2008;47:147–55.
25. Ibrahim A, Mbodji K, Hassan A, et al. Anti-inflammatory and antiangiogenic effect of long chain n-3 polyunsaturated fatty acids in intestinal microvascular endothelium. Clin Nutr 2011;30:678–87.
26. Wang D, Wang H, Brown J, et al. CXCL1 induced by prostaglandin E2promotes angiogenesis in colorectal cancer. J Exp Med 2006;203:941–51.
27. Aliberti J, Hieny S, Reis e Sousa C, et al. Lipoxin-mediated inhibition ofIL-12 production by DCs: a mechanism for regulation of microbial immunity. Nat Immunol 2002;3:76–82.
28. Wan M, Godson C, Guiry PJ, et al. Leukotriene B4/antimicrobial peptideLL-37 proinflammatory circuits are mediated by BLT1 and FPR2/ALX and are counterregulated by lipoxin A4 and resolvin E1. FASEB J 2011;25:1697–705.
29. Pizato N, Bonatto S, Piconcelli M, et al. Fish oil alters T-lymphocyte proliferation and macrophage responses in Walker 256 tumor-bearing rats. Nutrition 2006; 22:425–32.
30. Draper E, Reynolds CM, Canavan M, et al. Omega-3 fatty acids attenuate dendritic cell function via NF-[kappa]B independent of PPAR[gamma]. J Nutr Biochem 2011;22:784–90.
31. Harvey KA, Walker CL, Xu Z, et al. Oleic acid inhibits stearic acid-induced inhibition of cell growth and pro-inflammatory responses inhuman aortic endothelial cells. J Lipid Res 2010;51:3470–80.
32. Hassan A, Ibrahim A, Mbodji K, et al. An alpha-linolenic acid-rich formula reduces oxidative stress and inflammation by regulating NF-kappaB in rats with TNBS-induced colitis. J Nutr 2010;140:1714–21.
33. Marion-Letellier R, Butler M, Dechelotte P, et al. Comparison of cytokine modulation by natural peroxisome proliferator-activated receptor gamma ligands with synthetic ligands in intestinal-like Caco-2 cells and human dendritic cells—potential for dietary modulation of peroxisome proliferator-activated receptor gamma in intestinal inflammation. Am J Clin Nutr 2008;87:939–48.
34. Kliewer SA, Sundseth SS, Jones SA, et al. Fatty acids and eicosanoids regulate gene expression through direct interactions with peroxisome proliferator-activated receptors alpha and gamma. Proc Natl Acad Sci U S A 1997;94:4318–23.
35. Miura S, Imaeda H, Shiozaki H, et al. Increased proliferative response of lymphocytes from intestinal lymph during long chain fatty acid absorption. Immunology 1993;78(1):142–6.

36. Hoshimoto A, Suzuki Y, Katsuno T, et al. Caprylic acid and medium-chain triglyc-erides inhibit IL-8 gene transcription in Caco-2 cells: comparison with the potent histone deacetylase inhibitor trichostatin A. Br J Pharmacol 2002;136(2):280–6.

37. Mazzucchelli L, Hauser C, Zgraggen K, et al. Expression of interleukin-8 gene in inflammatory bowel disease is related to the histological grade of active inflam-mation. Am J Pathol 1994;144(5):997–1007.

38. Jansson J, Willing B, Lucio M, et al. Metabolomics reveals metabolic biomarkers of Crohn's disease. PLoS One 2009;4:e6386.

39. Hekmatdoost A, Feizabadi MM, Djazayery A, et al. The effect of dietary oils on cecal microflora in experimental colitis in mice. Indian J Gastroenterol 2008;27: 186–9.

40. Knoch B, Nones K, Barnett MPG, et al. Diversity of caecal bacteria is altered in interleukin-10 gene-deficient mice before and after colitis onset and when fed polyunsaturated fatty acids. Microbiology 2010;156:3306–16.

41. Zhao L, Kwon MJ, Huang S, et al. Differential modulation of Nods signaling path-ways by fatty acids in human colonic epithelial HCT116cells. J Biol Chem 2007; 282:11618–28.

42. Lee JY, Plakidas A, Lee WH, et al. Differential modulation of Toll-like receptors by fatty acids: preferential inhibition by n-3 polyunsaturated fatty acids. J Lipid Res 2003;44:479–86.

43. Weatherill AR, Lee JY, Zhao L, et al. Saturated and polyunsaturated fatty acids reciprocally modulate dendritic cell functions mediated through TLR4. J Immunol 2005;174:5390–7.

44. de La Serre CB, Ellis CL, Lee J, et al. Propensity to high-fat diet-induced obesity in rats is associated with changes in the gut microbiota and gut inflammation. Am J Physiol Gastrointest Liver Physiol 2010;299:G440–8.

45. Suzuki T, Hara H. Dietary fat and bile juice, but not obesity, are responsible for the increase in small intestinal permeability induced through the suppression of tight junction protein expression in LETO and OLETF rats. Nutr Metab (Lond) 2010;7:19.

46. Hou JK, Lee D, Lewis J. Diet and inflammatory bowel disease: review of patient-targeted recommendations. Clin Gastroenterol Hepatol 2014;12(10):1592–600.

47. Devkota S, Wang Y, Musch MW, et al. Dietary-fat-induced taurocholic acid pro-motes pathobiont expansion and colitis in Il10-/- mice. Nature 2012;487(7405): 104–8.

48. Ji Y, Sakata Y, Tso P. Nutrient-induced inflammation in the intestine. Curr Opin Clin Nutr Metab Care 2011;14(4):315–21.

49. Keita AV, Söderholm JD. The intestinal barrier and its regulation by neuroim-mune factors. Neurogastroenterol Motil 2010;22(7):718–33.

50. Chapman-Kiddell CA, Davies PS, Gillen L, et al. Role of diet in the development of inflammatory bowel disease. Inflamm Bowel Dis 2010;16:137–51.

51. de Silva PS, Olsen A, Christensen J, et al. An association between dietary arachidonic acid, measured in adipose tissue, and ulcerative colitis. Gastroen-terology 2010;139:1912–7.

52. Hart AR, Luben R, Olsen A, et al. Diet in the aetiology of ulcerative colitis: a Eu-ropean prospective cohort study. Digestion 2008;77:57–64.

53. John S, Luben R, Shrestha SS, et al. Dietary n-3 polyunsaturated fatty acids and the aetiology of ulcerative colitis: a UK prospective cohort study. Eur J Gastro-enterol Hepatol 2010;22:602–6.

54. IBD in EPIC Study Investigators, Tjonneland A, Overvad K, Bergmann MM, et al. Linoleic acid, a dietary n-6 polyunsaturated fatty acid, and the aetiology of

ulcerative colitis: a nested case-control study within a European prospective cohort study. Gut 2009;58(12):1606–11.

55. Amre DK, D'Souza S, Morgan K, et al. Imbalances in dietary consumption of fatty acids, vegetables, and fruits are associated with risk for Crohn's disease in children. Am J Gastroenterol 2007;102:2016–25.

56. Sakamoto N, Kono S, Wakai K, et al. Dietary risk factors for inflammatory bowel disease: a multicenter case-control study in Japan. Inflamm Bowel Dis 2005;11: 154–63.

57. Kasper H, Sommer H. Dietary fiber and nutrient intake in Crohn's disease. Am J Clin Nutr 1979;32:1898–901.

58. Thornton JR, Emmett PM, Heaton KW. Diet and Crohn's disease: characteristics of the pre-illness diet. Br Med J 1979;2:762–4.

59. Tragnone A, Valpiani D, Miglio F, et al. Dietary habits as risk factors for inflammatory bowel disease. Eur J Gastroenterol Hepatol 1995;7:47–51.

60. Geerling BJ, Dagnelie PC, Badart-Smook A, et al. Diet as a risk factor for the development of ulcerative colitis. Am J Gastroenterol 2000;95:1008–13.

61. Sharon P, Ligumsky M, Rachmilewitz D, et al. Role of prostaglandins in ulcerative colitis. Enhanced production during active disease and inhibition by sulfasalazine. Gastroenterology 1978;75:638–40.

62. Ananthakrishnan AN, Khalili H, Konijeti GG, et al. Long-term intake of dietary fat and risk of ulcerative colitis and Crohn's disease. Gut 2014;63:776–84.

63. Feagan BG, Sandborn WJ, Mittmann U, et al. Omega-3 free fatty acids for the maintenance of remission in Crohn disease: the EPIC randomized controlled trials. JAMA 2008;299:1690–7.

64. Turner D, Shah PS, Steinhart AH, et al. Maintenance of remission in inflammatory bowel disease using omega-3 fatty acids (fish oil): a systematic review and meta-analyses. Inflamm Bowel Dis 2011;17:336–45.

65. Maslowski KM, Mackay CR. Diet, gut microbiota and immune responses. Nat Immunol 2011;12:5–9h.

66. Roberts CL, Keita AV, Duncan SH, et al. Translocation of Crohn's disease Escherichia coli across M-cells: contrasting effects of soluble plant fibres and emulsifiers. Gut 2010;59:1331–9.

67. Ananthakrishnan AN, Khalili H, Konijeti GG, et al. A prospective study of long-term dietary fiber and risk of Crohn's disease and ulcerative colitis. Gastroenterology 2013;145:970–7.

68. Li F, Liu X, Wang W, et al. Consumption of vegetables and fruit and the risk of inflammatory bowel disease: a meta-analysis. Eur J Gastroenterol Hepatol 2015;27(6):623–30.

69. Stein AC, Cohen RD. Dietary fiber intake and Crohn's disease. Gastroenterology 2014;146(4):1133.

70. Ardesia M, Ferlazzo G, Fries W. Vitamin D and inflammatory bowel disease. Biomed Res Int 2015;2015:470805.

71. Ooi JH, Li Y, Rogers CJ, et al. Vitamin D regulates the gut microbiome and protects mice from dextran sodium sulfate-induced colitis. J Nutr 2013;143(10): 1679–86.

72. Del Pinto R, Pietropaoli D, Chandar AK, et al. Association between inflammatory bowel disease and vitamin D deficiency: a systematic review and meta-analysis. Inflamm Bowel Dis 2015;21:2708–17.

73. Ulitsky A, Ananthakrishnan AN, Naik A, et al. Vitamin D deficiency in patients with inflammatory bowel disease: association with disease activity and quality of life. JPEN J Parenter Enteral Nutr 2011;35:308–16.

74. Ananthakrishnan AN, Cagan A, Gainer VS, et al. Higher plasma vitamin D is associated with reduced risk of Clostridium difficile infection in patients with inflammatory bowel diseases. Aliment Pharmacol Ther 2014;39:1136–42.

75. Ananthakrishnan AN, Cagan A, Gainer VS, et al. Normalization of plasma 25-hydroxy vitamin D is associated with reduced risk of surgery in Crohn's disease. Inflamm Bowel Dis 2013;19:1921–7.

76. Ananthakrishnan AN, Cheng SC, Cai T, et al. Association between reduced plasma 25-hydroxy vitamin D and increased risk of cancer in patients with inflammatory bowel diseases. Clin Gastroenterol Hepatol 2014;12:821–7.

77. Gubatan J, Mitsuhashi S, Zenlea T, et al. Low serum vitamin D during remission increases risk of clinical relapse in patients with ulcerative colitis. Clin Gastroenterol Hepatol 2017;15(2):240–6.e1.

78. Miheller P, Muzes G, Hritz I, et al. Comparison of the effects of 1,25 dihydroxyvitamin D and 25 hydroxyvitamin D on bone pathology and disease activity in Crohn's disease patients. Inflamm Bowel Dis 2009;15(11):1656–62.

79. Jørgensen SP, Agnholt J, Glerup H, et al. Clinical trial: vitamin D3 treatment in Crohn's disease—a randomized double-blind placebo-controlled study. Aliment Pharmacol Ther 2010;32(3):377–83.

80. Yang L, Weaver V, Smith JP, et al. Therapeutic effect of vitamin D supplementation in a pilot study of Crohn's patients. Clin Transl Gastroenterol 2013;4:e33.

81. Stein AC, Gaetano JN, Jacobs J, et al. Northern latitude but not season is associated with increased rates of hospitalizations related to inflammatory bowel disease: results of a multi-year analysis of a national cohort. PLoS One 2016;11(8): e0161523.

82. Voigt RM, Forsyth CB, Green SJ, et al. Circadian rhythm and the gut microbiome. Int Rev Neurobiol 2016;131:193–205.

83. Feldman. Sleisenger and Fordtran's gastrointestinal and liver disease. Tenth edition. Elsevier; 2016.

84. Vagianos K, Bector S, McConnell J, et al. Nutrition assessment of patients with inflammatory bowel disease. JPEN J Parenter Enteral Nutr 2007;31:311–9.

85. Ojuawo A, Keith L. The serum concentrations of zinc, copper and selenium in children with inflammatory bowel disease. Cent Afr J Med 2002;48:116–9.

86. Alkhouri RH, Hashmi H, Baker RD, et al. Vitamin and mineral status in patients with inflammatory bowel disease. J Pediatr Gastroenterol Nutr 2013;56:89–92.

87. McClain C, Soutor C, Zieve L. Zinc deficiency: a complication of Crohn's disease. Gastroenterology 1980;78:272–9.

88. Siva S, Rubin DT, Gulotta G, et al. Zinc deficiency is associated with poor clinical outcomes in patients with inflammatory bowel disease. Inflamm Bowel Dis 2017; 23(1):152–7.

89. Weisshof R, Chermesh I. Micronutrient deficiencies in inflammatory bowel disease. Curr Opin Clin Nutr Metab Care 2015;18(6):576–81.

90. Dogan B, Suzuki H, Herlekar D, et al. Inflammation-associated adherent-invasive Escherichia coli are enriched in pathways for use of propanediol and iron and M-cell translocation. Inflamm Bowel Dis 2014;20(11):1919–32.

91. Jaeggi T, Kortman GA, Moretti D, et al. Iron fortification adversely affects the gut microbiome, increases pathogen abundance and induces intestinal inflammation in Kenyan infants. Gut 2015;64(5):731–42.

92. Tobacman JK. Review of harmful gastrointestinal effects of carrageenan in animal experiments. Environ Health Perspect 2001;109(10):983–94.

93. Bhattacharyya S, Shumard T, Xie H, et al. A randomized trial of the effects of the no-carrageenan diet on ulcerative colitis disease activity. Nutr Healthy Aging 2017;4(2):181–92.

94. Martino JV, Van Limbergen J, Cahill LE. The role of carrageenan and carboxy-methyl cellulose in the development of intestinal inflammation. Front Pediatr 2017;(5):96.

95. Bhattacharyya S, Xue L, Devkota S, et al. Carrageenan-induced colonic inflam-mation is reduced in Bcl10 null mice and increased in IL-10-deficient mice. Me-diators Inflamm 2013;2013:397642.

96. Nickerson KP, Chanin R, McDonald C. Deregulation of intestinal anti-microbial defense by the dietary additive, maltodextrin. Gut Microbes 2015;6(1):78–83.

97. Nickerson KP, McDonald C. Crohn's disease-associated adherent-invasive Es-cherichia coli adhesion is enhanced by exposure to the ubiquitous dietary poly-saccharide maltodextrin. PLoS One 2012;7(12):e52132.

98. Söderholm JD, Olaison G, Peterson KH, et al. Augmented increase in tight junc-tion permeability by luminal stimuli in the non-inflamed ileum of Crohn's disease. Gut 2002;50(3):307–13.

99. Chassaing B, Koren O, Goodrich JK, et al. Dietary emulsifiers impact the mouse gut microbiota promoting colitis and metabolic syndrome. Nature 2015; 519(7541):92–6.

100. Swidsinski A, Ung V, Sydora BC, et al. Bacterial overgrowth and inflammation of small intestine after carboxymethyl cellulose ingestion in genetically susceptible mice. Inflamm Bowel Dis 2009;15(3):359–64.

101. Dziechciarz P, Horvath A, Shamir R, et al. Meta-analysis: enteral nutrition in active Crohn's disease in children. Aliment Pharmacol Ther 2007;26(6):795–806.

102. Zachos M, Tondeur M, Griffiths AM. Enteral nutritional therapy for induction of remission in Crohn's disease. Cochrane Database Syst Rev 2007;(1):CD000542.

103. Lochs H, Dejong C, Hammarqvist F, et al. ESPEN guidelines on enteral nutrition: gastroenterology. Clin Nutr 2006;25(2):260–74.

104. Gerasimidis K, Bertz M, Hanske L, et al. Decline in presumptively protective gut bacterial species and metabolites are paradoxically associated with disease improvement in pediatric Crohn's disease during enteral nutrition. Inflamm Bowel Dis 2014;20(5):861–71.

105. Kaakoush NO, Day AS, Leach ST, et al. Effect of exclusive enteral nutrition on the microbiota of children with newly diagnosed Crohn's disease. Clin Transl Gastroenterol 2015;6:e71.

106. Afzal NA, Van Der Zaag-Loonen HJ, Arnaud-Battandier F, et al. Improvement in quality of life of children with acute Crohn's disease does not parallel mucosal healing after treatment with exclusive enteral nutrition. Aliment Pharmacol Ther 2004;20:167–72.

107. Fell JM, Paintin M, Arnaud-Battandier F, et al. Mucosal healing and a fall in mucosal pro-inflammatory cytokine mRNA induced by a specific oral polymeric diet in paediatric Crohn's disease. Aliment Pharmacol Ther 2000;14:281–9.

108. Bannerjee K, Camacho-Hubner C, Babinska K, et al. Anti-inflammatory and growth-stimulating effects precede nutritional restitution during enteral feeding in Crohn disease. J Pediatr Gastroenterol Nutr 2004;38:270–5.

109. Verma S, Brown S, Kirkwood B, et al. Polymeric versus elemental diet as primary treatment in active Crohn's disease: a randomized, double-blind trial. Am J Gas-troenterol 2000;95(3):735–9.

110. Hwang C, Ross V, Mahadevan U. Popular exclusionary diets for inflammatory bowel disease: the search for a dietary culprit. Inflamm Bowel Dis 2014;20(4): 732–41.

111. Nakayuenyongsuk W, Christofferson M, Nguyen K, et al. Diet to the rescue: cessation of pharmacotherapy after initiation of exclusive enteral nutrition (EEN) followed by strict and liberalized specific carbohydrate diet (SCD) in Crohn's disease. Dig Dis Sci 2017. [Epub ahead of print].

112. Sigall-Boneh R, Pfeffer-Gik T, Segal I, et al. Partial enteral nutrition with a Crohn's disease exclusion diet is effective for induction of remission in children and young adults with Crohn's disease. Inflamm Bowel Dis 2014;20(8):1353–60.

113. Riordan AM, Hunter JO, Cowan RE, et al. Treatment of active Crohn's disease by exclusion diet: East Anglian multicentre controlled trial. Lancet 1993;342(8880): 1131–4.

114. Yamamoto T, Shiraki M, Nakahigashi M, et al. Enteral nutrition to suppress postoperative Crohn's disease recurrence: a five-year prospective cohort study. Int J Colorectal Dis 2013;28(3):335–40.

115. Hirai F, Ishihara H, Yada S, et al. Effectiveness of concomitant enteral nutrition therapy and infliximab for maintenance treatment of Crohn's disease in adults. Dig Dis Sci 2013;58(5):1329–34.

116. Nguyen DL, Palmer LB, Nguyen ET, et al. Specialized enteral nutrition therapy in Crohn's disease patients on maintenance infliximab therapy: a meta-analysis. Therap Adv Gastroenterol 2015;8(4):168–75.

117. Haas SV, Haas MP. Management of celiac disease. Lippincott; 1951.

118. Gottschall E. Breaking the vicious cycle, 2012 edition. Baltimore (ON): The Kirkton Press; 2012.

119. Suskind DL, Wahbeh G, Cohen SA, et al. Patients perceive clinical benefit with the specific carbohydrate diet for inflammatory bowel disease. Dig Dis Sci 2016; 61(11):3255–60.

120. Kakodkar S, Mikolaitis SL, Engen P, et al. The effect of the specific carbohydrate diet (SCD) on gut bacterial fingerprints in inflammatory bowel disease. Gastroenterology 2012;142:S395.

121. Kakodkar S, Mikolaitis S, Engen P, et al. The bacterial microbiome of inflammatory bowel disease patients on the Specific Carbohydrate Diet (SCD). Gastroenterology 2013;144:S552.

122. Kakodkar S, Farooqui AJ, Mikolaitis SL, et al. The specific carbohydrate diet for inflammatory bowel disease: a case series. J Acad Nutr Diet 2015;115(8): 1226–32.

123. Obih C, Wahbeh G, Lee D, et al. Specific carbohydrate diet for pediatric inflammatory bowel disease in clinical practice within an academic IBD center. Nutrition 2016;32(4):418–25.

124. Burgis JC, Nguyen K, Park KT, et al. Response to strict and liberalized specific carbohydrate diet in pediatric Crohn's disease. World J Gastroenterol 2016; 22(6):2111–7.

125. Cohen SA, Gold BD, Oliva S, et al. Clinical and mucosal improvement with specific carbohydrate diet in pediatric Crohn disease. J Pediatr Gastroenterol Nutr 2014;59(4):516–21.

126. Olendzki BC, Silverstein TD, Persuitte GM, et al. An anti-inflammatory diet as treatment for inflammatory bowel disease: a case series report. Nutr J 2014; 13:5.

127. Crohn's & Colitis Foundation. First-ever national study of dietary interventions to treat Crohn's disease receives funding. Available at: http://www.ccfa.org/news/dietstudy.html. Accessed May 1, 2017.

128. Rao SS, Yu S, Fedewa A. Systematic review: dietary fibre and FODMAP-restricted diet in the management of constipation and irritable bowel syndrome. Aliment Pharmacol Ther 2015;41:1256.

129. Simren M, Axelsson J, Gillberg R, et al. Quality of life in inflammatory bowel disease in remission: the impact of IBS-like symptoms and associated psychological factors. Am J Gastroenterol 2002;97:389–96.

130. Gearry RB, Irving PM, Barrett JS, et al. Reduction of dietary poorly absorbed short-chain carbohydrates (FODMAPs) improves abdominal symptoms in patients with inflammatory bowel disease-a pilot study. J Crohns Colitis 2009; 3(1):8–14.

131. Cooke RA. Pig Bel. Perspect Pediatr Pathol 1979;5:137–52.

132. Mutlu EA, Susan Mikolaitis S, Sedghi S, et al. Dietary treatment of Crohn's disease: a randomized, placebo-controlled, double-blinded clinical trial. Am J Gastroenterol 2016;150(4 Supplement 1):S778.

133. Seok J, Warren HS, Cuenca AG, et al. Inflammation and Host Response to Injury, Large Scale Collaborative Research Program. Genomic responses in mouse models poorly mimic human inflammatory diseases. Proc Natl Acad Sci U S A 2013;110(9):3507–12.

Probiotics in Inflammatory Bowel Disease

Bincy P. Abraham, MD, MS[a,b], Eamonn M.M. Quigley, MD, FRCP, FACP, MACG, FRCPI[b,*]

KEYWORDS

- Microbiome • Microbiota • Probiotic • Inflammatory bowel disease
- Ulcerative colitis • Crohn disease • Inflammation • Pouchitis

KEY POINTS

- A substantial body of evidence points to key role for microbiome-host interactions in the pathogenesis of inflammatory bowel disease (IBD).
- Data from animal models support potent antiinflammatory effects for several specific commensal/probiotic strains.
- Well-designed studies of probiotics in IBD in humans remain scanty.
- Available evidence supports a role for probiotics in pouchitis and mild/moderate ulcerative colitis but not in Crohn disease.
- Novel approaches to the modulation of the microbiota in the management of IBD hold promise and are being explored.

INTRODUCTION

Probiotics are widely used by patients with inflammatory bowel disease (IBD) and frequently recommended by their physicians, usually as adjunctive therapy.[1] However, despite their popularity and a widespread perception of safety, the evidence base to support such extensive usage is thin. This statement is not to deny a substantial theoretic basis for the use of therapies, such as probiotics, that modulate the gut microbiota in IBD. The role of the gut microbiota in IBD has been extensively reviewed by Abigail R. Basson and colleagues' article, "Complementary and Alternative

Disclosure: E.M.M. Quigley holds stock in and patents with Alimentary Health and has served as an advisor/consultant to Alimentary Health, Biocodex, Bionutrec, Commonwealth Laboratories, Danone, Pharmasierra, Procter and Gamble, Salix, and Yakult. B.P. Abraham has no relevant disclosures.

[a] Fondren Inflammatory Bowel Disease Program, Division of Gastroenterology and Hepatology, Houston Methodist Hospital, Weill Cornell Medical College, 6550 Fannin Street, SM 1201, Houston, TX 77030, USA; [b] Lynda K and David M Underwood Center for Digestive Disorders, Division of Gastroenterology and Hepatology, Houston Methodist Hospital, Weill Cornell Medical College, 6550 Fannin Street, SM 1201, Houston, TX 77030, USA
* Corresponding author.
E-mail address: equigley@houstonmethodist.org

Medicine (CAM) and Next-Generation CAM (NG-CAM) Strategies for Therapeutic Gut Microbiota Modulation in Inflammatory Bowel Disease," in this issue; suffice it to say that there is substantial, if not overwhelming, evidence for a fundamental role for the gut microbiota and its interactions with the host immune system in IBD.[2–4] A much quoted paradigm views IBD as representing the convergence of host genetics (governing both its immune response and the integrity of the gut barrier), the luminal environment (containing bacteria, viruses, and other microbes), and the external environment (represented by such factors as diet, exercise, and cigarette smoking).[5] Therefore the gut microbiota is now being explored as both the source of, and target for, new therapies in IBD.[6–8] Modulation of the microbiota by diet (including prebiotics); antibiotics; and, most recently, fecal microbiota transplant (FMT)[9–11] in IBD (discussed in Alexander S. Browne and Colleen R. Kelly's article, "Fecal Transplant in Inflammatory Bowel Disease"; and Charles N Bernstein's article, "The Brain-Gut Axis and Stress in IBD," in this issue) show the potential of therapies that, in one way or another, target commensal bacterial populations in IBD.[6–8]

PROBIOTICS: DEFINITION

Probiotics are defined as live microbial food ingredients that, when ingested in adequate amounts, alter the microflora and confer a health benefit to the host.[12–14] For now the definition of a probiotic demands that the organisms included in the preparation be live and assumes that any biological or clinical effects depend on bacterial viability; studies showing (albeit in in vitro or animal models) that dead organisms or bioactive molecules produced by bacteria, such as proteins, polysaccharides, nucleotides, or peptides, also exert biological effects that might be beneficial in IBD suggest that this definition may be broadened in the future.[6] Synbiotics, defined as a combination of a probiotic and a prebiotic, are intended to increase the survival and activity of proven probiotics in vivo, thereby promoting or enhancing the beneficial properties of both products. In vitro studies have shown that synbiotics exert antiinflammatory effects and some show antiproliferative properties.[15] The synbiotic literature is challenging to interpret because it often proves impossible to differentiate between benefits attributable to the prebiotic (as discussed in Heather E. Rasmussen and Bruce R. Hamaker's article, "Prebiotics and Inflammatory Bowel Disease," in this issue), the probiotic, or the interaction between them. Furthermore, the literature on synbiotics in IBD remains scanty.[16–18] For these reasons this article focuses exclusively on probiotics.

PROBIOTICS: MECHANISMS OF ACTION RELEVANT TO INFLAMMATORY BOWEL DISEASE

Many probiotics are derived from the commensal microbiota in the healthy human gut; their properties, understandably, mimic those of the homeostatic effects of the intact microbiota, and several are relevant to IBD.

First and foremost, a substantial literature attests to the antiinflammatory effects of probiotics which, in turn, reflect the immune tolerance that exists between the host and its microbiota. Studies show that probiotics alter the mucosal immune system through a process mediated by Toll-like receptors to promote T-helper 1 cell differentiation, thereby augmenting antibody production; increasing phagocytic and natural killer cell activity; inhibiting the nuclear factor kappa-light-chain-enhancer of activated B cells pathway; inducing T-cell apoptosis; upregulating antiinflammatory cytokines, such as interleukin (IL)-10 and transforming growth factor beta; and simultaneously reducing proinflammatory cytokines such as tumor necrosis factor alpha, interferon gamma, and IL-8.[6,19–24]

For some probiotic strains, such as *Bifidobacterium longum* spp *longum* 35624, the basis of these antiinflammatory effects have been elucidated in considerable detail.[25] Initial experiments with this strain in an animal model showed a potent antiinflammatory effect associated with a suppression of proinflammatory and preservation of antiinflammatory cytokines.[26] Subsequent work confirmed its ability, in contrast with pathogens[27,28] and other probiotic strains,[29] to generate an antiinflammatory response. This effect has been shown in normal human volunteers through the ability of the orally administered organism to lead to the increased levels, in serum, of the important antiinflammatory cytokine IL-10.[30] Furthermore, this same organism has been shown to reduce C-reactive protein levels in patients with ulcerative colitis (UC).[31] The immunologic and molecular basis for these effects have been elaborated in considerable detail and seem to be based on preferential engagement with dendritic cells (as antigen-presenting cells) leading to the induction of regulatory T cells rather than the activation on an inflammatory cascade.[28–30,32,33] These effects have also been shown to blunt the inflammatory response to a common pathogen, *Salmonella typhimurium*.[34] Most recently, the entire genome of this organism has been sequenced,[35] its exopolysaccharide coat molecularly characterized, and its role in the antiinflammatory effects of this organism elucidated.[36] Laboratory experiments involving this organism show several points: first, the importance of complete characterization of probiotic strains; second, the specificity of probiotic effects; and, third, the level of detail that should be the norm in any interrogation of a putative probiotic's antiinflammatory profile. In an intriguing experiment that showed how specific probiotic effects are, the cassette coding the exopolysaccharide code of this bacterium was knocked out and this transformed what was an antiinflammatory organism into one that now evoked an inflammatory response.[36]

Faecalibacterium prausnitzii has been identified as protective against IBD in humans, as shown by its suppression among patients with this disease.[37] This bacterium induces IL-10 in human and murine dendritic cells[38] and prevents the development of chronic inflammation.[39]

Second, probiotics improve (or restore) barrier function (disruption of which is thought to be another key factor in the pathogenesis of IBD[40])[39,41,42] by inhibiting apoptosis of intestinal epithelial cells[43] and promoting synthesis of proteins that are critical components of tight junctions (and thereby reducing paracellular permeability[44–46] and augmenting the mucus layer).[47]

Third, and again reflecting the properties of normal commensals, probiotics beneficially modulate the composition of the microbiota by inhibiting the growth of potentially pathogenic bacteria through the production of bacteriocins and the creation of a more acidic milieu that is inimical to proinflammatory bacteria but promotes the growth of beneficial species such as lactobacilli and bifidobacteria.[48–51] Probiotics increase bacterial diversity and decrease fungal diversity, and can also increase production of fatty acids that have antiinflammatory and anticarcinogenic properties.[51–54]

In addition, effects of probiotics on such physiologic processes as visceral sensation[55,56] may ameliorate symptoms in IBD and central nervous system effects could positively affect comorbid phenomena such as depression.[57,58]

PROBIOTICS IN THE MANAGEMENT OF INFLAMMATORY BOWEL DISEASE

The impact of probiotics on UC, Crohn disease, and pouchitis has been the subject of several systematic reviews and meta-analyses.[59–68] Before discussing the conclusions of these studies, several issues need to be addressed. First, combining diverse species and strains in a single analysis suggests that they are homogeneous, which they are not; second, populations of patients with UC or Crohn disease are remarkably heterogeneous; and, third, when critically reviewed, the overall methodological quality of the meta-analyses and systematic reviews on probiotics in IBD and pouchitis was low to moderate.[68] Nevertheless, the conclusions of these systematic and narrative reviews have been remarkably consistent; little evidence for efficacy in Crohn disease, modest and inconsistent data on UC, and good support for the use of probiotics in pouchitis. This article now examines the evidence for each of these conditions, dealing separately in each case with the induction and maintenance of remission.

Crohn Disease

Induction of remission

For induction of remission in CD, 2 open-label studies showed improvement in Crohn Disease Activity Index scores. However, taken together, these 2 studies included a total of only 14 patients; 1 study used *Lactobacillus rhamnosus* GG[69] and the other a combination of *Lactobacillus* and *Bifidobacterium* species.[70] However, a placebo-controlled trial involving only 11 patients who initially received concurrent antibiotic and steroid therapy for a week and were then randomized to placebo or *Lactobacillus* GG showed no difference between the groups in the time to relapse of Crohn disease. However, only 5 out of the 11 patients completed the study.[71]

Maintenance of remission

In the maintenance of remission in Crohn disease, a study involving the use of *Lactobacillus rhamnosus* GG in children showed no benefit compared with placebo, and was terminated early because of lack of efficacy and difficulty in recruitment.[72] In the largest and highest-quality study to date, Fedorak and colleagues[73] studied the impact of the probiotic cocktail VSL#3 on endoscopic relapse rates 90 and 365 days following surgery for Crohn disease. Although no statistical differences in endoscopic recurrence rates were noted at day 90 (the primary end point) between patients who received VSL#3 and patients who received placebo, lower mucosal levels of inflammatory cytokines and a lower rate of recurrence among patients who received VSL#3 for the entire 365 days suggested that there might be some efficacy. In another large, well-designed, and appropriately powered trial, Bourreille and colleagues[74] randomized 165 patients with Crohn disease who had achieved remission with steroids or salicylates to the probiotic yeast *Saccharomyces boulardii* or placebo for 52 weeks; no differences in recurrence rates were observed between the two groups. This finding contrasts with earlier, much smaller, studies with this organism, which suggested benefit.[75–77]

These findings in these recent high-quality studies confirm those of earlier meta-analyses; namely, that there is no apparent benefit for probiotics in the maintenance of remission in Crohn disease based on clinical and/or endoscopic relapse rates.[60,63] Other studies of individual organisms, whether *L rhamnosus* GG,[70–72] *Lactobacillus johnsonii*,[78,79] or *Escherichia coli* Nissle 1917,[80] failed to show any impact on remission rates.

Ulcerative Colitis

Induction of remission

A 2007 Cochrane Review that evaluated the use of the probiotics *S boulardii* and VSL#3 in the induction of remission in mild to moderate UC included 4 studies involving a total of 244 patients and concluded that probiotics, in combination with conventional therapy, did not increase remission rates but did provide a modest benefit in terms of reducing disease activity.[61]

Two subsequent large studies suggested a favorable effect for VSL#3.[81,82] Both studies investigated the probiotic cocktail as an adjunct to standard therapy comprising either aminosalicylates or thiopurines. In the first of these studies, VSL#3 increased remission rates at 12 weeks, with remission being defined as the combination of a reduction in the Ulcerative Colitis Disease Activity Index (UCDAI) score by more than 50% and mucosal healing.[81] However, the ability to generalize from these results was constrained by both the short duration of the study and a large dropout rate of the placebo group.[81] The study by Tursi and colleagues[82] found no difference in remission rates between VSL#3 and placebo, based on the physician's global assessment and endoscopic scores, but did note some clinical effects, as shown by reductions in rectal bleeding and stool frequency scores. A much smaller study of 29 children with newly diagnosed UC in which VSL#3 was added to standard treatment comprising steroids and 5-aminosalicylic acid, reported a significantly higher remission rate of 93% for the combination therapy compared with only 36% for those who received standard therapy plus placebo.[83]

A Japanese randomized controlled trial (RCT) using a bifidobacteria-fermented milk, which contained *Bifidobacterium* strains and *Lactobacillus acidophilus*, also reported a significant reduction in endoscopic and histologic scores in UC compared with patients who received a placebo.[84] A large study that randomized 100 patients with active UC to ciprofloxacin or placebo for 1 week followed by *E coli* Nissle or placebo for 7 weeks as adjunctive treatments found that fewer patients on the probiotic achieved clinical remission, and that the probiotic group experienced the largest number of withdrawals.[85]

Although most probiotic studies have delivered the active agent orally, rectal administration has also been studied. One study that evaluated the use of *E coli* strain Nissle 1917, administered as an enema, in the treatment of acute proctitis or proctosigmoiditis did not show benefit compared with placebo[86]; in contrast, a study comparing placebo plus mesalamine with *Lactobacillus reuteri* ATCC 55730 administered as an enema with mesalamine showed greater improvements in clinical disease severity, inflammatory markers, and endoscopic findings in the probiotic group.[87]

At present, there is, therefore, insufficient evidence to recommend for or against the use of probiotics either alone or in combination with standard therapy for the induction of remission in UC.

Maintenance of remission

Evidence from several controlled trials using several different probiotics (*E coli* Nissle 1917, *S boulardii*, *Bifidobacterium breve* strain Yakult, and *Bifidobacterium bifidum* strain Yakult) have suggested a role for probiotics in the maintenance of remission in patients with mild to moderate UC, with most studies showing similar levels of efficacy and safety to standard 5-aminosalicylic acid regimens.[88] However, another study using the combination of *L acidophilus* La-5 and *Bifidobacterium animalis* subspecies *lactis* BB-12 experienced less favorable results.[89]

Three RCTs using *E Coli* Nissle 1917 (a strain that is not available in the United States) showed that this probiotic organism was equivalent to low-dose mesalamine (1.2–1.5 g/d) in maintaining remission based on either quality-of-life scores, endoscopy, or histology.[90–92] Although there were no differences in time to relapse between the treatments, one study reported relapse rates in the region of 70% in both arms, suggesting the inclusion of a population with more severe UC.[90] In contrast, an open-label RCT comparing the probiotic *Lactobacillus* GG alone, mesalamine in a dose of 2.4 g/d, and the combination of *Lactobacillus* GG and mesalamine failed to show any difference in relapse or adverse event rates between the 3 groups over a 12-month period based on UCDAI scores.[93]

Small studies in children support the use of probiotics for maintenance of remission in UC. The addition of VSL#3 to standard therapy significantly decreased relapse rates compared with placebo (21.4% vs 73.3%) when given within a year of induction of remission in 29 children with UC,[83] whereas an open-label trial of VSL#3 given in addition to standard treatment reported a remission rate of 61% in 18 children with UC.[94]

Taken together, studies of probiotics in the induction and/or maintenance of remission in UC suggest a trend toward clinical benefit. Based on the available data, it is impossible to discern whether a specific probiotic species, strain, or preparation is superior to others in UC; further large, high-quality clinical trials are needed to better define the overall placement of probiotics in the management of UC and to delineate those strains that are optimal.

Pouchitis

Up to 60% of patients with UC with an ileal pouch anal anastomosis (IPAA) develop pouchitis.[95] That pouchitis can be successfully treated with antibiotics strongly suggests that the microbiome of the pouch plays a key role in the development of this inflammatory process.[96]

Induction of remission

One study evaluated the impact of *Lactobacillus* GG on the induction of remission in acute pouchitis and, although administration of the probiotic was shown to alter the pouch flora, there were no associated benefits in terms of symptoms or endoscopic findings compared with placebo.[97]

Maintenance of remission

Gionchetti and colleagues[98] showed convincingly that prophylactic therapy with the probiotic cocktail VSL#3 was highly effective in the primary prevention of pouchitis following an IPAA. The same formulation also proved far superior to placebo in maintaining remission in patients who had developed pouchitis and had been successfully treated with antibiotics; sustained remission was observed in 40% to 90% of those treated with the probiotic cocktail, compared with only 0% to 60% in those who received placebo.[99–101] The administration of VSL#3 has been associated with an increase in mucosal regulatory T cells, a reduction in the expression of the proinflammatory cytokine IL-1β messenger RNA in the mucosa,[101] an increase in bacterial diversity,[64,102] and a restoration of barrier integrity.[102]

A critical review of probiotic studies in pouchitis raised a note of caution. All studies had limitations: small size of study populations (15–40 patients), shorter duration of study (3–12 months), and a lack of uniformity in probiotic dosing.[65]

PROBIOTICS: QUALITY CONTROL

It is critical, at this juncture, to emphasize that no 2 probiotics are the same, despite commercial claims to the contrary. To be effective at their likely sites of action, probiotics need to be able to survive stomach acid, bile, and digestive enzymes and to be viable for the duration of their shelf lives; many products on supermarket shelves do not meet even these most basic standards. Many more have never been subjected to clinical evaluation in any disease category and base their claims on an extrapolation from other strains, which is an inappropriate strategy.

PROBIOTICS: SAFETY

Probiotics are generally regarded as safe.[103–105] Furthermore, their record in patients with IBD, a population that may be susceptible to intestinal translocation and, thus, systemic sepsis, has been reassuring. Of concern was a case of systemic dissemination leading to sepsis in a newborn given *E coli* strain Nissle 1917 for viral gastroenteritis.[106] Although probiotics and prebiotics have a long safety record, there may still be risks in certain disease populations. Particular vigilance is recommended; for example, among patients with immunodeficiency, those with a severe attack of acute pancreatitis, or those who have central vein lines in situ.[6,103–105,107] Because probiotic strains usually do not colonize the adult intestine, they must be taken indefinitely for continued effects; long-term maintenance studies are needed to assess both efficacy and safety in IBD.

PROBIOTICS: THE FUTURE

Despite the existence of a compelling narrative that supports a critical role for the gut microbiota in IBD and a large volume of laboratory data showing impressive beneficial effects of various bacterial strains in animal models of IBD, the IBD probiotic clinical portfolio is far from convincing. Several factors may contribute to this disappointment: the limitations of animal models, differences in probiotic dosage, and a failure to account for the multiple phenotypes that IBD manifests in clinical practice. Clinicians may simply be targeting the wrong patients. How can it be done better?

First and foremost, better designed and appropriately powered studies are needed in appropriately phenotyped populations. Although various abnormalities in the gut microbiota have been described in IBD, results have not been consistent[2–6,108,109]; it is hoped that large, longitudinal studies will clarify relationships between microbiota and phenotype and IBD. One strategy that may emerge from such studies is the replenishment of deficient species or strains (eg, *F prausnitzii*); the era of individualized medicine may be nigh.

It may also be possible to expand the probiotic concept into so-called pharmabiotics, a concept that includes not only live organisms but also dead ones, genetically modified bacteria, bacterial components, and bacterial products.[110–112] Clinicians can also learn from the emerging experience with FMT[9]; specifically, the question of what bacterial species are essential for a successful FMT in IBD.

SUMMARY/DISCUSSION

Despite the undoubted role of the microbiota in IBD and the attractiveness of probiotics as a therapeutic intervention, the extant literature on these therapies is far from impressive and has many limitations. Furthermore, generic issues relating to quality control continue to bedevil what is essentially a lightly regulated market. Many probiotic products on sale in supermarkets and pharmacies have not been adequately tested for the viability of their bacteria over the durations of their recommended shelf lives nor has their precise composition been rigorously defined. Significant confounders, such as diet and concomitant medications (including antibiotics, proton pump inhibitors, and antidiarrheals) have often not been adequately controlled for. The net result is that, given the thin database, firm recommendations on the use of probiotics in IBD are not possible at this time.

It is, therefore, clear that more randomized clinical trials involving larger patient populations and of adequate duration are needed to properly evaluate the benefits of these products and to evaluate the optimal strain, dosing, formulation, and route of administration in each of the major subtypes of IBD. Such studies should also seek to define the patients who are most likely to respond to these interventions; are responses dictated by disease location and phenotype? Could a baseline study of the microbiota predict responders or even allow clinicians to define the optimal therapy for a given individual? Longitudinal studies of the impact of probiotics on the microbiota would also be of great interest. Studies of the microbiota in IBD should, ideally, include a detailed examination of the juxtamucosal, as well as the fecal, microbiome.

Could interventions that modulate the microbiota prevent the de novo development of IBD? This possibility seems to be present in the case of pouchitis[98] but has not been tested in the more prevalent manifestations of IBD. Long-term studies of this strategy are possible among individuals at increased risk for the development of IBD, such as those with a strong family history or who have been exposed to known environmental risk factors such as early antibiotic use; smoking; and high-fat, low-fiber diets. With regard to risk factors for relapse in IBD, *Clostridium difficile* has been repeatedly identified as a major cause; could the prophylactic administration of a probiotic prevent the development of *C difficile*–related infections and IBD relapses in susceptible individuals?

REFERENCES

1. Cheifetz AS, Gianotti R, Luber R, et al. Complementary and alternative medicines used by patients with inflammatory bowel diseases. Gastroenterology 2017;152:415–29.

2. Kostic AD, Xavier RJ, Gevers D. The microbiome in inflammatory bowel disease: current status and the future ahead. Gastroenterology 2014;146:1489–99.

3. Babickova J, Gardlik R. Pathological and therapeutic interactions between bacteriophages, microbes and the host in inflammatory bowel disease. World J Gastroenterol 2015;21:11321–30.

4. Sartor RB, Wu GD. Roles for intestinal bacteria, viruses, and fungi in pathogenesis of inflammatory bowel diseases and therapeutic approaches. Gastroenterology 2017;152:327–39.

5. Leone V, Chang EB, Devkota S. Diet, microbes, and host genetics: the perfect storm in inflammatory bowel diseases. J Gastroenterol 2013;48:315–21.

6. Shanahan F, Quigley EM. Manipulation of the microbiota for treatment of IBS and IBD–challenges and controversies. Gastroenterology 2014;146:1554–63.

7. Bejaoui M, Sokol H, Marteau P. Targeting the microbiome in inflammatory bowel disease: critical evaluation of current concepts and moving to new horizons. Dig Dis 2015;33(Suppl 1):105–12.

8. Hansen JJ, Sartor RB. Therapeutic manipulation of the microbiome in IBD: current results and future approaches. Curr Treat Options Gastroenterol 2015;13: 105–20.

9. Anderson JL, Edney RJ, Whelan K. Systematic review: faecal microbiota transplantation in the management of inflammatory bowel disease. Aliment Pharmacol Ther 2012;36:503–16.

10. Scaldaferri F, Pecere S, Petito V, et al. Efficacy and mechanisms of action of fecal microbiota transplantation in ulcerative colitis: pitfalls and promises from a first meta-analysis. Transplant Proc 2016;48:402–7.

11. Moayyedi P, Surette MG, Kim PT, et al. Fecal microbiota transplantation induces remission in patients with active ulcerative colitis in a randomized controlled trial. Gastroenterology 2015;149:102–9.

12. Howarth GS, Wang H. Role of endogenous microbiota, probiotics and their biological products in human health. Nutrients 2013;5:58–81.
13. FAO/WHO. Guidelines for the evaluation of probiotics in food. Report of a joint FAO/WHO working group on drafting guidelines for the evaluation of probiotics in food. London: World Health Organization; 2002.
14. Hill C, Guarner F, Reid G, et al. Expert consensus document. The International Scientific Association for Probiotics and Prebiotics consensus statement on the scope and appropriate use of the term probiotic. Nat Rev Gastroenterol Hepatol 2014;11:506–14.
15. Grimoud J, Durand H, de Souza S, et al. In vitro screening of probiotics and synbiotics according to anti-inflammatory and anti-proliferative effects. Int J Food Microbiol 2010;144:42–50.
16. Laurell A, Sjöberg K. Prebiotics and synbiotics in ulcerative colitis. Scand J Gastroenterol 2017;52:477–85.
17. Kaila M, Isolauri E, Soppi E, et al. Enhancement of the circulating antibody secreting cell response in human diarrhea by a human Lactobacillus strain. Pediatr Res 1992;32:141–4.
18. Ogawa T, Asai Y, Tamai R, et al. Natural killer cell activities of synbiotic *Lactobacillus casei* ssp. *casei* in conjunction with dextran. Clin Exp Immunol 2006;143:103–9.
19. Petrof EO, Kojima K, Ropeleski MJ, et al. Probiotics inhibit nuclear factor-kappaB and induce heat shock proteins in colonic epithelial cells through proteasome inhibition. Gastroenterology 2004;127:1474–87.
20. Di Marzio L, Russo FP, D'Alo S, et al. Apoptotic effects of selected strains of lactic acid bacteria on a human T leukemia cell line are associated with bacterial arginine deiminase and/or sphingomyelinase activities. Nutr Cancer 2001;40:185–96.
21. Maassen CB, van Holten-Neelen C, Balk F, et al. Strain-dependent induction of cytokine profiles in the gut by orally administered *Lactobacillus* strains. Vaccine 2000;18:2613–23.
22. Morita H, He F, Fuse T, et al. Adhesion of lactic acid bacteria to caco-2 cells and their effect on cytokine secretion. Microbiol Immunol 2002;46:293–7.
23. Ma D, Forsythe P, Bienenstock J. Live *lactobacillus reuteri* is essential for the inhibitory effect on tumor necrosis factor alpha-induced interleukin-8 expression. Infect Immun 2004;72:5308–14.
24. West CE, Jenmalm MC, Prescott SL. The gut microbiota and its role in the development of allergic disease: a wider perspective. Clin Exp Allergy 2015;45:43–53.
25. Konieczna P, Akdis CA, Quigley EM, et al. Portrait of an immunoregulatory Bifidobacterium. Gut Microbes 2012;3:261–6.
26. McCarthy J, O'Mahony L, O'Callaghan L, et al. Double blind, placebo controlled trial of two probiotic strains in interleukin 10 knockout mice and mechanistic link with cytokine balance. Gut 2003;2:975–80.
27. O'Hara AM, O'Regan P, Fanning A, et al. Functional modulation of human intestinal epithelial cell responses by *Bifidobacterium infantis* and *Lactobacillus salivarius*. Immunology 2006;118:202–15.
28. O'Mahony L, O'Callaghan L, McCarthy J, et al. Differential cytokine response from dendritic cells to commensal and pathogenic bacteria in different lymphoid compartments in humans. Am J Physiol Gastrointest Liver Physiol 2006;290:G839–45.

29. Gad M, Ravn P, Søborg DA, et al. Regulation of the IL-10/IL-12 axis in human dendritic cells with probiotic bacteria. FEMS Immunol Med Microbiol 2011;63: 93–107.

30. Konieczna P, Groeger D, Ziegler M, et al. Bifidobacterium infantis 35624 administration induces Foxp3 T regulatory cells in human peripheral blood: potential role for myeloid and plasmacytoid dendritic cells. Gut 2012;61:354–66.

31. Groeger D, O'Mahony L, Murphy EF, et al. *Bifidobacterium infantis* 35624 modulates host inflammatory processes beyond the gut. Gut Microbes 2013;4: 325–39.

32. O'Mahony C, Scully P, O'Mahony D, et al. Commensal-induced regulatory T cells mediate protection against pathogen-stimulated NF-kappaB activation. PLoS Pathog 2008;4:e1000112.

33. Konieczna P, Ferstl R, Ziegler M, et al. Immunomodulation by *Bifidobacterium infantis* 35624 in the murine lamina propria requires retinoic acid-dependent and independent mechanisms. PLoS One 2013;8:e62617.

34. Scully P, Macsharry J, O'Mahony D, et al. *Bifidobacterium infantis* suppression of Peyer's patch MIP-1α and MIP-1β secretion during *Salmonella* infection correlates with increased local CD4+CD25+ T cell numbers. Cell Immunol 2013; 281:134–40.

35. Altmann F, Kosma P, O'Callaghan A, et al. Genome analysis and characterisation of the exopolysaccharide produced by *Bifidobacterium longum* subsp. *longum* 35624™. PLoS One 2016;11:e0162983.

36. Schiavi E, Gleinser M, Molloy E, et al. The surface-associated exopolysaccharide of *Bifidobacterium longum* 35624 plays an essential role in dampening host proinflammatory responses and repressing local TH17 responses. Appl Environ Microbiol 2016;82:7185–96.

37. Cao Y, Shen J, Ran ZH. Association between *Faecalibacterium prausnitzii* reduction and inflammatory bowel disease: a meta-analysis and systematic review of the literature. Gastroenterol Res Pract 2014;2014:872725.

38. Rossi O, van Berkel LA, Chain F, et al. *Faecalibacterium prausnitzii* A2-165 has a high capacity to induce IL-10 in human and murine dendritic cells and modulates T cell responses. Sci Rep 2016;6:18507.

39. Martín R, Miquel S, Chain F, et al. *Faecalibacterium prausnitzii* prevents physiological damages in a chronic low-grade inflammation murine model. BMC Microbiol 2015;15:67.

40. Vindigni SM, Zisman TL, Suskind DL, et al. The intestinal microbiome, barrier function, and immune system in inflammatory bowel disease: a tripartite pathophysiological circuit with implications for new therapeutic directions. Therap Adv Gastroenterol 2016;9:606–25.

41. Lomasney KW, Cryan JF, Hyland NP. Converging effects of a *Bifidobacterium* and *Lactobacillus* probiotic strain on mouse intestinal physiology. Am J Physiol Gastrointest Liver Physiol 2014;307:G241–7.

42. Srutkova D, Schwarzer M, Hudcovic T, et al. *Bifidobacterium longum* CCM 7952 promotes epithelial barrier function and prevents acute DSS-induced colitis in strictly strain-specific manner. PLoS One 2015;10:e0134050.

43. Yan F, Polk DB. Probiotic bacterium prevents cytokine-induced apoptosis in intestinal epithelial cells. J Biol Chem 2002;277:50959–65.

44. Ahrne S, Hagslatt ML. Effect of lactobacilli on paracellular permeability in the gut. Nutrients 2011;3:104–17.

45. Lomasney KW, Houston A, Shanahan F, et al. Selective influence of host micro-biota on cAMP-mediated ion transport in mouse colon. Neurogastroenterol Motil 2014;26:887–90.

46. Souza ÉL, Elian SD, Paula LM, et al. *Escherichia coli* strain Nissle 1917 amelio-rates experimental colitis by modulating intestinal permeability, the inflammatory response and clinical signs in a faecal transplantation model. J Med Microbiol 2016;65:201–10.

47. Mack DR, Ahrne S, Hyde L, et al. Extra-cellular MUC3 mucin secretion follows adherence of *Lactobacillus* strains to intestinal epithelial cells in vitro. Gut 2003;52:827–33.

48. Shiba T, Aiba Y, Ishikawa H, et al. The suppressive effect of bifidobacteria on *Bacteroides vulgatus*, a putative pathogenic microbe in inflammatory bowel dis-ease. Microbiol Immunol 2003;47:371–8.

49. Servin AL. Antagonistic activities of lactobacilli and bifidobacteria against micro-bial pathogens. FEMS Microbiol Rev 2004;28:405–40.

50. Sartor RB. Therapeutic manipulation of the enteric microflora in inflammatory bowel diseases: antibiotics, probiotics, and prebiotics. Gastroenterology 2004;126:1620–33.

51. Constante M, Fragoso G, Lupien-Meilleur J, et al. Iron supplements modulate colon microbiota composition and potentiate the protective effects of probiotics in dextran sodium sulfate-induced colitis. Inflamm Bowel Dis 2017;23:753–66.

52. Kuhbacher T, Ott SJ, Helwig U, et al. Bacterial and fungal microbiota in relation to probiotic therapy (VSL#3) in pouchitis. Gut 2006;55:833–41.

53. Ewaschuk JB, Walker JW, Diaz H, et al. Bioproduction of conjugated linoleic acid by probiotic bacteria occurs in vitro and in vivo in mice. J Nutr 2006;136: 1483–7.

54. Collado MC, Surono IS, Meriluoto J, et al. Potential probiotic characteristics of *Lactobacillus* and *Enterococcus* strains isolated from traditional dadih fer-mented milk against pathogen intestinal colonization. J Food Prot 2007;70: 700–5.

55. McKernan DP, Fitzgerald P, Dinan TG, et al. The probiotic *Bifidobacterium infan-tis* 35624 displays visceral antinociceptive effects in the rat. Neurogastroenterol Motil 2010;22:1029–35.

56. Johnson AC, Greenwood-Van Meerveld B, McRorie J. Effects of *Bifidobacterium infantis* 35624 on post-inflammatory visceral hypersensitivity in the rat. Dig Dis Sci 2011;56:3179–86.

57. Emge JR, Huynh K, Miller EN, et al. Modulation of the microbiota-gut-brain axis by probiotics in a murine model of inflammatory bowel disease. Am J Physiol Gastrointest Liver Physiol 2016;310:G989–98.

58. Desbonnet L, Garrett L, Clarke G, et al. Effects of the probiotic *Bifidobacterium infantis* in the maternal separation model of depression. Neuroscience 2010; 170:1179–88.

59. Naidoo K, Gordon M, Fagbemi AO, et al. Probiotics for maintenance of remis-sion in ulcerative colitis. Cochrane Database Syst Rev 2011;(12):CD007443.

60. Rolfe VE, Fortun PJ, Hawkey CJ, et al. Probiotics for maintenance of remission in Crohn's disease. Cochrane Database Syst Rev 2006;(4):CD004826.

61. Mallon P, McKay D, Kirk S, et al. Probiotics for induction of remission in ulcera-tive colitis. Cochrane Database Syst Rev 2007;(4):CD005573.

62. Zigra PI, Maipa VE, Alamanos YP. Probiotics and remission of ulcerative colitis: a systematic review. Neth J Med 2007;65:411–8.

63. Rahimi R, Nikfar S, Rahimi F, et al. A meta-analysis on the efficacy of probiotics for maintenance of remission and prevention of clinical and endoscopic relapse in Crohn's disease. Dig Dis Sci 2008;53:2524–31.

64. Veerappan GR, Betteridge J, Young PE. Probiotics for the treatment of inflammatory bowel disease. Curr Gastroenterol Rep 2012;14:324–33.

65. Ghouri YA, Richards DM, Rahimi EF, et al. Systematic review of randomized controlled trials of probiotics, prebiotics, and synbiotics in inflammatory bowel disease. Clin Exp Gastroenterol 2014;7:473–87.

66. Fujiya M, Ueno N, Kohgo Y. Probiotic treatments for induction and maintenance of remission in inflammatory bowel diseases: a meta-analysis of randomized controlled trials. Clin J Gastroenterol 2014;7:1–13.

67. Shen J, Zuo ZX, Mao AP. Effect of probiotics on inducing remission and maintaining therapy in ulcerative colitis, Crohn's disease, and pouchitis: meta-analysis of randomized controlled trials. Inflamm Bowel Dis 2014;20:21–35.

68. Dong J, Teng G, Wei T, et al. Methodological quality assessment of meta-analyses and systematic reviews of probiotics in inflammatory bowel disease and pouchitis. PLoS One 2016;11:e0168785.

69. Gupta P, Andrew H, Kirschner BS, et al. Is Lactobacillus GG helpful in children with Crohn's disease? Results of a preliminary, open-label study. J Pediatr Gastroenterol Nutr 2000;31:453–7.

70. Fujimori S, Tatsuguchi A, Gudis K, et al. High dose probiotic and prebiotic co-therapy for remission induction of active Crohn's disease. J Gastroenterol Hepatol 2007;22:1199–204.

71. Schultz M, Timmer A, Herfarth HH, et al. Lactobacillus GG in inducing and maintaining remission of Crohn's disease. BMC Gastroenterol 2004;4:5.

72. Bousvaros A, Guandalini S, Baldassano RN, et al. A randomized, double-blind trial of Lactobacillus GG versus placebo in addition to standard maintenance therapy for children with Crohn's disease. Inflamm Bowel Dis 2005;11:833–9.

73. Fedorak RN, Feagan BG, Hotte N, et al. The probiotic VSL#3 has anti-inflammatory effects and could reduce endoscopic recurrence after surgery for Crohn's disease. Clin Gastroenterol Hepatol 2015;13:928–35.

74. Bourreille A, Cadiot G, Le Dreau G, et al, FLORABEST Study Group. Saccharomyces boulardii does not prevent relapse of Crohn's disease. Clin Gastroenterol Hepatol 2013;11:982–7.

75. Plein K, Hotz J. Therapeutic effects of Saccharomyces boulardii on mild residual symptoms in a stable phase of Crohn's disease with special respect to chronic diarrhea – a pilot study. Z Gastroenterol 1993;31:129–34.

76. Guslandi M, Mezzi G, Sorghi M, et al. Saccharomyces boulardii in maintenance treatment of Crohn's disease. Dig Dis Sci 2000;45:1462–4.

77. Garcia Vilela E, De Lourdes De Abreu Ferrari M, Oswaldo Da Gama Torres H, et al. Influence of Saccharomyces boulardii on the intestinal permeability of patients with Crohn's disease in remission. Scand J Gastroenterol 2008;43:842–8.

78. Marteau P, Lemann M, Seksik P, et al. Ineffectiveness of Lactobacillus johnsonii LA1 for prophylaxis of postoperative recurrence in Crohn's disease: a randomised, double blind, placebo controlled GETAID trial. Gut 2006;55:842–7.

79. Van Gossum A, Dewit O, Louis E, et al. Multicenter randomized-controlled clinical trial of probiotics (Lactobacillus johnsonii, LA1) on early endoscopic recurrence of Crohn's disease after ileo-caecal resection. Inflamm Bowel Dis 2007;13:135–42.

80. Malchow HA. Crohn's disease and *Escherichia coli*: a new approach to therapy to maintain remission of colonic Crohn's disease. J Clin Gastroenterol 1997;25: 653–8.
81. Sood A, Midha V, Makharia GK, et al. The probiotic preparation, VSL#3 induces remission in patients with mild-to-moderately active ulcerative colitis. Clin Gastroenterol Hepatol 2009;7:1202–9.
82. Tursi A, Brandimarte G, Papa A, et al. Treatment of relapsing mild-to-moderate ulcerative colitis with the probiotic VSL#3 as adjunctive to a standard pharmaceutical treatment: a double-blind, randomized, placebo-controlled study. Am J Gastroenterol 2010;105:2218–27.
83. Miele E, Pascarella F, Giannetti E, et al. Effect of a probiotic preparation (VSL#3) on induction and maintenance of remission in children with ulcerative colitis. Am J Gastroenterol 2009;104:437–43.
84. Kato K, Mizuno S, Umesaki Y, et al. Randomized placebo-controlled trial assessing the effect of bifidobacteria-fermented milk on active ulcerative colitis. Aliment Pharmacol Ther 2004;20:1133–41.
85. Petersen A, Mirsepasi H, Halkjaer S, et al. Ciprofloxacin and probiotic *Escherichia coli* Nissle add-on treatment in active ulcerative colitis: a double blind randomized placebo controlled clinical trial. J Crohns Colitis 2014;8:1498–505.
86. Matthes H, Krummenerl T, Giensch M, et al. Clinical trial: probiotic treatment of acute distal ulcerative colitis with rectally administered *Escherichia coli* Nissle 1917 (EcN). BMC Complement Altern Med 2010;10:13.
87. Oliva S, Di Nardo G, Ferrari F, et al. Randomised clinical trial: the effectiveness of *Lactobacillus reuteri* ATCC 55730 rectal enema in children with active distal ulcerative colitis. Aliment Pharmacol Ther 2012;35:327–34.
88. Shanahan F, Collins SM. Pharmabiotic manipulation of the microbiota in gastrointestinal disorders, from rationale to reality. Gastroenterol Clin North Am 2010; 39:721–6.
89. Wildt S, Nordgaard I, Hansen U, et al. A randomised double-blind placebo-controlled trial with *Lactobacillus acidophilus* La-5 and *Bifidobacterium animalis* subsp. *lactis* BB-12 for maintenance of remission in ulcerative colitis. J Crohns Colitis 2011;5:115–21.
90. Kruis W, Schutz E, Fric P, et al. Double-blind comparison of an oral *Escherichia coli* preparation and mesalazine in maintaining remission of ulcerative colitis. Aliment Pharmacol Ther 1997;11:853–8.
91. Rembacken BJ, Snelling AM, Hawkey PM, et al. Non-pathogenic *Escherichia coli* versus mesalazine for the treatment of ulcerative colitis: a randomised trial. Lancet 1999;354:635–9.
92. Kruis W, Fric P, Pokrotnieks J, et al. Maintaining remission of ulcerative colitis with the probiotic *Escherichia coli* Nissle 1917 is as effective as with standard mesalazine. Gut 2004;53:1617–23.
93. Zocco MA, dal Verme LZ, Cremonini F, et al. Efficacy of *Lactobacillus* GG in maintaining remission of ulcerative colitis. Aliment Pharmacol Ther 2006;23: 1567–74.
94. Huynh HQ, deBruyn J, Guan L, et al. Probiotic preparation VSL#3 induces remission in children with mild to moderate acute ulcerative colitis: a pilot study. Inflamm Bowel Dis 2009;15:760–8.
95. Sandborn WJ. Pouchitis following ileal pouch-anal anastomosis: definition, pathogenesis, and treatment. Gastroenterology 1994;107:1856–60.
96. Ruseler-van Embden JG, Schouten WR, van Lieshout LM. Pouchitis: result of microbial imbalance? Gut 1994;35:658–64.

97. Kuisma J, Mentula S, Jarvinen H, et al. Effect of *Lactobacillus rhamnosus* GG on ileal pouch inflammation and microbial flora. Aliment Pharmacol Ther 2003;17: 509–15.

98. Gionchetti P, Rizzello F, Helwig U, et al. Prophylaxis of pouchitis onset with probiotic therapy: a double-blind, placebo-controlled trial. Gastroenterology 2003; 124:1202–9.

99. Gionchetti P, Rizzello F, Venturi A, et al. Oral bacteriotherapy as maintenance treatment in patients with chronic pouchitis: a double-blind, placebo-controlled trial. Gastroenterology 2000;119:305–9.

100. Mimura T, Rizzello F, Helwig U, et al. Once daily high dose probiotic therapy (VSL#3) for maintaining remission in recurrent or refractory pouchitis. Gut 2004;53:108–14.

101. Pronio A, Montesani C, Butteroni C, et al. Probiotic administration in patients with ileal pouch-anal anastomosis for ulcerative colitis is associated with expansion of mucosal regulatory cells. Inflamm Bowel Dis 2008;14:662–8.

102. Landy J, Hart A. Commentary: the effects of probiotics on barrier function and mucosal pouch microbiota during maintenance treatment for severe pouchitis in patients with ulcerative colitis. Aliment Pharmacol Ther 2013;38:1405–6.

103. Sanders ME, Akkermans LM, Haller D, et al. Safety assessment of probiotics for human use. Gut Microbes 2010;1:164–85.

104. Whelan K, Myers CE. Safety of probiotics in patients receiving nutritional support: a systematic review of case reports, randomized controlled trials, and non-randomized trials. Am J Clin Nutr 2010;91:687–703.

105. Shanahan F. A commentary on the safety of probiotics. Gastroenterol Clin North Am 2012;41:869–76.

106. Guenther K, Straube E, Pfister W, et al. Severe sepsis after probiotic treatment with *Escherichia coli* Nissle 1917. Pediatr Infect Dis J 2010;29:188–9.

107. Besselink MG, van Santvoort HC, Buskens E, et al, Dutch Acute Pancreatitis Study Group. Probiotic prophylaxis in predicted severe acute pancreatitis: a randomised, double-blind, placebo-controlled trial. Lancet 2008;371:651–9.

108. Gong D, Gong X, Wang L, et al. Involvement of reduced microbial diversity in inflammatory bowel disease. Gastroenterol Res Pract 2016;2016:6951091.

109. Knoll RL, Forslund K, Kultima JR, et al. Gut microbiota differs between children with inflammatory bowel disease and healthy siblings in taxonomic and functional composition: a metagenomic analysis. Am J Physiol Gastrointest Liver Physiol 2017;312:G327–39.

110. Bermúdez-Humarán LG, Motta JP, Aubry C, et al. Serine protease inhibitors protect better than IL-10 and TGF-β anti-inflammatory cytokines against mouse colitis when delivered by recombinant lactococci. Microb Cell Fact 2015;14:26.

111. Shigemori S, Shimosato T. Applications of genetically modified immunobiotics with high immunoregulatory capacity for treatment of inflammatory bowel diseases. Front Immunol 2017;8:22.

112. Van Tol EAF, Holt L, Ling Li F, et al. Bacterial cell wall polymers promote intestinal fibrosis by direct stimulation of myofibroblasts. Am J Physiol 1999;277:G245–55.

Prebiotics and Inflammatory Bowel Disease

Heather E. Rasmussen, PhD, RDN[a],*, Bruce R. Hamaker, PhD[b]

KEYWORDS

• Inflammatory bowel disease • Ulcerative colitis • Crohn disease • Prebiotics • Fiber

KEY POINTS

• Inflammatory bowel disease risk factors include poor diet, and corresponding low intake of dietary fiber, specifically prebiotics, which is fermented by the gut microbiota.
• Dietary fibers, many of which are potential prebiotics, have hundreds to thousands of unique chemical structures that may promote bacteria or bacterial groups to provide beneficial health effects.
• In vitro and in vivo animal models provide some support for the use of prebiotics for inflammatory bowel disease through inflammation reduction.
• Studies using prebiotics in patients with inflammatory bowel disease are limited and focus on only a select few prebiotic substances.

INTRODUCTION

Prebiotics are fermentable carbohydrates that vary greatly in chemical structure, giving rise to digestion by specific gut microbiota and eliciting discrete beneficial functions. Although hundreds to thousands of fermentable dietary fibers, which are potential prebiotic substances, exist in nature, use of prebiotics in research is often limited to a few distinct structural types. Research centered on prebiotic interventions to beneficially modify the gut milieu is increasing and includes modifying microbiota, improving intestinal barrier function, and producing beneficial metabolites for both local and systemic health benefit. Despite increasing use, limited data exist for prebiotic benefit for certain conditions, including inflammatory bowel disease (IBD). This

Disclosures: B.R. Hamaker is a part owner of Nutrabiotix Inc, a company that develops fibers with prebiotic capacity. Dr B.R. Hamaker's involvement in this company has no influence on his statements regarding prebiotic effectiveness for inflammatory bowel disease.
[a] Department of Clinical Nutrition, Rush University Medical Center, 1700 W Van Buren Street, Suite 425, Chicago, IL 60612, USA; [b] Department of Food Science, Purdue University, 745 Agriculture Mall Drive, West Lafayette, IN 47907, USA
* Corresponding author.
E-mail address: Heather_Rasmussen@rush.edu

article reviews prebiotic types and the various ways in which they modify the gastrointestinal tract related to IBD. The use of select prebiotics in IBD is described in detail, highlighting their potential effectiveness, as well as the lack of evidence, for their clinical use. Recommendations for future research are made.

PREBIOTICS: DEFINITION AND STRUCTURE

The term prebiotics has, over time, undergone some changes in its definition, although it still adheres to the concept of carbohydrates that make their way to the large intestine where they are fermented and promote beneficial bacteria.[1] At the time of the original definition in the 1990s, a focus was put on oligosaccharides, and larger soluble fibers, because it was found that certain of such carbohydrates promoted 2 genera of beneficial bacteria, namely *Bifidobacterium* and *Lactobacillus*.[2] The term prebiotics became synonymous with oligosaccharides, such as fructooligosaccharides (FOS) and galactooligosaccharides (GOS), as they were accepted in the scientific, although not necessarily the regulatory, community to promote a healthy colon through the favoring of these bacteria. It was true, too, that other dietary carbohydrates promote 1 or both of *Bifidobacterium* spp and *Lactobacillus* spp, and in the scientific literature examples can be found that also are claimed as prebiotic, such as resistant starch and β-glucans. However, as more was learned regarding other relevant beneficial colonic bacteria and the importance of maintaining a favorable gut ecosystem for health, it has become apparent that the concept of prebiotics has a broader, and perhaps more complicated, role in gut health.

Prebiotics are found within the larger class of carbohydrates known as dietary fiber. These carbohydrates include all plant carbohydrates taken in the diet, plus lignin, and although fibers can be broken down into various subfractions, in the current discussion fiber may best be divided into fermentable and nonfermentable fibers. Because prebiotics are all fermentable, a case could be made for a beneficial effect of all fermentable fibers and that they promote beneficial bacteria. Hence, the concept of prebiotics could potentially take in many types of fermentable fibers comprising both oligosaccharides and polysaccharides. In contrast, nonfermentable fibers are recognized for their water-holding property and laxation capacity, although it is not known whether nonfermentable fibers could also induce an environment in the colon in which beneficial bacteria might flourish.

Perhaps what is not well recognized by scientists and clinicians specializing in gastrointestinal health and the gut microbiome is the broad and complex range of dietary fiber chemical and physical structures that exist (see the review by Hamaker and Tuncil,[3] 2014). All dietary fibers, and therefore prebiotics, are composed of 1 or more sugar units (eg, glucose, fructose, galactose, arabinose) or sugar acids (eg, galacturonic and glucuronic acid) that are linked via glycosidic bonds. Although dietary fibers are chemically and physically classified in various ways, for the purpose of the current discussion related to IBD, it is perhaps useful to think of them as (1) plant cell wall polysaccharides of the cereals (mostly composed of cellulose, arabinoxylans, β-glucans, but also small amounts of pectin and even inulin in wheat), legumes (cellulose, pectin, galactans), tubers (cellulose, pectin), and fruits and vegetables (mostly composed of cellulose, pectins, xyloglucans); (2) plant storage oligosaccharides and polysaccharides, such as starch (those entering the large intestines being resistant starch) and inulin; (3) plant exudates (eg, gum arabic); and (4) animal-based carbohydrates (eg, galactooligosaccharides, chitin/chitosan). As discussed here, most prebiotics used in human studies for patients with IBD are in the oligosaccharide and inulin classes: classes 2 and 4, respectively. Plant polysaccharides can have complicated chemical structures (**Fig. 1** for the example of pectin),[3] which gut bacteria can use through specialized abilities to access and metabolize certain structural components.

Down to the strain level, colonic bacteria have encoded in their genomes the ability to degrade certain carbohydrates they encounter and to absorb and metabolize the simple sugars released. The authors have proposed that there is high specificity of bacteria for carbohydrate chemical and physical structures and that beneficial bacteria can potentially be favored through fiber selection.[3]

PREBIOTIC FUNCTION

Prebiotic, or fermentable dietary fiber, function in the colon depends on several factors, including obvious ones like fiber type and structure, as well as an individual's gut microbiota community members and structure. Also relevant to prebiotic function are such things as cross-feeding, bacteriocins, and phage communities that influence how fibers are used. However, it is likely that prebiotic dietary fibers can shift the gut microbiome and have a beneficial effect on health, because the bacteria evolved under dietary stresses and were selected for, in significant part, based on their ability to access carbohydrates and use them efficiently for their maintenance and growth.

Fermentable dietary fibers function in the colon by providing essential food to the microbiota. Because individual bacteria, and groups or consortia of bacteria, have different abilities to use carbohydrates and must compete with other bacteria for them, there is a growing recognition that mixtures of fibers are more likely to promote growth of a wider range of bacteria than single fibers. Along with this, there is a generally accepted concept that more diverse bacterial communities are better for health than less diverse ones.[4] Much still needs to be learned regarding fibers and their action in the colon, and what mixtures are best suited for the microbiome and health, although some things are known. In addition to the function of FOS, GOS, and inulin in promoting *Bifidobacterium* and *Lactobacillus*, certain other beneficial genera and groups of bacteria have been studied in relation to fiber types for their promotion.

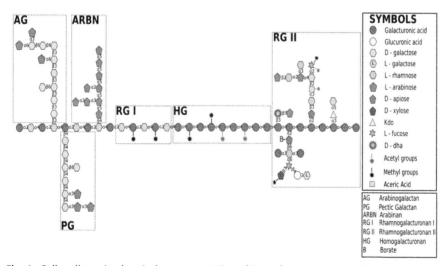

Fig. 1. Cell wall pectin chemical structure. AG, arabinogalactan; ARBN, arabinan; B, borate; HG, homogalacturonan; PG, pectic galactan; RG I, rhamnogalacturonan I; RG II, rhamnogalacturonan II. (*Data from* Hamaker BR, Tuncil YE. A perspective on the complexity of dietary fiber structures and their potential effect on the gut microbiota. J Mol Biol 2014;426(23):3842; with permission.)

The *Clostridium* clusters IV and IVa bacteria have drawn interest because they are associated with the mucosal layer of the gut epithelium, and contain several of the butyrogenic bacteria in the colon (ie, *Faecalibacterium prausnitzii, Eubacterium rectales, Roseburia infantalis*); there is also some evidence that insoluble (and fermentable) fibers favor these groups.[3,5,6]

INFLAMMATORY BOWEL DISEASE

IBD is increasing, both in the United States and in less-developed countries.[7,8] The disease is characterized by immune activation in the gastrointestinal tract, causing inflammation and damage to the mucosa or submucosa. Ulcerative colitis (UC) differs from Crohn disease (CD) in presentation, with disease activity focused on the colon and rectum in UC and intermittent disease activity throughout the gastrointestinal tract in CD. IBD is characterized by both activated innate and adaptive immune responses, with response varying by IBD type.[9] Although a T-helper 1–type response is thought to be predominant in CD and a T-helper 2–type response in UC, the stimulation and deregulation of these pathways in each type of IBD is more complex and not so clearly delineated.[10]

The cause of IBD is multifaceted, and a combination of genetic predisposition and environmental stimuli promote IBD. Genetic susceptibility to IBD is greater in CD; genes involved in signaling between the immune system and microbiota have been associated with IBD susceptibility (eg, nucleotide-binding oligomerization domain–containing protein 2 [NOD2], interleukin [IL]-23R, IL-10). An immune response in genetically predisposed individuals can be triggered by environmental stimuli through the modern lifestyle; sometimes these are otherwise innocuous. For example, drugs (eg, antibiotics, nonsteroidal antiinflammatory drugs), as well as infectious agents, stress, and diet, may all contribute to IBD.[11] Also, environmental stimuli can have opposing effects on IBD disease type; cigarette smoking increases CD risk but may be protective in UC. Some of these environmental stimuli may modify gut microbiota, creating an environment that is more susceptible to IBD development.

WHAT IS THE INVOLVEMENT OF MICROBIOTA IN INFLAMMATORY BOWEL DISEASE?

The gastrointestinal microbiota is composed of bacteria, viruses, and fungi, but the manipulation of just the bacterial component of the microbiota is the focus of the IBD literature to date. All components of the microbiota intimately interact with the host immune system, including communication between bacterial species and dendritic cells (DCs) to drive differentiation of T cells toward either an effector or regulatory T-cell response. In the context of IBD, it is not clear whether the microbiota drive changes in the host immune system or the host changes the microbiota through aberrant immune activation; likely it is a combination of the two interactions that contributes to IBD susceptibility.

The involvement of the gut microbiota in IBD was recently reviewed.[12,13] Evidence of the influence of the microbiota/immune system interaction on IBD is convincing; however, alterations in specific microbiota that increase IBD disease risk or disease course are not completely clear. Overall, patients with IBD have less microbial diversity and increased mucosal bacteria than healthy individuals.[12,14] Individual bacterial species also may differ between those with IBD and healthy individuals, with more adherent-invasive *Escherichia coli* and Enterobacteriaceae, among others,[12] in those with IBD. In addition, several taxa may be decreased, including *Bifidobacterium* and *F prausnitizii*.[12,15–17] CD recurrence has been associated with low levels of *F prausnitizii*.[18]

Although differences in microbiota composition between healthy individuals and those with IBD provide insight into microbiota's potential role in IBD, this does not indicate how, or whether, these differences contribute an altered intestinal milieu. Differing metabolites were found in fecal samples between patients with CD and healthy concordant twins.[19] Compared with healthy subjects, fecal butyrate concentrations were lower in those with IBD compared with healthy controls.[20] Maintenance or improvement in butyrate concentrations is especially important because butyrate is a primary energy source for the colonic mucosa, contributes to gut epithelial barrier integrity, and shows antiinflammatory activity.[21] More literature on the contribution of microbial metabolites to IBD disease course is warranted.

DIETARY STRATEGIES TO MINIMIZE PROGRESSION AND SYMPTOMS OF INFLAMMATORY BOWEL DISEASE: IS THERE A NICHE FOR PREBIOTICS?

Management of IBD through medication (eg, aminosalicylates, antibiotics, anti–tumor necrosis factor alpha therapy, and corticosteroids) is often needed to control disease activity; however, medication management is not always effective. This lack of efficacy may lead to uncontrolled inflammation and complications such as rectal bleeding, bowel obstruction, and intestinal resection, the occurrence of which depends on IBD type. These complications, along with intermittent diarrhea, may lead to malnutrition and weight loss. Whereas/although nutritional inadequacy, may be addressed by elemental diets or parenteral nutrition; recommendations for IBD when in remission or in less active disease suggest dietary fiber manipulation as a component of treatment.

Low-fiber diets are recommended for acute exacerbation or strictures. This minimization of fiber intake may be detrimental to encouraging a beneficial microbial environment. However, during remission, a high-fiber diet is warranted to maintain normal bowel habit, minimize gastrointestinal symptoms, and promote a healthy intestinal milieu. These recommendations focus largely on the inclusion of dietary fiber in the context of a diet high in fruits, vegetables, and whole grains. However, dietary fiber intake in the United States is inadequate (17 g/d),[22] as it is in other countries around the world. Thus, supplementation with select fibers that target specific bacteria and other components of gut health is warranted. As highlighted earlier, a structure-function relationship exists with prebiotics, suggesting that a specific prebiotic could be identified to target enhancement of a desired specific bacterial strain based on examining these structure-function relationships. However, on the whole, this has not been thoughtfully considered when selecting prebiotics, nor has it been fully researched. In addition, because uncertainty surrounds the specific bacterial taxa and metabolites that differ between both healthy individuals and those with IBD, as well as between those with UC and CD, it is currently difficult to accurately identify specific dietary modifiers for IBD because the targets of modification are not clearly known. Despite this, investigators have attempted to provide prebiotic interventions in both animal models and in humans.

USE OF PREBIOTICS IN IN VITRO AND ANIMAL MODELS AS A FOUNDATION FOR THE USE IN HUMANS WITH INFLAMMATORY BOWEL DISEASE

A few studies have examined the effect of potential prebiotic fibers using in vitro fermentation of microbiota from patients with IBD. Rose and colleagues[23] (2010) showed the effect of a fabricated butyrate-producing fiber on the microbiota communities of patients with IBD with inactive CD and active UC. The test fiber was an alginate-based starch-entrapped microsphere, and application in vitro fermentation system resulted in slower fermentation than FOS, but with similar butyrate levels; a maintenance of low pH better than FOS; and a reduction in patients with inactive CD of potentially harmful gut bacteria (species of *Bacteroides*, *Enterococcus*, *Fusobacterium*, and *Veillonella*) compared with FOS.

In recent studies in our laboratory at Purdue University on in vitro fecal fermentation assessment of dietary fibers on patients with CD and UC, many patients had microbiota with low capacity to generate short-chain fatty acids (SCFAs), which correlated with the loss of the Bacteroidetes phylum. Patients with CD and UC microbiota had lower diversity than healthy controls. It seemed that the severity of dysbiosis dictates the SCFA production with fiber supplementation. When fed in vitro a mixture of fibers containing equal amounts of FOS, β-glucan, pectin, and arabinoxylan (soluble), there was a promotion of SCFAs and gas production in the CD group that was better than when any single fiber was given. In the fiber mixture group, the *Bacteroides* genus was increased, although there was no significant pattern of microbiota change related to the fiber mixture among the individuals with CD and UC. *Bacteroides* was increased by all the fibers. Thus, in vitro human fecal fermentation analysis seems to have potential in screening dietary fibers for prebiotic effect, but studies comparing in vitro with human intervention results must still be done.

In animals, there are several studies using mostly the dextran sodium sulfate model to induce UC in mice, which show a beneficial effect of prebiotics on gut bacteria. For instance, prebiotic fructans increased amounts of *Bifidobacterium* and *Lactobacillus* in colitis-induced mice.[24,25] Larrosa and colleagues[26] (2009) studied the potential prebiotic effect of the noncarbohydrate phenolic compound, resveratrol, in rats with DSS-induced colitis and found increased levels of *Bifidobacterium* and *Lactobacillus*, and lower amounts of *E coli* and Enterobacteriaceae. In addition, in a mouse model of colitis, FOS increased luminal *Bifidobacterium* and reduced disease activity.[27]

Overall, there is a good indication of prebiotic effect resulting in improvements in microbiota community structure in IBD-type conditions. A more systematic approach toward understanding how prebiotics could optimally be used through the aforementioned, as well as additional, approaches is desired (eg, with maximum effect on creating favorable microbiota shifts, with concomitant low levels of bloating and discomfort).

USE OF PREBIOTICS IN HUMANS WITH INFLAMMATORY BOWEL DISEASE: ARE THEY EFFECTIVE?

In human studies reporting treatment outcomes in patients with IBD, degree of disease activity is assessed through biomarkers (eg, C-reactive protein, fecal calprotectin, IL-10), established indices (Crohn disease activity index [CDAI] or Harvey-Bradshaw index [HBI]), or self-report of specific outcomes such as gastrointestinal symptoms or quality-of-life improvement. In addition, and germane to this topic, microbiota composition and metabolite production (eg, SCFAs) can be measured to identify the prebiotic capacity of the supplement, as well as to provide a potential mechanism for disease improvement.

As discussed here, prebiotics are often specific carbohydrate structures that may be categorized as a type of dietary fiber. Although several researchers have shown that dietary fiber from whole foods and specific high-fiber dietary patterns can influence IBD outcomes,[28,29] no studies have been done that examine the impact of specific prebiotic-containing whole foods on IBD. Thus, evaluation of the literature to determine the impact of prebiotics on IBD is limited to prebiotic supplementation (**Table 1**).

Table 1
Human intervention studies administering prebiotics in individuals with inflammatory bowel disease

	Study Design/ Intervention Duration	Sample	Prebiotic	Clinical Outcomes	Molecular/Microbial Outcomes
Fructans					
Lindsay et al,[30] 2006	One group, open label 3 wk	Moderately active CD (HBI >5) n = 10	15 g FOS (70% oligofructose, 30% inulin)	Decrease in HBI (9.8 [3.1] to 6.9 [3.4], $P = .01$) Decrease in CADI (250.9 [77.8] to 220.6 [127.8], $P = .39$) Increase in patient and physician global assessment scores, $P < .01$ Increased borborygmi, $P = .049$, and flatulence severity, $P = .009$	Increase in fecal *Bifidobacterium*, $P = .005$; no change in mucosal *Bifidobacterium*, $P = .76$ Increase in mucosal *Bifidobacterium* in those who entered disease remission (n = 4), $P = .03$ No change in CRP, $P = .12$ Increase in IL-10–positive CD11c + DC (30.1% [38%] to 53.3% [33%], $P = .06$) Increase in DC TLR4 expression (36.8% [32%] to 75.4% [7.9%], $P < .001$)

(continued on next page)

Table 1
(continued)

	Study Design/Intervention Duration	Sample	Prebiotic	Clinical Outcomes	Molecular/Microbial Outcomes
Benjamin et al,[32] 2011	Double-blind RCT 4 wk	Active CD (CDAI ≥220 plus increased inflammation) n = 103	15 g FOS (70% DP <10, 30% DP >10) 15 g maltodextrin control	No difference in clinically significant decrease in CDAI (22% FOS and 39% placebo, $P = .067$) No difference in those achieving clinical remission (11% FOS and 20% placebo, $P = .19$) More flatulence ($P = .004$), borborygmi ($P = .029$), and abdominal pain ($P = .048$), than placebo at treatment end	No difference in *Bifidobacterium* ($P = .20$) or *F prausnitzii* ($P = .95$) between groups after treatment No difference in CRP ($P = .32$) or fecal calprotectin ($P = .09$) between groups after treatment Increase in IL-10-positive CD11c + DC intensity ratio (1.3 [0.6] to 2.0 [1.6], $P = .04$)
De Preter et al,[33] 2013	Double-blind RCT 4 wk	Inactive or moderately active CD (HBI 0–12) n = 67	10 g 1:1 OF-IN 10 g maltodextrin control	Decrease in HBI from 4 to 3 ($P = .048$) in prebiotic group, no change in placebo; decrease from 7 to 5 in moderately active patients with CD ($P = .02$) 32% dropout rate in prebiotic group vs 12% in placebo because of side effects, $P = .07$	Increase in *Bifidobacterium longum* ($P = .03$) and decrease in *Ruminococcus gnavus* ($P = .03$) Disease activity correlated with *B longum* ($r = 0.894$, $P = .02$) in patients with active CD Increase in relative concentration of acetaldehyde ($P = .001$) and butyrate ($P = .001$) in OF-IN group

Casellas et al,[34] 2007	Double-blind RCT 2 wk	Mild to moderate UC (index of Rachmilewitz 6–19) n = 19	12 g oligofructose-enriched inulin 12 g maltodextrin	Decrease in clinical disease activity in both groups ($P<.05$), no difference between groups Decrease in dyspepsia scores with oligofructose-enriched inulin ($P<.05$)	Decrease in fecal calprotectin with oligofructose-enriched inulin ($P<.05$) No change in inflammatory mediator release ($P>.05$)
Germinated Barley					
Kanauchi et al,[35] 2003	One group, open label 24 wk	Mild to moderate UC n = 21	20–30 g germinated barley (48% protein, 35% fiber, 9% lipid)	Reduction in total clinical activity index score and in 2 of the 6 components (blood in stool, nocturnal diarrhea)[a]	No difference in biochemical parameters[b] Decrease in erythema, granularity, and erosion[a]
Plantago ovata					
Fernandez-Banares et al,[38] 1999	Open-label RCT 1 y	UC in remission n = 105	20 g P ovata seeds 1.5 g mesalamine 20 g P ovata seeds plus mesalamine	Treatment effect not associated with probability of relapse, $P = .67$	Increase in fecal butyrate in those taking P ovata seeds, $P = .018$[c]
Fujimori et al,[39] 2009	3-group, randomized trial 4 wk	UC in remission n = 120	2×10^9 CFU B longum 4.0 g psyllium 2×10^9 CFU B longum plus 4.0 g psyllium	Improvement in bowel function subcomponent of IBDQ, $P = .04$	No change in C-reactive protein, $P>.05$

Abbreviations: CRP, C-reactive protein; IBDQ, IBD quality-of-life questionnaire; OF-IN, oligofructose/inulin; RCT, randomized controlled trial; TLR, Toll-like receptor.

[a] P value not reported.
[b] Biochemical parameters measured were not reported.
[c] n = 7, specific treatment group not reported.

Mixed results exist for supplementation of fructan-based prebiotics. A 1-group, open-label study supplemented 15 g of FOS for 3 weeks in 10 patients with CD.[30] Supplementation reduced the HBI score, increased fecal *Bifidobacterium* concentrations, and increased the percentage of IL-10–positive DCs. However, fluorescence in situ hybridization was used to assess changes in microbiota, a method that may not be directly comparable with more common sequencing methods used currently. In addition, the placebo response could have contributed to benefits attributed to the FOS supplement.[31] In a follow-up study by the same group, patients with CD were enrolled in a placebo-controlled randomized controlled trial (RCT) to test the effectiveness of 15 g of FOS on CD disease activity.[32] No differences in clinical response existed between groups. In addition, no change in fecal *Bifidobacterium* or *F prausnitzii* was seen with FOS intake, but the proportion of IL-6–positive DCs decreased and the proportion of IL-10 DCs increased with treatment. De Preter and colleagues[33] conducted a double-blind, parallel-group RCT using 10 g of fructan (1:1 inulin to oligofructose) versus a maltodextrin control. In the prebiotic group, butyrate was significantly increased from baseline, and HBI decreased in the entire sample as well as in patients with moderately active disease. In addition, Casellas and colleagues[34] conducted a study with a mixture of inulin and oligofructose (BENEO Synergy 1) and reported decreases in fecal calprotectin in patients with mild to moderately active UC. Importantly, side effects were common in 3 of these studies, contributing to increased dropout in 2. Although most saw a beneficial change in clinical disease activity indices, improvement in molecular outcomes were not consistent between studies.

Although fructan-containing compounds are the most well-known prebiotics, other fibers may have prebiotic capacity and thus may benefit patients with IBD. One such example is germinated barley. Composed of not only fiber (cellulose, hemicellulose, and lignin), malted barley in the form used in IBD studies (termed germinated barley foodstuff, GBF) contains protein and lipid as major and minor components, respectively, of the dietary compound. Several studies by the same researchers reported a benefit of this compound for patients with UC.[35–37] In one study (see **Table 1**), these researchers provided patients with UC with 20 to 30 g of GBF for 24 weeks.[35] Total clinical activity index score, as well as 2 subcomponents, were reduced with GBF intake; however, the magnitude of change was not clearly reported. Images of the colon and rectum indicated improvement in erythema, granularity, and erosion. Importantly, the study was open label with no control group and thus could not account for the natural change in disease activity over the study duration. In addition, this study did not assess microbiota or metabolites. Also, GBF was stated to be well tolerated, but no supporting data were presented.

In addition, *Plantago ovata* (psyllium) has been used in patients with UC to identify the impact on remission maintenance.[38,39] Supplementation of 20 g of *P ovata* seeds a day resulted in no difference in remission maintenance compared with mesalamine. Fecal butyrate levels increased with *P ovata* intake; however, data were presented on only 7 subjects, and it was not stated from which group these subjects originated (see **Table 1**).[38] In addition, Fujimori and colleagues[39] did not have a control group and thus any change seen with prebiotic treatment (change in bowel function–related quality of life) is difficult to interpret in the context of prebiotic effectiveness.

In addition to studies providing prebiotics, several investigators have supplemented with synbiotics, a combination of prebiotics and probiotics, with benefit for inflammation[39,40] and improvement in endoscopic score.[41] These studies are not reviewed here because the probiotic component is likely to influence gut microbiota and other measured outcomes, thus obscuring the effect of the prebiotic alone.

Limitations of current studies specifically reporting prebiotic intake in patients with IBD include inconsistency in outcomes, methods used to assess these outcomes, and variations in disease activity. Thus far, identification of a prebiotic that consistently addresses assumedly detrimental changes in microbiota in patients with IBD (eg, lower *F prausnitzii*) has not been done in humans. Also, dietary intake was not assessed, thus it is not known whether variation in diet could have affected outcomes. In addition to the lack of available evidence, assumptions about prebiotic consumption to benefit patients with IBD are many. First, IBD risk likely originates early in life; supplementing with prebiotics may modify IBD disease activity, but it is far more effective to create an environment amenable to ideal microbiota development early in life, whether through prebiotic supplementation or modification of other environmental stimuli. Although not emphasized earlier, CD and UC are heterogeneous diseases; it is possible that 1 prebiotic type will not be effective for both CD and UC. In addition to tailoring the prebiotic to the disease type and stage, it is possible that a mixture of prebiotic fibers will be most useful to enhance the functional capacity of a variety of bacteria that may have health benefits for patients with IBD.

SUMMARY

Prebiotics are fermentable carbohydrates with the ability to modify gut microbiota and subsequent metabolites to improve gut health. Results from in vitro and animal studies provide some support for the use of prebiotics to modify a variety of factors, including intestinal-derived inflammation, a key contributor to IBD pathogenesis. Although these studies support prebiotic use in patients with IBD, few prospective, controlled human trials exist. In the studies that have been completed, the prebiotic used varies, making it impossible to provide consensus on its effectiveness. In addition, limited studies exist including functional analyses. It is important to further identify alternative prebiotics with low-bloating characteristics with minimal gas production to provide a tolerable fiber for beneficial modulation of the microbiota, metabolite production, and inflammation reduction. In addition, more needs to be known about mechanisms behind IBD and the specific bacteria involved before targeted prebiotics can be effective.

REFERENCES

1. Hutkins RW, Krumbeck JA, Bindels LB, et al. Prebiotics: why definitions matter. Curr Opin Biotechnol 2016;37:1–7.
2. Gibson GR, Fuller R. Aspects of in vitro and in vivo research approaches directed toward identifying probiotics and prebiotics for human use. J Nutr 2000;130(2S Suppl):391S–5S.
3. Hamaker BR, Tuncil YE. A perspective on the complexity of dietary fiber structures and their potential effect on the gut microbiota. J Mol Biol 2014;426(23): 3838–50.
4. Sonnenburg ED, Sonnenburg JL. Starving our microbial self: the deleterious consequences of a diet deficient in microbiota-accessible carbohydrates. Cell Metab 2014;20(5):779–86.
5. Flint HJ, Bayer EA, Rincon MT, et al. Polysaccharide utilization by gut bacteria: potential for new insights from genomic analysis. Nat Rev Microbiol 2008;6(2): 121–31.
6. Van den Abbeele P, Gerard P, Rabot S, et al. Arabinoxylans and inulin differentially modulate the mucosal and luminal gut microbiota and mucin-degradation in humanized rats. Environ Microbiol 2011;13(10):2667–80.

7. Kappelman MD, Rifas-Shiman SL, Kleinman K, et al. The prevalence and geographic distribution of Crohn's disease and ulcerative colitis in the united states. Clin Gastroenterol Hepatol 2007;5(12):1424–9.
8. Loftus EV Jr. Clinical epidemiology of inflammatory bowel disease: incidence, prevalence, and environmental influences. Gastroenterology 2004;126(6): 1504–17.
9. Sartor RB. Mechanisms of disease: pathogenesis of Crohn's disease and ulcerative colitis. Nat Clin Pract Gastroenterol Hepatol 2006;3(7):390–407.
10. de Mattos BR, Garcia MP, Nogueira JB, et al. Inflammatory bowel disease: an overview of immune mechanisms and biological treatments. Mediators Inflamm 2015;2015:493012.
11. Bernstein CN, Shanahan F. Disorders of a modern lifestyle: reconciling the epidemiology of inflammatory bowel diseases. Gut 2008;57(9):1185–91.
12. Sheehan D, Shanahan F. The gut microbiota in inflammatory bowel disease. Gastroenterol Clin North Am 2017;46(1):143–54.
13. Shanahan F, Quigley EM. Manipulation of the microbiota for treatment of IBS and IBD-challenges and controversies. Gastroenterology 2014;146(6):1554–63.
14. Kostic AD, Xavier RJ, Gevers D. The microbiome in inflammatory bowel disease: current status and the future ahead. Gastroenterology 2014;146(6):1489–99.
15. Quevrain E, Maubert MA, Michon C, et al. Identification of an anti-inflammatory protein from *Faecalibacterium prausnitzii*, a commensal bacterium deficient in Crohn's disease. Gut 2016;65(3):415–25.
16. Joossens M, Huys G, Cnockaert M, et al. Dysbiosis of the faecal microbiota in patients with Crohn's disease and their unaffected relatives. Gut 2011;60(5):631–7.
17. Sokol H, Seksik P, Furet JP, et al. Low counts of *Faecalibacterium prausnitzii* in colitis microbiota. Inflamm Bowel Dis 2009;15(8):1183–9.
18. Sokol H, Pigneur B, Watterlot L, et al. *Faecalibacterium prausnitzii* is an anti-inflammatory commensal bacterium identified by gut microbiota analysis of Crohn disease patients. Proc Natl Acad Sci U S A 2008;105(43):16731–6.
19. Jansson J, Willing B, Lucio M, et al. Metabolomics reveals metabolic biomarkers of Crohn's disease. PLoS One 2009;4(7):e6386.
20. Marchesi JR, Holmes E, Khan F, et al. Rapid and noninvasive metabonomic characterization of inflammatory bowel disease. J Proteome Res 2007;6(2):546–51.
21. Hamer HM, Jonkers D, Venema K, et al. Review article: the role of butyrate on colonic function. Aliment Pharmacol Ther 2008;27(2):104–19.
22. US Department of Agriculture, Agricultural Research Service. Nutrient intakes from food: mean amounts consumed per individual, by gender and age, what we eat in America, NHANES 2013-2014. 2014. Available at: www.ars.usda.gov/ba/bhnrc/fsrg. Accessed June 1, 2017.
23. Rose DJ, Venema K, Keshavarzian A, et al. Starch-entrapped microspheres show a beneficial fermentation profile and decrease in potentially harmful bacteria during in vitro fermentation in faecal microbiota obtained from patients with inflammatory bowel disease. Br J Nutr 2010;103(10):1514–24.
24. Hoentjen F, Welling GW, Harmsen HJ, et al. Reduction of colitis by prebiotics in HLA-B27 transgenic rats is associated with microflora changes and immunomodulation. Inflamm Bowel Dis 2005;11(11):977–85.
25. Lara-Villoslada F, de Haro O, Camuesco D, et al. Short-chain fructooligosaccharides, in spite of being fermented in the upper part of the large intestine, have anti-inflammatory activity in the TNBS model of colitis. Eur J Nutr 2006;45(7):418–25.

26. Larrosa M, Yanez-Gascon MJ, Selma MV, et al. Effect of a low dose of dietary resveratrol on colon microbiota, inflammation and tissue damage in a DSS-induced colitis rat model. J Agric Food Chem 2009;57(6):2211–20.
27. Cherbut C, Michel C, Lecannu G. The prebiotic characteristics of fructooligosaccharides are necessary for reduction of TNBS-induced colitis in rats. J Nutr 2003; 133(1):21–7.
28. Chiba M, Abe T, Tsuda H, et al. Lifestyle-related disease in Crohn's disease: relapse prevention by a semi-vegetarian diet. World J Gastroenterol 2010; 16(20):2484–95.
29. James SL, Christophersen CT, Bird AR, et al. Abnormal fibre usage in UC in remission. Gut 2015;64(4):562–70.
30. Lindsay JO, Whelan K, Stagg AJ, et al. Clinical, microbiological, and immunological effects of fructo-oligosaccharide in patients with Crohn's disease. Gut 2006; 55(3):348–55.
31. Su C, Lichtenstein GR, Krok K, et al. A meta-analysis of the placebo rates of remission and response in clinical trials of active Crohn's disease. Gastroenterology 2004;126(5):1257–69.
32. Benjamin JL, Hedin CR, Koutsoumpas A, et al. Randomised, double-blind, placebo-controlled trial of fructo-oligosaccharides in active Crohn's disease. Gut 2011;60(7):923–9.
33. De Preter V, Joossens M, Ballet V, et al. Metabolic profiling of the impact of oligofructose-enriched inulin in Crohn's disease patients: a double-blinded randomized controlled trial. Clin Transl Gastroenterol 2013;4:e30.
34. Casellas F, Borruel N, Torrejon A, et al. Oral oligofructose-enriched inulin supplementation in acute ulcerative colitis is well tolerated and associated with lowered faecal calprotectin. Aliment Pharmacol Ther 2007;25(9):1061–7.
35. Kanauchi O, Mitsuyama K, Homma T, et al. Treatment of ulcerative colitis patients by long-term administration of germinated barley foodstuff: multi-center open trial. Int J Mol Med 2003;12(5):701–4.
36. Kanauchi O, Iwanaga T, Mitsuyama K. Germinated barley foodstuff feeding. A novel neutraceutical therapeutic strategy for ulcerative colitis. Digestion 2001; 63(Suppl 1):60–7.
37. Hanai H, Kanauchi O, Mitsuyama K, et al. Germinated barley foodstuff prolongs remission in patients with ulcerative colitis. Int J Mol Med 2004;13(5):643–7.
38. Fernandez-Banares F, Hinojosa J, Sanchez-Lombrana JL, et al. Randomized clinical trial of *Plantago ovata* seeds (dietary fiber) as compared with mesalamine in maintaining remission in ulcerative colitis. Spanish Group for the Study of Crohn's Disease and Ulcerative Colitis (GETECCU). Am J Gastroenterol 1999;94(2): 427–33.
39. Fujimori S, Gudis K, Mitsui K, et al. A randomized controlled trial on the efficacy of synbiotic versus probiotic or prebiotic treatment to improve the quality of life in patients with ulcerative colitis. Nutrition 2009;25(5):520–5.
40. Furrie E, Macfarlane S, Kennedy A, et al. Synbiotic therapy (*Bifidobacterium longum*/synergy 1) initiates resolution of inflammation in patients with active ulcerative colitis: a randomised controlled pilot trial. Gut 2005;54(2):242–9.
41. Ishikawa H, Matsumoto S, Ohashi Y, et al. Beneficial effects of probiotic *Bifidobacterium* and galacto-oligosaccharide in patients with ulcerative colitis: a randomized controlled study. Digestion 2011;84(2):128–33.

Vitamins and Minerals in Inflammatory Bowel Disease

Fayez K. Ghishan, MD[a], Pawel R. Kiela, DVM, PhD[a,b],*

KEYWORDS

- Crohn disease • Ulcerative colitis • Diet • Nutrition • Deficiency • Supplementation

KEY POINTS

- Vitamin and mineral deficiencies are common among inflammatory bowel disease (IBD) patients and warrant supplementation to restore recommended values.
- Those deficiencies likely contribute to the disease severity and associated comorbidities.
- There is a need for more evidence-based approaches supported by well-designed clinical trials to document the optimal supplementation level and to assess the benefits of supplementation exceeding the recommended daily allowance.

INTRODUCTION: FIXING DEFICIENCIES OR OVERSUPPLEMENTATION?

The role of diet in the pathogenesis of inflammatory bowel disease (IBD) remains an open topic despite the advances in the understanding of the gastrointestinal pathophysiology microbiology and mucosal immunology. A shift from a more aboriginal food to the highly refined and processed western diet, and the associated change in gut microbiome, as contributing environmental factors has been suggested by many nutritional studies.[1] The observed increased risk of autoimmune disease diagnosis among children and second-generation immigrants from regions of the world with low IBD incidence to developed countries with higher incidence of IBD also suggests the role of change in dietary habits.[2] Whereas singularly pointing to diet or dietary constituents as the main culprit that precipitates or promotes this complex disease has been very difficult, studying nutritional deficiencies, inherently associated with the course of IBD, is feasible and has been systematically done for decades.[3,4]

Complementary and alternative medicine (CAM) encompasses a vast array of treatment options, including dietary interventions. In IBD patients, they are aimed at eliminating food triggers and improving nutrition, and include supplementation of

[a] Department of Pediatrics, University of Arizona, Tucson, AZ, USA; [b] Department of Immunobiology, University of Arizona, Tucson, AZ, USA
* Corresponding author. Department of Pediatrics, University of Arizona, 1501 North Campbell Avenue, Room 6351, Tucson, AZ 85724.
E-mail address: pkiela@peds.arizona.edu

Gastroenterol Clin N Am 46 (2017) 797–808
http://dx.doi.org/10.1016/j.gtc.2017.08.011
0889-8553/17/© 2017 Elsevier Inc. All rights reserved.

vitamins and other micronutrients and macronutrients. Nutritional interventions are an integral part of clinical practice, although evidence from clinical studies is relatively uncommon and frequently suffers from inadequate design and/or small numbers of subjects. In some instances, for example, vitamin D_3, supplementation with doses far exceeding the recommended daily allowances has been proposed.[5] Considering the size of the US supplement industry (estimated at as much as $37 billion),[6] wide general use of over-the-counter supplements, including vitamins and minerals, and high rate of CAM use among patients with gastrointestinal disorders and IBD in particular,[7] it is important to consider the efficacy of vitamin and mineral supplements, especially in the context of alleviating the primary and secondary symptoms of disease.

The mechanisms responsible for nutritional deficiencies are not always clear and could be related to decreased intake, malabsorption, or excess losses. Increased metabolic demand related to the active inflammatory process should also be taken into consideration. Micronutrient and vitamin deficiencies are relatively common among IBD patients, especially in Crohn disease (CD) with active small bowel disease, or patients undergoing intestinal resection. Those deficiencies have been subject to several excellent reviews,[3,4,8] a comprehensive recent monograph on nutritional management of IBD,[9] and are discussed relatively briefly in this article. This article briefly describes the state of knowledge regarding vitamin and mineral deficiencies, and presents and discusses the studies related to the efficacy of selected vitamin and mineral supplements in preclinical models of IBD and in clinical trials.

VITAMIN A

Serum retinol concentrations are typically used to identify vitamin A deficiency risk. Based on this factor alone, a high proportion of adult and pediatric IBD patients has been diagnosed with deficiency.[10–12] da Rocha and colleagues[13] published a case report of retinol deficiency and night blindness in a CD patient with repeated small bowel resections. Sufficiency and normal eyesight was restored by regular parenteral vitamin A administration.[13] However, serum retinol concentrations do not begin to decline until liver reserves of vitamin A are close to exhaustion, thus it is plausible that different assessment of vitamin A status that accounts for hepatic storage, would yield higher numbers of vitamin A-deficient IBD patients. Indeed, when Soares-Mota and colleagues[14] measured relative dose response in serum retinol after ingestion of retinyl palmitate as an indirect indicator of the hepatic retinol storage, a higher percentage of CD patients was diagnosed with insufficiency compared with measurement of steady-state serum level of retinol (37% vs 29%, respectively). Although no association was found between vitamin A status assessed this way with ileal disease, ileal resection, disease duration, or C-reactive protein (CRP) level, CD patients with vitamin A deficiency had significantly lower body mass index and body fat than those with normal levels.[14]

Retinoic acid, a metabolite of retinol, plays key roles in maintaining mucosal immune homeostasis by supporting the tolerogenic dendritic cells (DCs), balancing Th17 and regulatory T cell responses, gut homing of the innate lymphoid cells, and immunoglobulin-A class switching in B cells.[15] In rodent IBD models, vitamin A deficiency exacerbates inflammation, and supplementation offers protection.[16–19] Human studies with vitamin A or retinoic acid supplementation are sparse and disappointing. Wright and colleagues[20] showed no benefit of 50,000 U twice daily in a double-blind study involving 68 subjects with CD. In another small study by Norrby and colleagues,[21] 150,000 U of vitamin A daily led to no measurable improvement in 8 subjects with severe CD.

Perhaps those failures are in part due to the pleiotropy of the effects of vitamin A and its metabolites on the mucosal immune system. Effectiveness of vitamin A supplementation may be potentially limited due to reduced expression of aldehyde dehydrogenase 1 family member (A2ALDH1a2), a pivotal enzyme in the synthesis of all-trans retinoic acid (atRA) from retinol in DCs[22] and/or increased activity of atRA-catabolizing enzyme, CYP26A1.[23–25] It is, nevertheless, prudent to supplement vitamin A in confirmed cases of deficiency to at least meet the recommended dietary allowance (RDA) of 900 μg (3000 IU) daily for adult men and 700 μg (2300 IU) daily for adult women.

VITAMIN B1 (THIAMINE)

Thiamine (mainly thiamine pyrophosphate) is indispensable for carbohydrate metabolism, mitochondrial adenosine triphosphate (ATP) production, and reduction of cellular oxidative stress. Low intracellular levels of thiamine lead to acute energy failure, propensity for oxidative stress, and mitochondrial abnormalities. Symptoms of thiamine deficiency, which may be associated with diet rich in highly refined carbohydrates (polished rice, white flour, white sugar) or during general malnutrition (eg, anorexia), range from nonspecific fatigue, irritability, poor memory, sleep disturbances, or abdominal discomfort among others, to severe neurologic deficits, such as beriberi, Wernicke encephalopathy, Korsakoff psychosis, or their combination (Wernicke-Korsakoff syndrome). Case reports have been published that include severe optic neuropathy and oculomotor palsy in UC patients that were correctable by high doses of vitamin B1,[26] and clinical and radiological diagnosis of Wernicke's encephalopathy in CD patients on parenteral nutrition.[27,28]

The role of thiamine in general energy metabolism suggested a potential role for intracellular thiamine deficiency in the pathogenesis of IBD-associated fatigue. In a pilot study with 12 subjects with CD with normal blood thiamine and thiamine pyrophosphate, Costantini and Pala[29] showed that 600 to 1,500 mg of thiamine daily completely alleviated symptoms of fatigue in 10 out of 12 subjects, with the remaining 2 also reporting significant improvement.

BIOTIN

Humans are not able to synthesize biotin (vitamin B7, also referred to as vitamin H), which must be obtained from dietary sources or bacterial synthesis by gut microbiota. Biotin functions as cofactor for 5 carboxylases critical in the fatty acid, glucose, and amino acid metabolism; cellular energy metabolism; and the regulation of cellular oxidative stress. Biotin deficiency, among other consequences, has been implicated in immune dysfunction,[30] although the effects of supplementation are not easily interpretable. Wiedmann and colleagues[31,32] showed that daily supplementation with 2150 μg of biotin for 21 days (RDA is 300 μg daily) enhanced T helper (Th)-1 and inhibited Th2 responses in restimulated peripheral blood mononuclear cells (PBMCs). This may indicate a divergent response in CD (worsening) and UC patients (improvement of symptoms) should they increase their daily intake to such levels. In vitro, biotin deficiency promoted nuclear factor-kappa beta (NF-κβ) activation and tumor necrosis factor (TNF) expression in murine macrophages,[33] and an enhanced inflammatory response was recently shown in biotin-deficient human monocyte-derived dendritic cells.[34] However, biotin deficiency has not been conclusively demonstrated in IBD, with inconsistent reports published.[35–37]

VITAMIN B6

Pyridoxal 5'-phosphate (PLP) is the biologically active form of vitamin B6 and serves as a cofactor for more than 140 biochemical reactions involved in a vast array of metabolic pathways.[38] Although severe vitamin B6 deficiency is uncommon, mild insufficiency (plasma PLP <20 nmol/L) is observed in 10% to 16% of the adult US population.[39] In mammals, food and gut commensal bacteria are the 2 main sources of vitamin B6. PLP tends to be generally reduced in patients with inflammatory conditions and is inversely correlated with CRP concentration.[40] Restoring normal levels in patients with inflammation requires higher dietary intake.[41] Saibeni and colleagues[42] showed that subjects with active CD and UC have significantly lower plasma PLP concentrations than subjects with quiescent disease or healthy controls. However, the relationship between inflammation and B6 level is not straightforward. In mice, short-term (2-week) B6 and B12 deprivation reduced the severity of dextran sodium sulphate (DSS)-induced colitis and the investigators attributed these unexpected results to B6 deficiency alone.[43] In interleukin (IL)-10$^{-/-}$ mice with chronic colitis, a bell-shaped response curve was shown; that is, reduced inflammation at both deficiency and oversupplementation as compared with a normal B6 status after 12-week dietary intervention. The investigators suggested that reduced inflammation in supplemented animals may be the result of reduced local colonic levels of sphinosine-1-phosphate (S1P), a potent chemoattractant, a phenomenon potentially related to the role of PLP as a cofactor of the S1P-metabolizing enzymes: serine C-palmitoyltransferase and S1P lyase.[44]

VITAMIN B12 AND FOLIC ACID

These 2 nutrients are especially known for their role in erythropoiesis and association with IBD-associated anemia. Vitamin B12 (cobalamin) and folate have crucial roles in nucleic acid synthesis and erythropoiesis. During their differentiation, erythroblasts require both vitamins for proliferation, and their deficiency leads to macrocytosis, erythroblast apoptosis, and anemia. Although several reports showed higher prevalence of B12 deficiency in CD than in healthy controls, a meta-analysis (3732 subjects) by Battat and colleagues[45] concluded that there is insufficient evidence in the literature to suggest an association, regardless of the ileal involvement. However, consistent with the ileum being the primary site of B12 absorption, ileal resection of greater than 30 cm in Crohn subjects were found to predispose to deficiency and warrant treatment.[45] Although similar meta-analysis of folate deficiency has not been performed, Bermejo and colleagues[46] reported that the prevalence is higher among subjects with CD (22.2%) than in subjects with UC (4.3%), and was associated with disease severity, but not ileal resection. The recent guidelines of the European Crohn's and Colitis Organisation (ECCO) recommend checking for cobalamin and folate level at least once per year or when macrocytosis is present, especially in patients not receiving thiopurines, which may directly elevate mean corpuscular volume. Although folate deficiency and elevated homocysteine have been suggested to contribute to IBD-associated colon cancer, contradicting data from preclinical studies with folic acid supplementation were published. Carrier and colleagues[47] used a complex model of UC-associated colon cancer with IL-2 and β2-microglobulin double knockout mice and showed a significantly lower incidence of high-grade lesions in the folate-supplemented group (8 mg/kg diet for 32 weeks). However, the same dose in 12-week treatment regime in DSS-azoxymethane (AOM) model of colitis-associated cancer showed no measurable effect on tumor formation or colonic microbiome composition.[48]

IRON

Iron is an essential element for blood production and is responsible for reversible oxygen binding in the hemoglobin. The incidence of iron deficiency anemia (IDA) and the associated fatigue is high in IBD patients with prevalence reported in 36% to 76% of patients.[49] The etiologic factors of IDA in IBD patients include inadequate intake, chronic blood loss caused by mucosal ulcerations, and anemia of chronic inflammation secondary to impairment of transepithelial iron absorption in the gut. The latter is associated with IL-6 driven increase in hepatic hepcidin, which binds to ferroportin on enterocytes (also monocytes and macrophages) and leads to its internalization and lysosomal degradation, thus resulting in intracellular iron sequestration.

Oral iron supplementation is the primary mode of preventing IDA secondary to blood loss or inadequate intake, with multiple and equally effective forms of iron available. Most frequently used forms are ferrous fumarate, ferrous sulfate, and ferrous gluconate, which contain 33%, 20%, and 12% of elemental iron, respectively, and are frequently combined with vitamin C to enhance absorption. For IBD patients, the Centers for Disease Control and Prevention recommends 30 mg/d of elemental iron for IDA prophylaxis, and 50 to 60 mg/d for treatment. However, oral supplementation in IBD may be ineffective in the settings of normocytic anemia of chronic inflammation. It may also be poorly tolerated with adverse effects, such as epigastric pain, nausea, flatulence, and diarrhea, which lead to poor adherence to treatment. High doses and excess of nonabsorbed iron in IBD may also be toxic to the epithelium because it undergoes Fenton reaction with hydrogen peroxide and increases inflammatory response. The efficacy of oral iron is low in patients with high levels of CRP and, in general, oral supplementation is considered safer and more effective in IBD patients with inactive or mild disease. Newer oral preparations, such as ferric maltol, a combination of iron and maltol (3-hydroxy-2-methyl-4-pyrone), offer a viable alternative to the more mainstream forms of iron in mild-to-moderate IBD without resorting to intravenous therapy, even in patients who do not tolerate oral ferrous products.[50] However, ferric maltol is not yet available as an over-the-counter supplement. Intravenous iron infusions offer another alternative in which oral preparations are ineffective or are poorly tolerated. Because free iron is toxic, all intravenous iron contains carbohydrates that bind the elemental iron to prevent reactions. ECCO guidelines recommend intravenous iron to be considered the first line of treatment in patients with clinically active IBD, previous intolerance to oral iron, hemoglobin lower than 10 g/dL, or in patients with documented need for erythropoiesis-stimulating agents.[51]

VITAMIN D₃ AND CALCIUM

Vitamin D is an essential nutrient with wide systemic effects. Regulation of the innate and adaptive immune responses and regulation of calcium homeostasis and bone metabolism are of particular importance in IBD due to immune dysregulation and inflammation-associated loss of bone mineral density prevalent among IBD patients. Vitamin D3 (cholecalciferol) is the natural form of vitamin D active in humans and is provided in diet and synthesized in the skin via UV-B exposure and thermal conversion. After 2 hydroxylation steps in the liver and kidney, $1,25(OH)_2\,D_3$ becomes the most biologically active form of D_3. Clinically measured $25(OH)D_3$ is considered a better marker of dietary intake or absorption, hepatic stores and conversion, and general systemic availability. Although the guidelines are somewhat fluid, blood levels of $25(OH)D_3$ less than 20 ng/mL are considered as a deficiency, with 30 to 100 ng/mL considered optimal. Concentrations of greater than or equal to 150 ng/mL have been associated with toxicity. Among all nutritional deficiencies in IBD, vitamin D_3

received the most attention with relatively consistent reports of prevalent deficiency or insufficiency.[52,53] Vitamin D_3 deficiency is considered to be an etiologic factor behind impaired epithelial calcium absorption and bone metabolism,[54] as well as potential defects in the function of innate immune system (eg, phagocyte bacterial killing) and dysregulation of the adaptive immune responses.[55]

Restoring normal levels is imperative in clinical care and has been associated with beneficial clinical outcomes.[56,57] Both vitamin D_2 (ergocalciferol) and D_3 (cholecalciferol) are available and used as supplements, although the overall biological activity of ergocalciferol was estimated to be no more than 30% of cholecalciferol. Thus, cholecalciferol or natural sources of vitamin D_3 (especially oily fish like salmon, mackerel, herring, and cod liver) are the preferred forms of supplementation. Current vitamin D intake recommendations of the Institute of Medicine suggest 1000 to 2000 IU/d in healthy adults, a dose embraced by the Endocrine Society's Clinical Practice Guidelines, which also considered 10,000 IU/d to be safe. Although there are no strict developed guidelines for IBD patients, an annual screening of $25(OH)D_3$ is recommended, especially in patients on steroid therapy. Supplementation of 600 IU/d and 800 IU/d has been considered adequate in patients with normal D_3 levels who are between 1 and 70 years old, and greater than 70 years, respectively. In adults at risk for deficiency (in the insufficiency range), a daily intake of 1000 IU/d is recommended and 6000 IU/d or 50,000 IU once a week in patient with identified deficiency has been proposed. These values were developed largely with normalizing the serum levels of $25(OH)D_3$ as a primary outcome measure. The effectiveness of D_3 supplementation on bone health and inflammation in IBD is not uniformly beneficial in clinical studies. For example, the effects of vitamin D_3 alone or in combination with calcium and bisphosphonates on bone mineral density in IBD patients yielded inconclusive data, ranging from significant[58] or limited benefits.[59] In pediatric IBD patients conflicting data have been reported.[60,61] More systematic studies in pediatric and adult IBD patients need to be conducted to identify factors determining the clinical response to vitamin D and Ca^{2+} supplementation, the form and route of administered vitamin D, with careful monitoring of the parameters of bone mass, bone turnover, and mineral homeostasis. The need for such systematic approach is further justified by identification of at least a subset of IBD patients with inappropriate hypercalcitriolemia, which is elevated serum $1,25(OH)_2D_3$.[62,63] The authors' group has suggested that because cytokines associated with active inflammation, such as IL-1β, IL-6, and TNFα, may act synergistically with vitamin D_3 to negatively regulate bone turnover, high-dose vitamin D_3 supplementation in active IBD may not improve bone density or even lead to a paradoxic bone mineral density (BMD) loss[64] and that in patients at clear risk of osteopenia or osteoporosis or with proven osteopenia or osteoporosis, vitamin D_3 be withheld until remission is achieved.[54,65] This would also be consistent with vitamin D_3 supplementation as a means of relapse prevention, which has clinical support in published studies.[66,67] Although long-term high-dose D_3 supplementation has been shown in some studies to significantly reduce disease score in active IBD (eg, Yang and colleagues[68]), the effects on the bone are typically not assessed in those inflammation-centric studies.

VITAMIN K

Vitamin K is a group of structurally related fat-soluble compounds. Vitamin K_1, also known as phylloquinone, is particularly abundant in green leafy vegetables due to its involvement in photosynthesis. Both animals and their gut bacteria convert vitamin K_1 into K_2 isoforms known as menaquinones. Menaquinones differ in length from

1 to 14 repeats of 5-carbon units in the isoprenoid side chain of the molecules, are designated as MK2 though MK14, and differ in their apparent biological effects. Three synthetic types of vitamin K are known: vitamins K_3, K_4, and K_5

Vitamin K is the essential cofactor in the process of carboxylation of glutamic acid residues in many vitamin K–dependent proteins involved in blood coagulation, bone metabolism, prevention of vascular mineralization, and regulation of many other cellular functions. Early and limited study by Krasinski and colleagues[69] showed relatively high prevalence of vitamin K deficiency in CD and UC, but not celiac patients, without an identified bleeding disorder.

Bone formation by osteoblasts requires vitamin K–dependent post-translational gamma-carboxylation of glutamate residues on osteocalcin, matrix Gla protein, and protein S, whereas bone resorption is inhibited by vitamin K via inhibition of the synthesis of prostaglandin E2 by osteoclast. Consistent with the effects of vitamin K on bone metabolism, several clinical studies suggested that in CD patients, vitamin K deficiency contributes to low BMD.[70–72] However, a more recent clinical study in CD patients with vitamin K insufficiency supplemented with 1000 µg of phylloquinone (K_1) daily for 12 months (along with calcium and vitamin D_3) failed to demonstrate measurable effects on bone metabolism. It is plausible that conversion of K_1 to potentially more efficacious menaquinones (K_2) by the inflamed host and gut microbiome is altered. Although other forms, such as menatetrenone (MK)-4, have been shown to be effective in postmenopausal bone loss, they have not yet been tested in IBD patients. Interestingly, MK-4 has been shown to reduce the symptoms of DSS-induced colitis in mice, suggesting that it may also work as an immune modulator.[73]

ZINC

Zinc is an essential mineral that plays pivotal roles in many aspects of cellular metabolism, such as supporting catalytic activity of approximately 100 enzymes, modulation of immune function, protein synthesis, wound healing, DNA synthesis, cell division, and improvement of intestinal barrier function. Assessment of zinc status in patients is not straightforward because it lacks storage mechanisms and significantly fluctuates with intake. With that in mind, it has been estimated that 15% of IBD patients are affected by zinc deficiency.[74] A recent study showed that zinc deficiency in patients with CD and UC was associated with poor clinical outcomes: increased risk of subsequent hospitalizations, surgeries, and disease-related complications.[75] The investigators showed that these outcomes improve with normalization of zinc, and suggested close monitoring and replacement of zinc in IBD patients as needed. Current RDA is 11 mg/d and 8 mg/d of elemental zinc for male patients and female patients, respectively, but higher doses have been recommended or used in IBD: from 40 mg/d for 10 days to 110 mg 3 times a day for 8 weeks in CD patients in remission.[76] Chronic IBD-associated diarrhea is an additional indication for zinc supplementation. High-dose and long-tern supplementation with zinc should be used with caution, however. The upper limit (highest daily intake above which side effects or toxicity may occur) for this mineral is set to 40 mg/d, and zinc can interfere with iron and copper absorption, exacerbating their potential deficiencies. In turn, supplementation with calcium or folate and can reduce zinc absorption. Two most common supplemental forms zinc sulfate (23% of elemental zinc) and zinc gluconate (13% elemental zinc).

SUMMARY

Insufficient intake, impaired absorption via inflamed or otherwise functionally impaired epithelia, and increased metabolic needs all contribute to vitamin and mineral deficiencies, which are relatively common among IBD patients. Although good clinical practice should include surveillance for micronutrient deficiencies and, in respective cases, a relevant treatment and supplementation, in many cases, doses needed to restore normal levels are not consistent with nutritional recommendations for healthy individuals. Better evidence-based guidelines are required to established appropriate doses. In some cases, pharmacologic doses, regardless of the confirmed deficiency, may offer benefits, although more clinical evidence to support these approaches is still needed.

REFERENCES

1. Dolan KT, Chang EB. Diet, gut microbes, and the pathogenesis of inflammatory bowel diseases. Mol Nutr Food Res 2017;61(1).
2. Benchimol EI, Mack DR, Guttmann A, et al. Inflammatory bowel disease in immigrants to Canada and their children: a population-based cohort study. Am J Gastroenterol 2015;110(4):553–63.
3. Weisshof R, Chermesh I. Micronutrient deficiencies in inflammatory bowel disease. Curr Opin Clin Nutr Metab Care 2015;18(6):576–81.
4. Massironi S, Rossi RE, Cavalcoli FA, et al. Nutritional deficiencies in inflammatory bowel disease: therapeutic approaches. Clin Nutr 2013;32(6):904–10.
5. Hlavaty T, Krajcovicova A, Payer J. Vitamin D therapy in inflammatory bowel diseases: who, in what form, and how much? J Crohns Colitis 2015;9(2):198–209.
6. Bradley J. NBJ: 'The US supplement industry is $37 billion, not $12 billion. 2015; Available at: http://www.nutraingredients-usa.com/Markets/NBJ-The-US-supplement-industry-is-37-billion-not-12-billion. Accessed March 27,2017.
7. Rossi RE, Whyand T, Murray CD, et al. The role of dietary supplements in inflammatory bowel disease: a systematic review. Eur J Gastroenterol Hepatol 2016; 28(12):1357–64.
8. Hwang C, Ross V, Mahadevan U. Micronutrient deficiencies in inflammatory bowel disease: from A to zinc. Inflamm Bowel Dis 2012;18(10):1961–81.
9. Ashwin N. Ananthakrishnan, editor. Nutritional management of inflammatory bowel diseases: a comprehensive guide. New York: Springer Science+Business Media; 2016.
10. Hashemi J, Asadi J, Amiriani T, et al. Serum vitamins A and E deficiencies in patients with inflammatory bowel disease. Saudi Med J 2013;34(4):432–4.
11. Alkhouri RH, Hashmi H, Baker RD, et al. Vitamin and mineral status in patients with inflammatory bowel disease. J Pediatr Gastroenterol Nutr 2013;56(1):89–92.
12. Main AN, Mills PR, Russell RI, et al. Vitamin A deficiency in Crohn's disease. Gut 1983;24(12):1169–75.
13. da Rocha Lima B, Pichi F, Lowder CY. Night blindness and Crohn's disease. Int Ophthalmol 2014;34(5):1141–4.
14. Soares-Mota M, Silva TA, Gomes LM, et al. High prevalence of vitamin A deficiency in Crohn's disease patients according to serum retinol levels and the relative dose-response test. World J Gastroenterol 2015;21(5):1614–20.
15. Erkelens MN, Mebius RE. Retinoic acid and immune homeostasis: a balancing act. Trends Immunol 2017;38(3):168–80.
16. Reifen R, Nur T, Ghebermeskel K, et al. Vitamin A deficiency exacerbates inflammation in a rat model of colitis through activation of nuclear factor-kappa B and collagen formation. J Nutr 2002;132(9):2743–7.

17. Okayasu I, Hana K, Nemoto N, et al. Vitamin A inhibits development of dextran sulfate sodium-induced colitis and colon cancer in a mouse model. Biomed Res Int 2016;2016:4874809.

18. Kang SG, Wang C, Matsumoto S, et al. High and low vitamin A therapies induce distinct FoxP3+ T-cell subsets and effectively control intestinal inflammation. Gastroenterology 2009;137(4):1391–402.e1–6.

19. Collins CB, Aherne CM, Kominsky D, et al. Retinoic acid attenuates ileitis by restoring the balance between T-helper 17 and T regulatory cells. Gastroenterology 2011;141(5):1821–31.

20. Wright JP, Mee AS, Parfitt A, et al. Vitamin A therapy in patients with Crohn's disease. Gastroenterology 1985;88(2):512–4.

21. Norrby S, Sjodahl R, Tagesson C. Ineffectiveness of vitamin A therapy in severe Crohn's disease. Acta Chir Scand 1985;151(5):465–8.

22. Laffont S, Siddiqui KR, Powrie F. Intestinal inflammation abrogates the tolerogenic properties of MLN CD103+ dendritic cells. Eur J Immunol 2010;40(7):1877–83.

23. Bhattacharya N, Yuan R, Prestwood TR, et al. Normalizing microbiota-induced retinoic acid deficiency stimulates protective cd8(+) t cell-mediated immunity in colorectal cancer. Immunity 2016;45(3):641–55.

24. Sanders TJ, McCarthy NE, Giles EM, et al. Increased production of retinoic acid by intestinal macrophages contributes to their inflammatory phenotype in patients with Crohn's disease. Gastroenterology 2014;146(5):1278–88.e1-2.

25. DePaolo RW, Abadie V, Tang F, et al. Co-adjuvant effects of retinoic acid and IL-15 induce inflammatory immunity to dietary antigens. Nature 2011; 471(7337):220–4.

26. van Noort BA, Bos PJ, Klopping C, et al. Optic neuropathy from thiamine deficiency in a patient with ulcerative colitis. Doc Ophthalmol 1987;67(1–2):45–51.

27. Shin IS, Seok H, Eun YH, et al. Wernicke's encephalopathy after total parenteral nutrition in patients with Crohn's disease. Intest Res 2016;14(2):191–6.

28. Zeljko K, Darija VB, Dina LK, et al. Wernicke's encephalopathy during parenteral nutrition in a Crohn's disease patient. Nutrition 2011;27(4):503–4.

29. Costantini A, Pala MI. Thiamine and fatigue in inflammatory bowel diseases: an open-label pilot study. J Altern Complement Med 2013;19(8):704–8.

30. Kuroishi T. Regulation of immunological and inflammatory functions by biotin. Can J Physiol Pharmacol 2015;93(12):1091–6.

31. Wiedmann S, Eudy JD, Zempleni J. Biotin supplementation increases expression of genes encoding interferon-gamma, interleukin-1beta, and 3-methylcrotonyl-CoA carboxylase, and decreases expression of the gene encoding interleukin-4 in human peripheral blood mononuclear cells. J Nutr 2003;133(3):716–9.

32. Wiedmann S, Rodriguez-Melendez R, Ortega-Cuellar D, et al. Clusters of biotin-responsive genes in human peripheral blood mononuclear cells. J Nutr Biochem 2004;15(7):433–9.

33. Kuroishi T, Endo Y, Muramoto K, et al. Biotin deficiency up-regulates TNF-alpha production in murine macrophages. J Leukoc Biol 2008;83(4):912–20.

34. Agrawal S, Agrawal A, Said HM. Biotin deficiency enhances the inflammatory response of human dendritic cells. Am J Physiol Cell Physiol 2016;311(3): C386–91.

35. Matsusue S, Kashihara S, Takeda H, et al. Biotin deficiency during total parenteral nutrition: its clinical manifestation and plasma nonesterified fatty acid level. JPEN J Parenter Enteral Nutr 1985;9(6):760–3.

36. Fernandez-Banares F, Abad-Lacruz A, Xiol X, et al. Vitamin status in patients with inflammatory bowel disease. Am J Gastroenterol 1989;84(7):744–8.

37. Kuroki F, Iida M, Tominaga M, et al. Multiple vitamin status in Crohn's disease. Correlation with disease activity. Dig Dis Sci 1993;38(9):1614–8.

38. Mooney S, Leuendorf JE, Hendrickson C, et al. Vitamin B6: a long known compound of surprising complexity. Molecules 2009;14(1):329–51.

39. Prevention CfDCa. Second national report on biochemical indicators of diet and nutrition in the U.S. population. 2012. Available at: https://www.cdc.gov/nutritionreport/index.html. Accessed March 27, 2017.

40. Friso S, Jacques PF, Wilson PW, et al. Low circulating vitamin B(6) is associated with elevation of the inflammation marker C-reactive protein independently of plasma homocysteine levels. Circulation 2001;103(23):2788–91.

41. Morris MS, Sakakeeny L, Jacques PF, et al. Vitamin B-6 intake is inversely related to, and the requirement is affected by, inflammation status. J Nutr 2010;140(1):103–10.

42. Saibeni S, Cattaneo M, Vecchi M, et al. Low vitamin B(6) plasma levels, a risk factor for thrombosis, in inflammatory bowel disease: role of inflammation and correlation with acute phase reactants. Am J Gastroenterol 2003;98(1):112–7.

43. Benight NM, Stoll B, Chacko S, et al. B-vitamin deficiency is protective against DSS-induced colitis in mice. Am J Physiol Gastrointest Liver Physiol 2011;301(2):G249–59.

44. Selhub J, Byun A, Liu Z, et al. Dietary vitamin B6 intake modulates colonic inflammation in the IL10-/- model of inflammatory bowel disease. J Nutr Biochem 2013;24(12):2138–43.

45. Battat R, Kopylov U, Szilagyi A, et al. Vitamin B12 deficiency in inflammatory bowel disease: prevalence, risk factors, evaluation, and management. Inflamm Bowel Dis 2014;20(6):1120–8.

46. Bermejo F, Algaba A, Guerra I, et al. Should we monitor vitamin B12 and folate levels in Crohn's disease patients? Scand J Gastroenterol 2013;48(11):1272–7.

47. Carrier J, Medline A, Sohn KJ, et al. Effects of dietary folate on ulcerative colitis-associated colorectal carcinogenesis in the interleukin 2- and beta(2)-microglobulin-deficient mice. Cancer Epidemiol Biomarkers Prev 2003;12(11 Pt 1):1262–7.

48. MacFarlane AJ, Behan NA, Matias FM, et al. Dietary folate does not significantly affect the intestinal microbiome, inflammation or tumorigenesis in azoxymethane-dextran sodium sulphate-treated mice. Br J Nutr 2013;109(4):630–8.

49. Stein J, Hartmann F, Dignass AU. Diagnosis and management of iron deficiency anemia in patients with IBD. Nat Rev Gastroenterol Hepatol 2010;7(11):599–610.

50. Stallmach A, Buning C. Ferric maltol (ST10): a novel oral iron supplement for the treatment of iron deficiency anemia in inflammatory bowel disease. Expert Opin Pharmacother 2015;16(18):2859–67.

51. Dignass AU, Gasche C, Bettenworth D, et al. European consensus on the diagnosis and management of iron deficiency and anaemia in inflammatory bowel diseases. J Crohns Colitis 2015;9(3):211–22.

52. Del Pinto R, Pietropaoli D, Chandar AK, et al. Association between inflammatory bowel disease and vitamin D deficiency: a systematic review and meta-analysis. Inflamm Bowel Dis 2015;21(11):2708–17.

53. Sadeghian M, Saneei P, Siassi F, et al. Vitamin D status in relation to Crohn's disease: meta-analysis of observational studies. Nutrition 2016;32(5):505–14.

54. Ghishan FK, Kiela PR. Advances in the understanding of mineral and bone metabolism in inflammatory bowel diseases. Am J Physiol Gastrointest Liver Physiol 2011;300(2):G191–201.

55. Hewison M. Vitamin D and immune function: an overview. Proc Nutr Soc 2012; 71(1):50–61.
56. Ananthakrishnan AN, Cagan A, Gainer VS, et al. Normalization of plasma 25-hydroxy vitamin D is associated with reduced risk of surgery in Crohn's disease. Inflamm Bowel Dis 2013;19(9):1921–7.
57. Ananthakrishnan AN, Khalili H, Higuchi LM, et al. Higher predicted vitamin D status is associated with reduced risk of Crohn's disease. Gastroenterology 2012; 142(3):482–9.
58. Vogelsang H, Ferenci P, Resch H, et al. Prevention of bone mineral loss in patients with Crohn's disease by long-term oral vitamin D supplementation. Eur J Gastroenterol Hepatol 1995;7(7):609–14.
59. Bartram SA, Peaston RT, Rawlings DJ, et al. A randomized controlled trial of calcium with vitamin D, alone or in combination with intravenous pamidronate, for the treatment of low bone mineral density associated with Crohn's disease. Aliment Pharmacol Ther 2003;18(11–12):1121–7.
60. Benchimol EI, Ward LM, Gallagher JC, et al. Effect of calcium and vitamin D supplementation on bone mineral density in children with inflammatory bowel disease. J Pediatr Gastroenterol Nutr 2007;45(5):538–45.
61. Hradsky O, Soucek O, Maratova K, et al. Supplementation with 2000 IU of cholecalciferol is associated with improvement of trabecular bone mineral density and muscle power in pediatric patients with IBD. Inflamm Bowel Dis 2017;23(4): 514–23.
62. Abreu MT, Kantorovich V, Vasiliauskas EA, et al. Measurement of vitamin D levels in inflammatory bowel disease patients reveals a subset of Crohn's disease patients with elevated 1,25-dihydroxyvitamin D and low bone mineral density. Gut 2004;53(8):1129–36.
63. Rudnicki M, Frolich A, Transbol I. Inappropriate hypercalcitriolemia in ileum-resected patients with Crohn's disease. Miner Electrolyte Metab 1992;18(1):52–5.
64. Larmonier CB, McFadden RM, Hill FM, et al. High vitamin D3 diet administered during active colitis negatively affects bone metabolism in an adoptive T cell transfer model. Am J Physiol Gastrointest Liver Physiol 2013;305(1):G35–46.
65. Kiela PR, Ghishan FK. Metabolic bone disease in patients with inflammatory bowel disease. Pract Gastroenterol 2012;XXXVI(9):16–26.
66. Jorgensen SP, Agnholt J, Glerup H, et al. Clinical trial: vitamin D3 treatment in Crohn's disease - a randomized double-blind placebo-controlled study. Aliment Pharmacol Ther 2010;32(3):377–83.
67. Miheller P, Muzes G, Hritz I, et al. Comparison of the effects of 1,25 dihydroxyvitamin D and 25 hydroxyvitamin D on bone pathology and disease activity in Crohn's disease patients. Inflamm Bowel Dis 2009;15(11):1656–62.
68. Yang L, Weaver V, Smith JP, et al. Therapeutic effect of vitamin d supplementation in a pilot study of Crohn's patients. Clin Transl Gastroenterol 2013;4:e33.
69. Krasinski SD, Russell RM, Furie BC, et al. The prevalence of vitamin K deficiency in chronic gastrointestinal disorders. Am J Clin Nutr 1985;41(3):639–43.
70. Schoon EJ, Muller MC, Vermeer C, et al. Low serum and bone vitamin K status in patients with longstanding Crohn's disease: another pathogenetic factor of osteoporosis in Crohn's disease? Gut 2001;48(4):473–7.
71. Duggan P, O'Brien M, Kiely M, et al. Vitamin K status in patients with Crohn's disease and relationship to bone turnover. Am J Gastroenterol 2004;99(11):2178–85.
72. Nowak JK, Grzybowska-Chlebowczyk U, Landowski P, et al. Prevalence and correlates of vitamin K deficiency in children with inflammatory bowel disease. Sci Rep 2014;4:4768.

73. Shiraishi E, Iijima H, Shinzaki S, et al. Vitamin K deficiency leads to exacerbation of murine dextran sulfate sodium-induced colitis. J Gastroenterol 2016;51(4): 346–56.
74. Vagianos K, Bector S, McConnell J, et al. Nutrition assessment of patients with inflammatory bowel disease. JPEN J Parenter Enteral Nutr 2007;31(4):311–9.
75. Siva S, Rubin DT, Gulotta G, et al. Zinc deficiency is associated with poor clinical outcomes in patients with inflammatory bowel disease. Inflamm Bowel Dis 2017; 23(1):152–7.
76. Sturniolo GC, Di Leo V, Ferronato A, et al. Zinc supplementation tightens "leaky gut" in Crohn's disease. Inflamm Bowel Dis 2001;7(2):94–8.

Herbs and Inflammatory Bowel Disease

Gregory M. Sebepos-Rogers, MRCP[a], David S. Rampton, PhD, FRCP[b],*

KEYWORDS

- Herbs • Herbal medicines • Ulcerative colitis • Crohn disease
- Inflammatory bowel disease

KEY POINTS

- Herbal products are widely used by patients with inflammatory bowel disease (IBD).
- Mostly small studies of varying quality have suggested that several different herbal preparations may have clinical efficacy in IBD.
- Larger and better designed clinical trials are needed to confirm the efficacy and safety of herbal preparations showing promise in preliminary studies.
- Contrary to widespread belief, herbal products are not necessarily safe.
- Patients and health care workers need to be aware of the limitations and risks associated with the use of herbal products.

INTRODUCTION

Given the common use of herbal products by patients with inflammatory bowel disease (IBD) an understanding of their potential efficacy and safety is essential for clinicians who manage the disease. (See Petros Zezos and Geoffrey C. Nguyen's article, "Use of Complementary and Alternative Medicine in Inflammatory Bowel Disease Around The World," in this issue.)

Many herbal medicine practices are based on ancient ideas or beliefs that ignore modern pathophysiological and pharmacologic concepts, and that historically have placed them outside the realm of scientific evaluation in clinical trials. Although some controlled studies of the effects of herbal preparations have been reported in recent years, much information relating to their possible therapeutic effectiveness remains anecdotal and uncontrolled. However, herbal medicine is readily accessible and is seen by many patients as a potential therapeutic strategy for a

Disclosure Statement: Neither author has any financial or commercial interest to declare.
[a] Department of Gastroenterology, Royal London Hospital, Barts Health NHS Trust, Whitechapel Road, London E1 1BB, UK; [b] Centre for Immunobiology, Blizard Institute, Barts and the London Queen Mary School of Medicine and Dentistry, University of London, 4 Newark Street, Whitechapel, London E1 2AT, UK
* Corresponding author. Endoscopy Unit, Royal London Hospital, London E1 1BB, UK.
E-mail address: d.rampton@qmul.ac.uk

Gastroenterol Clin N Am 46 (2017) 809–824
http://dx.doi.org/10.1016/j.gtc.2017.08.009
0889-8553/17/© 2017 Elsevier Inc. All rights reserved.

gastro.theclinics.com

wide range of reasons, including its use over several centuries, in different cultural and geographic regions; for example, Ayurvedic medicine and Traditional Chinese Medicine (TCM). Furthermore, the lack of clear safety alert signals for herbal products, in part due to the absence of any formal equivalent of drug registries in herbal medicine practice, can lead to lay interpretation of minimal risk being associated with their use.

This article reviews published evidence of the efficacy of herbal preparations in IBD, briefly outline their possible mechanisms of action and highlight the risk of side effects from the herbs used. It ends with a call for better regulation of the manufacture, distribution, and administration of herbal preparations.

EFFICACY OF HERBS IN INFLAMMATORY BOWEL DISEASE
Literature Review

The authors' literature review was compiled using a systematic search of the Medline database from 1966 to 2016. Reports of controlled clinical trials published either in English or with English abstracts were used. Search headings and keywords used were combinations of herbs, herbal therapy, botanic, traditional Chinese medicine, inflammatory bowel disease, colitis, Crohn disease, ulcerative colitis (UC), and proctitis.

Interpreting Trial Results

The difficulties associated with designing, executing, and interpreting trials of new conventional drugs in IBD are numerous[1] and have often been compounded in trials of herbal products. The herbal preparations under testing have often been poorly characterized and/or standardized. Trials have often been small, underpowered, unrandomized, unblinded, and inadequately or totally uncontrolled. Few studies have included subjects whose IBD has been adequately phenotyped. Outcome measures have sometimes been unconventional and unvalidated. Bias may have been introduced by failure to publish trials with negative outcomes. These issues have been emphasized in recent reviews.[2–5]

Moreover, rarely has a study in which an herbal preparation has shown an initial indication of efficacy been followed up by a large-scale, well-designed clinical trial to confirm the benefit suggested.[6] This may in part be a consequence of difficulties in obtaining the necessary funding and regulatory approval for herbal trials. For example, analytical dossiers of the multiple constituents of herbs are difficult and expensive to assemble; without them, however, regulatory approval for a trial may be unobtainable. Furthermore, given the expense entailed, commercial companies may be reluctant to fund clinical trials for a particular indication (in this context, IBD) of preparations that already have a successful market among the general public for other indications.

Review of Trial Outcomes

The authors found nearly 30 controlled clinical studies, as of December 2016, assessing the effects of herbal products in IBD. As shown in **Tables 1** and **2**, we have classified them into 4 subgroups: active UC (induction treatment), inactive UC (remission maintenance), active Crohn disease (induction treatment), and inactive Crohn disease (remission maintenance). For more extensive and detailed tables, readers are referred to other reviews.[2–5,7]

The overall assessment of the possible efficacy of each herbal product listed in see **Tables 1** and **2** takes into account the quality of the clinical trials investigating each herb, assessed by us and by Cheifetz and colleagues.[5] Factors considered in rating each trial included trial size, entry criteria, disease definition, concurrent therapies,

Table 1
Herbal preparations assessed in controlled trials in ulcerative colitis

Disease Activity at Inclusion	Herbal Product	Route	Number of Subjects	Comparator	Duration (weeks)	Likely Efficacy	Reference
Active	Aloe vera	Oral	44	Placebo	4	+	Langmead et al,[8] 2004
	Wheat grass juice	Oral	23	Placebo	4	+	Ben-Arye et al,[9] 2002
	Andrographis paniculata	Oral	120	Mesalamine	8	+/−	Tang et al,[10] 2011
	Andrographis paniculata	Oral	224	Placebo	8	+	Sandborn et al,[6] 2013
	Boswellia serrata	Oral	42, 30	Sulfasalazine	6	+/−	Gupta et al,[12] 2001; Gupta et al,[11] 1997
	Curcumin	Enemas	45	Placebo	8	+/−	Singla et al,[13] 2014
	Curcumin	Oral	50	Placebo	4	+	Lang et al,[14] 2015
	Germinated barley	Oral	20	Standard	4	+/−	Kanauchi et al,[15] 2002
	Xilei-san	Suppository	30	Placebo	26	+	Fukunga et al,[16] 2012
	Xilei-san	Enemas	35	Dexamethasone enemas	8	+	Zhang et al,[17] 2013
	Fufangkushen	Oral	340	Mesalamine	8	+/−	Gong et al,[18] 2012
	Bowman-Birk	Inhibitor oral	28	Placebo	12	+/−	Lichtenstein et al,[19] 2008
	Tormentil	Oral	16	Dose-ranging	3	+/−	Huber et al,[20] 2007
Inactive	Boswellia serrata	Oral	43	Standard	4	+/−	Pellegrini et al,[22] 2016
	Curcumin	Oral	89	Placebo	26	+	Hanai et al,[23] 2007
	Plantago ovata	Oral	105	Mesalamine	52	+/−	Fernandes-Benares et al,[24] 1999
	Germinated barley	Oral	59	Standard	52	+/−	Hanai et al,[25] 2004
	Evening primrose	Oral	43	Placebo	26	+/−	Greenfield et al,[26] 1993
	Myrrhinil-Intest	Oral	96	Mesalamine	26	+	Langhorst et al,[27] 2013
	Silymarin	Oral	80	Placebo	26	+/−	Rastergarpanah et al,[28] 2015

Further details are shown in the article and in tables in other reviews. The overall assessment of possible efficacy takes into account the quality of the trials of each herb (see article).
Data from Refs.[2–5,47]

Table 2
Herbal preparations assessed in controlled trials in Crohn disease

Disease Status at Inclusion	Herbal Product	Route	Number of subjects	Comparator	Duration	Likely Efficacy	Reference
Active	Wormwood	Oral	40	Placebo	10	+	Omer et al,[29] 2007
Active	Wormwood	Oral	20	Placebo	6	+	Krebs et al,[30] 2010
Active	Boswellia serrata	Oral	102	Mesalamine	8	+	Gerhardt et al,[31] 2001
Active	Cannabinoids	Cigarettes	21	Placebo	8	+/−	Holtmeier et al,[35] 2010
Inactive	Boswellia serrata	Oral	108	Placebo	52	−	Naftali et al,[34] 2013
Postoperative	Tripterygium wilfordii	Oral	39	Mesalamine	52	+	Ren et al,[36] 2013
Postoperative	Tripterygium wilfordii	Oral	90	Azathioprine	52	−	Zhu et al,[37] 2015
Inactive	Tripterygium wilfordii	Oral	198	Mesalamine	52	+/−	Sun et al,[38] 2015

Details are shown in the text and in tables in other reviews. The overall assessment of possible efficacy takes into account the quality of the trials of each herb (see article).
Data from Refs.[2-5,47]

randomization, blinding, comparator, inclusion of intention-to-treat (ITT) analysis, outcome measures, and trial duration.

TREATMENT OF ACTIVE ULCERATIVE COLITIS

Probably because trials are easier to design and execute in UC than in Crohn disease, many more studies of the effects of herbal preparations have been made in this type of IBD (see **Table 1**).

Aloe vera (Xanthorrhoeaceae)

Aloe vera has global historical use in traditional medicine for a wide range of purposes, primarily as a gel derived from the leaf pulp extract. Its multiple biologically active constituents include acetylated mannans, polymannans, anthraquinones, and lectins.

A randomized, double-blind, placebo-controlled trial on 44 subjects who were outpatients with mild to moderately active UC from 2 United Kingdom centers tested Aloe vera gel, in a dose of 100 mL orally twice daily for 4 weeks. The active gel produced a more frequent clinical response (47%; a composite of remission [simple clinical colitis activity index (SCCAI) $\leq$2] and improvement [SCCAI reduction $\geq$3]) than did placebo (14%; P = .048) on ITT analysis.[8] There was a nonsignificant trend to more frequent remission (37%) versus placebo (7%, P = .09). Within the Aloe vera cohort, median SCCAI (P = .01) and histologic score (P = .031) both decreased. There were no changes in C-reactive protein (CRP) in either group. The trial was limited by a small sample size and short follow-up designed to limit exposure to Aloe vera in its first application in IBD. There were no serious adverse effects.

Triticum aestivum (Wheat Grass Juice)

Triticum aestivum is a cultivated wheat that can be processed into liquid or powder. Wheat grass juice contains chlorophyll, phenols, and flavonoids, and has achieved lay popularity recently for generalized health benefit attributed to its rich nutrient content.

An Israeli tertiary center conducted a randomized double-blind, controlled trial on 23 subjects with active distal UC, comparing wheat grass juice (100 mL once daily) with placebo over 4 weeks.[9] A novel disease activity index (DAI) was used comprising stool frequency and rectal bleeding diary scores, endoscopic score, and physician's global assessment. On per protocol analysis, subjects given wheat grass juice showed greater improvements in rectal bleeding (P = .025), DAI score (P = .019), and physician's global assessment (P = .031), but not in stool frequency or sigmoidoscopic score, compared with placebo. The predominant side effect was nausea but that did not result in trial drop-out. Follow-up was short and no ITT analysis was provided.

Andrographis paniculata (Indian Echinacea)

Andrographis paniculata has been used as an herbal mixture in Asia and Scandinavia for respiratory infections and diarrhea. Extracts yield mainly diterpene lactones, including andrographolide. HMPL-004, a proprietary ethanol extract, has been evaluated in 2 manufacturer-funded trials.

The first was a multicenter Chinese, randomized, double-blind, parallel group pilot study.[10] Subjects (120) with mild to moderately active UC were evenly randomized to 1200 mg/d HMPL-004 and 4.5 g/d slow-release mesalamine. Although not powered to demonstrate noninferiority, the primary endpoint of a composite of clinical, endoscopic, and histologic changes in activity scores at 8 weeks showed no significant difference on ITT analysis between HMPL-004 and mesalamine (76% vs 82%). Subject dropout due to adverse events was low and similar in both groups.

A subsequent larger high-quality international, multicenter, randomized, placebo-controlled, double-blind study from the same group assessed 2 doses of HMPL-004 over 8 weeks in 224 subjects with mild to moderately active UC on stable doses of mesalamine or no treatment.[6] Subjects on the higher dose (1800 mg/d) showed a significantly greater response rate (59.5%; decrease in total Mayo score >3) than those on placebo (40%; $P = .018$). Mucosal healing rate at 8 weeks was significantly higher in subjects on high-dose HMPL-004 (50%) than on placebo (33%), but remission (total Mayo score ≤2) rates were similar (about 30%) in all 3 subject groups. Apart from rash, the adverse event rate on HMPL-004 was similar to placebo.

Boswellia serrata (Indian Frankincense)

Boswellia serrata is a traditional Ayurvedic remedy and a component of incense. An Indian group assessed B serrata as a gum resin (900 mg orally daily) in 2, nonrandomized studies compared with sulfasalazine (3 g/d) over 6 weeks in subjects with chronically active UC.[11,12] In both studies, there were no significant differences in remission rates, severity of symptoms, or safety between groups. However, power calculations and ITT analysis were not available, outcome measures were unvalidated, and follow-up was short.

Curcumin

Curcumin is a phytochemical derived from turmeric (Curcuma longa) with extensive historical use in both Indian and Chinese medicine systems. Two studies have assessed curcumin for induction of remission in UC.

A randomized, single-center pilot study in 45 subjects with mild-to-moderate distal disease on oral mesalamine compared curcumin enema (140 mg each night) to placebo enema over 8 weeks.[13] The study found no significant differences in clinical remission or response Ulcerative Colitis Disease Activity Index (UCDAI), or endoscopic activity, on ITT analysis, although on per protocol analysis subjects did significantly better on these measures when using curcumin versus placebo.

A subsequent randomized, multicenter, double-blind study of 50 oral and topical mesalamine-refractory subjects with active mild-to-moderate UC compared oral curcumin (3 g/d) with placebo.[14] After 4 weeks, there were significant differences for curcumin versus placebo in clinical remission (SCCAI ≤2), 53.8% and 0%, respectively ($P = .01$); clinical response (≥3 point reduction in SCCAI), 65.3% and 12.5%, respectively ($P<.001$); and endoscopic remission rates, 38% and 0%, respectively ($P = .043$).

Germinated Barley Foodstuff

Germinated barley foodstuff (GBF) is a prebiotic containing glutamine-rich protein and hemicellulose-rich fiber. A Japanese industry-associated group has assessed the preparation in both active and inactive (see later discussion) UC. In a very small open-label, controlled study in active UC, 11 subjects given GBF (20–30g) for 4 weeks as adjunctive treatment showed a greater decrease in clinical disease activity than 9 subjects given conventional therapy alone ($P<.05$).[15]

Xilei-San

Xilei-san is used in traditional Chinese medical practice for oral ulceration. The partly herbal constituents include watermelon frost, calcite, cow gallstone, peal powder, borax, borneol, indigo, and ammonium chloride.

A Japanese group conducted a single-center randomized, double-blind, controlled study in 30 subjects with ulcerative proctitis refractory to conventional topical therapy, comparing Xilei-san suppository (0.1 g/d) against placebo.[16] On per protocol analysis, induction of remission (colitis activity index [CAI] $\leq$4) at day 14 was more frequent with Xilei-san (45.5%) than with placebo (0%, P = .038). The primary endpoint of mainte-nance of remission at 180 days occurred in 82% subjects given Xilei-san compared with 17% subjects given placebo (P = .0009); in addition, significant improvements in endoscopic and histologic scores from baseline occurred in subjects on Xilei-san.

A later Chinese randomized, double-blind trial in subjects with mild, moderately active ulcerative proctitis, who were all on oral mesalamine, compared 8 weeks additional therapy with Xilei-san enemas (1 g/60 mL daily) versus dexamethasone enemas (5 mg/60 mL daily) in 35 subjects.[17] On per protocol analysis, clinical response rates were similar in the 2 groups (88% and 87%, respectively) at 4 weeks, as were sigmoidoscopic remission rates at 8 weeks (75% and 73%, respectively). Histologic scores significantly improved within each group at 8 weeks. At week 20, relapse rates were low (6% and 13%, respectively). Xilei-san was well-tolerated.

Fufangkushen Colon-Coated Capsule

Fufangkushen colon-coated capsule (FCC) is a newer composite drug of traditional Chinese medicine ingredients (*Sophora flavescentis, Sanguisorba officinalis L*, indigo naturalis, *Bletilla striata*, and *Glycyrrhiza uralensis*). FCC was evaluated in a multicenter, double-blind, double-dummy, controlled study in 340 subjects with active UC randomized 3:1 to FCC versus mesalamine 4 g orally daily over 8 weeks.[18] There was no difference in clinical response rates (total Mayo decrease $\geq$3) to FCC and mesalamine (72.5% vs 65.0%, respectively; P = .19). This was also the case for clinical remission (41%, 41%) and mucosal healing rates (55% vs 55%, respectively). No adverse events were reported. This large study merits replication.

Bowman-Birk Inhibitor Concentrate

Bowman-Birk inhibitor concentrate is a soy extract with high protease inhibitor activity. In a randomized, double-blind, placebo-controlled study in 28 subjects with active UC it was associated with nonsignificant trends to a greater decrease in Sutherland DAI (P = .067) and higher remission rate (P = .082) than placebo.[19]

Tormentil

Potentilla erecta is a plant whose root and aerial components have been used historically for a range of indications, which include abdominal cramps, diarrhea, and rectal bleeding. Tormentil extracts contain a mixture of tannins and flavonoids common to other herbs with antidiarrheal usage.

In an open-label, single-center, dose-finding study in 16 subjects who were outpatients with active UC, a tormentil extract (1200, 1800, 2400, or 3000 mg) was given daily for 3 weeks with intervening 4 week washout phases and dose escalation if the CAI remained greater than 5.[20] CAI and CRP improved on therapy in a dose-dependent manner. The extract was well-tolerated with mild upper gastrointestinal discomfort reported in one-third of subjects, none of whom withdrew. Although this study was small and uncontrolled, the dose dependency of tormentil's effects suggest that it is worthy of further evaluation.

Active Ulcerative Colitis: Conclusions

Most of the studies described suffered from methodological deficiencies limiting the conclusions that could be drawn from them. Nevertheless, on the evidence available, further trials to investigate the possible roles in active UC of *Aloe vera, Andrographis paniculata* (as HMPL-400), curcumin, and topical Xilei-san, as well as, perhaps, wheat grass juice, fufangkushen, and tormentil would seem worthwhile. An interesting trial of bilberry is not described here because it was uncontrolled, but its results suggest that a formal controlled trial is merited.[21]

MAINTENANCE OF INACTIVE ULCERATIVE COLITIS
Boswellia serrata (Indian Frankincense)

B serrata has been assessed in an industry-led, open-label study of quiescent UC in a novel drug delivery form (Casperome) in 22 subjects over 4 weeks[22] (see **Table 1**). Symptomatic and inflammatory indices, including fecal calprotectin, suggested significant improvement against baseline and compared with 21 control subjects on no supplementary therapy. The lack of validated endpoints and a study period of only 4 weeks, which is extremely short in a remission maintenance study, limit interpretation.

Curcumin

A randomized, double-blind, multicenter study compared curcumin with placebo in addition to sulfasalazine or mesalamine for maintenance of remission in UC.[23] Subjects (89) were randomized to curcumin (oral 1 g twice daily) or placebo for 6 months with 4.6% versus 20.5% ($P = .040$), respectively, relapsing over this period in per protocol analysis ($P = .049$ on ITT analysis). Unsurprisingly, these differences were not sustained at 12-month follow-up assessment. Curcumin also significantly improved clinical activity and endoscopic indices at 6 months, and was well tolerated.

Plantago ovata (Psyllium)

Plantago ovata is processed predominantly into seed form as a dietary fiber with lay use as a bulk laxative; it is likely also to act as a prebiotic (see later discussion). (See Heather E. Rasmussen and Bruce R. Hamaker's article, "Prebiotics and Inflammatory Bowel Disease," in this issue.)

A multicenter, open-label, randomized, controlled trial was conducted on 105 UC subjects in remission for 3 months or longer comparing *P ovata* seeds (20 g/d), low-dose mesalamine (1.5 g/d), and combination therapy.[24] Relapse rates at 12 months between the 3 groups were similar (40% vs 35% vs 30%, respectively; $P = .67$) although the trial was not powered for noninferiority assessment. Constipation and flatulence were predictable adverse events and may have compromised blinding.

Germinated Barley Foodstuff

A Japanese group reported, in a multicenter study that was neither randomized nor blinded, that GBF (20 g/d) given as an adjunct to mesalamine and/or corticosteroids produced a lower relapse rate (18%) over 12 months when given to 22 subjects with UC in remission (Rachmilewitz CAI $\leq$4) than did conventional therapy alone (46%; $P<.05$) in 37 such subjects.[25] GBF was well-tolerated and seemed to be safe.

Oenothera biennis (Super Evening Primrose Oil)

Evening primrose oil, a product of *Oenothera biennis*, was assessed in a placebo-controlled study in 43 subjects comparing fish oil (MaxEPA), super evening primrose oil, and olive oil for 6 months in addition to maintenance mesalamine.[26] Although evening primrose oil significantly improved stool consistency, there were no differences in other symptoms, or in endoscopic or histologic indices between the 3 groups. Blinding was suboptimal.

Myrrhinil-Intest (Myrrh, Chamomile, and Coffee Charcoal)

A randomized, double-blind, double-dummy noninferiority trial in 96 subjects with quiescent UC compared a mixture of myrrh, chamomile flower extract, and coffee charcoal with mesalamine 1.5 g/d over a 12-month period. This mixture is reported to have antidiarrheal and anti-inflammatory properties. There were no significant differences in relapse rates between the Myrrhinil-Intest (53%) and mesalamine (45%) groups, or in endoscopic indices and fecal biomarkers. No major adverse events were noted. Although the comparator was a rather low dose of mesalamine, this option may be worth evaluating in larger trials.[27]

Silymarin (Milk Thistle)

The weed, milk thistle, has been used medicinally for centuries, particularly for liver complaints. In a randomized, double-blinded, placebo-controlled study from Iran, 80 subjects with inactive UC were given silymarin 140 mg or placebo orally once daily for 6 months as adjuncts to their usual treatment.[28] Remission was maintained in 92% subjects on silymarin versus 72% ($P = .5$) on placebo or standard therapy. Silymarin, but not placebo, significantly improved the DAI used, serum hemoglobin, and erythrocyte sedimentation rate. This study merits replication with more conventional endpoints.

Inactive Ulcerative Colitis: Conclusions

Again, study designs in several instances limited the conclusions that could be drawn from them. The most promising preparations for further assessment would seem to be curcumin, and possibly Myrrhinil-Intest and milk thistle.

TREATMENT OF ACTIVE CROHN DISEASE
Artemisia absinthium (Wormwood)

The leaves and stems of Artemisia absinthium, commonly known as wormwood, are used all over the world for a range of medicinal purposes (see **Table 2**).

A randomized, double-blind, controlled trial in 40 subjects with active Crohn disease receiving a tapering dose of prednisolone assessed response to a wormwood herbal blend (500 mg 3 times daily orally) or placebo for 10 weeks. There was a significant improvement in response rate (Crohn's Disease Activity Index (CDAI) decrease >70) after 8 weeks (65%) versus placebo (0%).[29] Furthermore, at 20 weeks of follow-up, 90% subjects who had been on wormwood were steroid-free, as opposed to 20% in the placebo group. It has to be noted that the placebo response rate recorded at 8 weeks, in subjects on tapering prednisolone, was exceptionally low.

A subsequent smaller 6-week open-label, unblinded, randomized controlled trial by the same group on 20 subjects with Crohn disease showed an 80% clinical response and 60% remission rate in subjects given wormwood 750 mg 3 times daily, compared with 20% and 0%, respectively, in the placebo group. Wormwood, unlike placebo, also reduced serum tumor necrosis factor (TNF)-α levels.[30] In both studies, follow-up was short.

Boswellia serrata (Indian Frankincense)

A randomized, double-blind, noninferiority parallel-group study of 102 subjects with active Crohn disease compared B serrata extract H15 with high-dose mesalamine (4.5 g/d) over 8 weeks.[31] No significant difference between the 2 groups was seen in disease activity indices (CDAI) or remission rates (36% and 31%, respectively) and no serious adverse effects were reported. Follow-up was short. The investigators concluded efficacy for *B serrata* in view of its noninferiority to high-dose mesalamine, for which there is some evidence of effectiveness in active Crohn disease.[32]

Cannabis sativa

Cannabinoids are reported to have anti-inflammatory and antifibrotic effects.[33] An Israeli group undertook a randomized, placebo-controlled study in 21 subjects with active Crohn disease refractory to conventional treatment.[34] Subjects were given twice daily cigarettes containing 115 mg Δ9-tetrahydrocannabinol (THC) or placebo containing cannabis flowers from which the THC had been extracted. After 8 weeks, clinical remission (CDAI score <150) was achieved by 45% subjects on THC and 10% on placebo (10%, $P = .43$). Clinical response (decrease in CDAI score >100) occurred in 90% THC group versus 40% on placebo ($P = .028$). However, CRP was unchanged by THC and no other objective measures of disease activity were made. There were no serious adverse events, although subjects on THC noted improvements in sleep and appetite. Blinding failed and the primary endpoint was not met, perhaps because the study was underpowered. Furthermore, subjective elements of the CDAI could have been influenced by the mind-altering effects of THC. Nevertheless, the investigators concluded that further larger studies using a different THC formulation are merited: objective measures of disease activity would be essential.

Active Crohn Disease: Conclusions

As in the far more numerous trials of herbs in UC, the published reports each suffer from design weaknesses. However, wormwood and *B serrata* seem worthy of further trial in active Crohn disease.

MAINTENANCE OF INACTIVE CROHN DISEASE
Boswellia serrata

In a well-designed multicenter randomized, placebo-controlled, double-blind trial aiming to recruit 108 subjects in 22 German centers, a new *B serrata* extract (Boswelan, PS0201Bo) showed no advantage over placebo in maintaining remission at 52 weeks[35] (see **Table 2**). The extract was well-tolerated but also no better than placebo in relation to time to relapse or CDAI scores. The trial was terminated early.

Tripterygium wilfordii

Tripterygium wilfordii is a vine-like plant, of which the extracts are used in traditional Chinese medicine. It contains triptolide, a compound with anti-inflammatory properties. Its possible use for remission maintenance in Crohn disease has been assessed in 3 Chinese studies from the same center.

In the first, 39 subjects with postoperative Crohn disease in remission (CDAI ≤150) were randomized to receive polyglycosides of *T wilfordii* (poylyglycosides of Triptery-gium wilfordi (GTW), 1 mg/kg/d), or mesalamine 4 g orally daily for 52 weeks on a single-blind basis.[36] Clinical (5%) and endoscopic recurrences (21%) were less common in the GTW group than in those given mesalamine (24%, $P < .001$ and 53%, $P < .001$, respectively). Subjects on GTW showed improvements in Rutgeerts' endoscopic scores.

In the second, also unblinded, report, 90 subjects with Crohn disease who had undergone resection were randomized to *T wilfordii* 1.5 mg/kg/d or azathioprine 2.0 mg/kg/d.[37] Of these, 47 subjects completed the trial. Clinical recurrence rate at 52 weeks was similar in both groups (27% and 18%, respectively, $P = .45$), but endoscopic recurrence was more common in those on the herb (74% and 50%, respectively, $P = .03$).

In the third study from the same center, 198 subjects with medically induced remission were randomized but, again, not on a blinded basis, to receive mesalamine (3 g/d), or *T wilfordii* in low-dose (1.5 mg/kg/d) or high-dose (2.0 mg/kg/d) for 52 weeks.[38] Only 137 subjects completed the study. At week 52, fewer subjects on high-dose *T wilfordii* had relapsed (10%) than on low-dose *T wilfordii* (22%, $P = .047$) or mesalamine (29%, $P = .006$), at the expense of more side effects (30%, 28%, and 14%, respectively, $P < .05$); these included leukopenia and hepatic dysfunction.

These reports give conflicting results and further studies of *T wilfordii* in inactive and well-characterized Crohn disease should be undertaken on a fully blinded basis and at a different center.

Inactive Crohn Disease: Conclusions

T wilfordii seems worthy of further evaluation, but no other herbal products have shown potential for the prevention of relapse in patients with inactive Crohn disease.

POSSIBLE MODES OF ACTION OF HERBS IN INFLAMMATORY BOWEL DISEASE

One barrier to the acceptance of complementary and alternative medicine (CAM) by conventional doctors has been the apparent lack of any scientific explanation for their possible efficacy. Recently, however, mechanisms by which some herbal preparations may act have been investigated. A detailed description of the anti-inflammatory actions in vitro and in animal models of colitis of each of the preparations previously listed is beyond the scope of this article, and interested readers are referred to relevant review articles.[39–46] However, some general comments are worthwhile.

First, it should be noted that unpurified herbal preparations contain a wide range of biologically active compounds, some of which may have beneficial and others adverse effects. Extensive work of varying quality has suggested that, at least in vitro, individual chemicals derived from a variety of plants may have antibacterial, antioxidant, anti-cytokine, antispasmodic, nuclear factor-κB inhibiting, and/or neuromodulatory actions.[7] In vivo, the polysaccharide content of plant preparations means that they may also act as prebiotics, perhaps in part through intracolonic release of butyrate. (See Heather E. Rasmussen and Bruce R. Hamaker's article, "Prebiotics and Inflammatory Bowel Disease," in this issue.) It is clearly difficult, however, to extrapolate from a knowledge of the chemical composition and activities of an extract from a given plant in vitro to its possible efficacy (or safety) in vivo. This may vary, depending on the amounts of individual constituents in the extract (which may vary with the plant's geographic origin and the method of preparation of the extract), on interactions between individual constituents, and on their pharmacokinetics, of which little is known in most instances.

SIDE EFFECTS OF HERBAL THERAPIES IN INFLAMMATORY BOWEL DISEASE

Side effects of herbal preparations can be direct or indirect.

Direct Toxicity

There is a widely held popular view that because it is termed natural, herbal therapy is safe. This is a misconception, and toxicity from herbal therapies has included fatal liver and renal failure.[47,48] Unfortunately, there are no formal data on the incidence even of acute severe side effects, and knowledge of more subtle and possible longer term sequelae, such as mutagenicity and carcinogenicity, is still more scanty.

Toxic effects have also been associated with the deliberate inclusion of prescription medicines in some herbal preparations, including corticosteroids, fenfluramine, and glibenclamide.[49] Other toxic products found in some preparations have included mercury, arsenic, lead, human placenta (with a risk of transmitting hepatitis C or human immunodeficiency virus), and bat excreta.

In the context of IBD, all that can be said is that, in the trials described in this article, few serious adverse reactions to the wide range of herbal products evaluated were reported.[38] However, in the absence of any formal postmarketing surveillance of herbal products, side effects may be overlooked if or when they are used by larger numbers of patients, particularly if they do not inform their doctors that they are doing so.

Drug Interactions

Potentially dangerous interactions between herbal preparations and conventional drugs have been widely reported but are insufficiently recognized by many conventional practitioners.[50] In the context of UC, for example, St. John's wort, an herbal preparation with antidepressant properties, reduces blood levels of cyclosporine by enhancing the activity of cytochrome P450 enzymes.[47]

Indirect Adverse Effects

Perhaps more importantly than direct toxicity or drug interactions, use of herbal preparations may be complicated by indirect adverse effects. For example, patients with IBD initially consulting alternative practitioners may be wrongly diagnosed. Others may delay or forego appropriate conventional options in favor of ineffective unconventional ones; this may lead to late presentation to a gastroenterologist with severe or complicated IBD.

Regulation of Herbal Preparations

In most countries further legislation is needed to regulate both the quality of the herbal products available and the training, accreditation, and practice of CAM health care professionals who administer them. It is disturbing to the authors, for example, that in the European Union there is an explicit lower evidence threshold permitting marketing of herbal medicines if there is plausibility of efficacy based on long-standing use and experience.[51]

In relation to safety, the frequency with which adverse responses to herbal remedies are reported to the World Health Organization (WHO) monitoring center is small compared with that of conventional drugs.[52,53] A mandatory national and/or international systematic reporting scheme for the collection of adverse responses to herbs is highly desirable, if difficult to implement, above and beyond the voluntary reporting coordinated by the Uppsala Monitoring Center on behalf of the WHO, or through national structures such as the US Food and Drug Administration MedWatch scheme, given the limitations associated with spontaneous reports.[54–56] Any new regulatory framework also needs descriptions of good agricultural practice, good laboratory practice, good manufacturing practice, and good clinical practice.[57] Analytical techniques that provide reproducible and rapid verification of the chemical components of herbal products should help prevent their adulteration, either by similar but toxic plant species such as *Aristolochia*, or by chemicals such as heavy metals or steroids.

SUMMARY

A high proportion of patients with IBD have tried some form of herbal remedy, the type often being geographically and culturally determined. (See Petros Zezos and

Geoffrey C. Nguyen's article, "Use of Complementary and Alternative Medicine in Inflammatory Bowel Disease Around The World," in this issue.) Although patients use a wide range of herbal products, there is a lack of reliable data about the efficacy and safety of most of them in IBD. This is, in part, a consequence of the difficulties associated with funding clinical trials involving herbal preparations.

Because patients with IBD are frequently resorting to herbal preparations, it is imperative that efforts continue to evaluate their efficacy and safety, and to regulate more closely their quality and marketing. Finally, further education of patients, doctors, and other health care workers about any potential benefits and, conversely, the possible dangers of herbal products, is essential to minimize the risks and expense that their inappropriate use may entail.

REFERENCES

1. D'Haens G, Feagan B, Colombel J-F, et al. Challenges to the design, execution, and analysis of randomized controlled trials for inflammatory bowel disease. Gastroenterology 2012;143:1461–9.
2. Ng SC, Lam YT, Tsoi KK, et al. Systematic review: the efficacy of herbal therapy in inflammatory bowel disease. Aliment Pharmacol Ther 2013;38:854–63.
3. Langhorst J, Wulfert H, Lauche R, et al. Systematic review of complementary and alternative medicine treatments in inflammatory bowel diseases. J Crohns Colitis 2015;9(1):86–106.
4. Triantafyllidi A, Xanthos T, Papalois A, et al. Herbal and plant therapy in patients with inflammatory bowel disease. Ann Gastroenterol 2015;28:210–20.
5. Cheifetz AS, Gianotti R, Luber R, et al. Complementary and alternative medicines used by patients with inflammatory bowel disease. Gastroenterology 2017; 152(2):415–29.
6. Sandborn WJ, Targan SR, Byers VS, et al. *Andrographis paniculata* extract (HMPL-004) for active ulcerative colitis. Am J Gastroenterol 2013;108(1):90–8.
7. Langmead L, Rampton DS. Complementary medicine. In: Targan SR, Shanahan F, Karp LC, editors. Inflammatory bowel disease. Translating basic science into clinical practice. Oxford, UK: Wiley-Blackwell; 2010. p. 717–28.
8. Langmead L, Feakins RM, Goldthorpe S, et al. Randomised, double-blind, placebo-controlled trial of oral aloe vera gel for active ulcerative colitis. Aliment Pharmacol Ther 2004;19:739–47.
9. Ben-Arye E, Goldin E, Wengrower D, et al. Wheat grass juice in the treatment of active distal ulcerative colitis: a randomised double-blind placebo-controlled trial. Scand J Gastroenterol 2002;37:444–9.
10. Tang T, Targan SR, Li ZS, et al. Randomized clinical trial: herbal extract HMPL-004 in active ulcerative colitis – a double-blind comparison with sustained release mesalazine. Aliment Pharmacol Ther 2011;33:194–202.
11. Gupta I, Parihar A, Malhotra R, et al. Effects of *Boswellia serrata* gum resin in patients with ulcerative colitis. Eur J Med Res 1997;2:37–43.
12. Gupta I, Parihar A, Malhotra P, et al. Effects of gum resin of *Boswellia serrata* in patients with chronic colitis. Planta Med 2001;67:391–5.
13. Singla V, Mouli VP, Garg SK, et al. Induction with NCB-02 (curcumin) enema for mild-to-moderate distal ulcerative colitis – a randomised, placebo-controlled, pilot study. J Crohns Colitis 2014;8:208–14.
14. Lang A, Salomon N, Wu J, et al. Curcumin in combination with mesalamine induces remission in patients with mild-to-moderate ulcerative colitis in a randomised controlled trial. Clin Gastroenterol Hepatol 2015;13:1444–9.

15. Kanauchi O, Suga T, Tochihara M, et al. Treatment of ulcerative colitis by feeding with germinated barley foodstuff: first report of a multicenter open control trial. J Gastroenterol 2002;37(14):67–72.
16. Fukanaga K, Ohda Y, Hida N, et al. Placebo controlled evaluation of Xilei San, a herbal preparation in patients with intractable ulcerative proctitis. J Gastroenterol Hepatol 2012;27:1808–15.
17. Zhang F, Li Y, Xu F, et al. Comparison of Xilei-san, a Chinese herbal medicine, and dexamethasone in mild/moderate ulcerative proctitis: a double-blind randomized clinical trial. J Altern Complement Med 2013;19:838–42.
18. Gong Y, Zha Q, Li L, et al. Efficacy and safety of Fufangkushen colon-coated capsule in the treatment of ulcerative colitis compared with mesalazine: a double-blinded and randomized study. J Ethnopharmacol 2012;141:592–8.
19. Lichtenstein GR, Deren KK, Katz S, et al. Bowman-Birk inhibitor concentrate: a novel therapeutic agent for patients with active ulcerative colitis. Dig Dis Sci 2008;50:2191–3.
20. Huber R, Ditfurth AV, Amann F, et al. Tormentil for active ulcerative colitis: an open-label, dose-escalation study. J Clin Gastroenterol 2007;41:834–8.
21. Biedermann L, Mwinyi J, Scharl M, et al. Bilberry ingestion improves disease activity in mild to moderate ulcerative colitis – an open pilot study. J Crohns Colitis 2013;7:271–9.
22. Pellegrini L, Milano E, Franceshi F, et al. Managing ulcerative colitis in remission phase: usefulness of Casperome, an innovative lecithin-based delivery system of Boswellia serrata extract. Eur Rev Med Pharmacol Sci 2016;20:2695–700.
23. Hanai H, Iida T, Takeuchi K, et al. Curcumin maintenance therapy for ulcerative colitis: randomized multicentre, double-blind, placebo-controlled trial. Clin Gastroenterol Hepatol 2006;4:1502–6.
24. Fernandes-Benares F, Hinojosa J, Sanchez-Lombrana JL, et al. Randomized clinical trial of Plantago ovata seeds (dietary fiber) as compared with mesalamine in maintaining remission in ulcerative colitis. Spanish group for the study of Crohn's disease and ulcerative colitis. Am J Gastroenterol 1999;94:427–33.
25. Hanai H, Kanauchi O, Mitsuyama K, et al. Germinated barley foodstuff prolongs remission in patients with ulcerative colitis. Int J Mol Med 2004;13:643–7.
26. Greenfield SM, Green AT, Teare JP, et al. A randomized controlled study of evening primrose oil and fish oil in ulcerative colitis. Aliment Pharmacol Ther 1993;7: 159–66.
27. Langhorst J, Varnhagen I, Schneider SB, et al. Randomised clinical trial: a herbal preparation of myrrh, chamomile and coffee charcoal compared with mesalazine in maintaining remission in ulcerative colitis—a double-blind, double-dummy study. Aliment Pharmacol Ther 2013;38:490–500.
28. Rastergarpanah M, Malekzadeh R, Vahedi H, et al. A randomized, double blinded, placebo-controlled clinical trial of silymarin in ulcerative colitis. Chin J Integr Med 2015;21(12):902–6.
29. Omer B, Krebs S, Omer H, et al. Steroid-sparing effect of wormwood (Artemisia absinthium) in Crohn's disease: a double-blind placebo-controlled study. Phytomedicine 2007;14:87–95.
30. Krebs S, Omer TN, Omer B. Wormwood (Artemisia absinthium) suppresses tumour necrosis factor alpha and accelerates healing in patients with Crohn's disease – a controlled clinical trial. Phytomedicine 2010;17:305–9.
31. Gerhardt H, Seifert F, Buvari P, et al. Therapy of active Crohn disease with Boswellia serrata extract H 15. Z Gastroenterol 2001;39:11–7.

32. Lim WC, Wang Y, MacDonald JK, et al. Aminosalicylates for induction of remission or response in Crohn's disease. Cochrane Database Syst Rev 2016;(7):CD008870.

33. Zurier RB, Burstein SH. Cannabinoids, inflammation, and fibrosis. FASEB J 2016; 30(11):3682–9.

34. Naftali T, Bar-Lev Schleider L, Dotan I, et al. Cannabis induces a clinical response in patients with Crohn's disease: a prospective placebo-controlled study. Clin Gastroenterol Hepatol 2013;11(10):1276–80.

35. Holtmeier W, Zeuzem S, Preibeta J, et al. Randomized, placebo-controlled, double-blind trial of *Boswellia serrata* in maintaining remission of Crohn's disease: good safety profile but lack of efficacy. Inflamm Bowel Dis 2010;17:573–82.

36. Ren J, Wu Z, Liao N, et al. Prevention of postoperative recurrence of Crohn's disease: *Tripterygium wilfordii* in preventing postoperative versus mesalazine. J Int Med Res 2013;41:176–87.

37. Zhu W, Li Y, Gong J. *Tripterygium wilfordii Hook. f.* Versus azathioprine for prevention of postoperative recurrence in patients with Crohn's disease: a randomized clinical trial. Dig Liver Sci 2015;47:14–9.

38. Sun J, Shen X, Dong J. *Tripterygium wilfordii Hook F* as maintenance treatment for Crohn's disease. Am J Med Sci 2015;350(5):345–51.

39. Algieri F, Rodriguez-Nogales A, Rodriquez-Cabezas ME, et al. Botanical drugs as an emerging strategy in inflammatory bowel disease: a review. Mediators Inflamm 2015;2015:179616.

40. Triantafillidis JK, Triantafyllidi A, Vagianos C, et al. Favorable results from the use of herbal and plant products in inflammatory bowel disease: evidence from experimental animal studies. Ann Gastroenterol 2016;29(3):268–81.

41. Kishore V, Yarla NS, Bishayee A, et al. Multi-targeting Andrographolide and its natural analogs as potential therapeutic agents. Curr Top Med Chem 2017; 8(13):845–57.

42. Ammon HP. Modulation of the immune system by *Boswellia serrata* extracts and boswellic acids. Phytomedicine 2010;17(11):862–7.

43. Hanai H, Sugimoto K. Curcumin has bright prospects for the treatment of inflammatory bowel disease. Curr Pharm Des 2009;15(18):2087–94.

44. Ho WE, Peh HY, Chan TK, et al. Artemisinins: pharmacological actions beyond anti-malarial. Pharmacol Ther 2014;142(1):126–39.

45. Wong KF, Yuan Y, Luk JM. *Tripterygium wilfordii* bioactive compounds as anti-cancer and anti-inflammatory agents. Clin Exp Pharmacol Physiol 2012;39(3): 311–20.

46. Wen J, Teng B, Yang P, et al. The potential mechanism of Bawei Xileisan in the treatment of dextran sulfate sodium-induced ulcerative colitis in mice. J Ethnopharmacol 2016;188:31–8.

47. Langmead L, Rampton DS. Review article: herbal treatment in gastrointestinal and liver disease – benefits and dangers. Aliment Pharmacol Ther 2001;15: 1239–52.

48. Koretz RL, Rotblatt M. Complementary and alternative medicine in gastroenterology: the good, the bad and the ugly. Clin Gastroenterol Hepatol 2004;2:957–67.

49. Koretz RL, Rotblatt M. Safety of traditional Chinese medicines and herbal remedies. Curr Probl Pharmacovigilance 2004;30:10–1.

50. Ulbricht C, Chao W, Costa D, et al. Clinical evidence of herb-drug interactions: a systematic review by the natural standard research collaboration. Curr Drug Metab 2008;9(10):1063–120.

51. European Commission. Directive 2004/24/EC of the European Parliament and of the council of 31 March 2004 amending, as regards traditional herbal medicinal products, Directive 2001/83/EC on the community code relating to the medicinal products for human use. Off J Eur Union 2004;47(L136):85–90.

52. Tsutani K, Takuma H. Regulatory sciences in herbal medicine and dietary supplements. Yakugaku Zasshi 2008;128(6):867–80.

53. Shaw D, Graeme L, Pierre D, et al. Pharmacovigilance of herbal medicine. J Ethnopharmacol 2012;140(3):513–8.

54. Hazell L, Shakir SAW. Under reporting of adverse drug reactions: a systematic review. Drug Saf 2006;29:385–96.

55. Gardiner P, Sarma DN, Dog TL, et al. The state of dietary supplement adverse event reporting in the United States. Pharmacoepidemiol Drug Saf 2008;17(10): 962–70.

56. Frankos VH, Street DA, O'Neill RK. FDA regulation of dietary supplements and requirements regarding adverse event reporting. Clin Pharmacol Ther 2010;87(2): 239–44.

57. Kroes BH. The legal framework governing the quality of (traditional) herbal medicinal products in the European Union. J Ethnopharmacol 2014;158:449–53.

Fecal Transplant in Inflammatory Bowel Disease

 CrossMark

Alexander S. Browne, MD, Colleen R. Kelly, MD*

KEYWORDS

• FMT • IBD • Ulcerative colitis • Crohn disease • Fecal transplant • Dysbiosis

KEY POINTS

- Patients with IBD have differences in the composition of their microbiome compared to healthy individuals, but it is unclear whether this dysbiosis is a cause or consequence of chronic inflammation.
- Studies have explored whether manipulation of the gut microbiome through FMT might be an effective treatment for IBD since it has proven to be so effective CDI.
- Two of the three RCTs published on the use of FMT in UC achieved their primary end point of clinical remission; no RCTs have been done in CD patients.
- Hopefully the numerous ongoing trials investigating FMT in IBD will help clarify the efficacy of this modality as a treatment option.

Crohn disease (CD) and ulcerative colitis (UC) are chronic relapsing and remitting inflammatory diseases of the gastrointestinal tract that affect both the pediatric and adult populations. The incidence of inflammatory bowel disease (IBD) is increasing in the United States. There are currently about 1.6 million people in the United States living with IBD, with as many as 70,000 new cases of IBD diagnosed each year.[1] The incidence of IBD is also increasing in Asia, Africa, the Middle East, and South America, which may, in part, be caused by the rapid industrialization of these countries over the last 20 to 30 years.[2] The exact pathogenesis of CD and UC is still unknown but it is postulated that environmental factors and a dysregulated immune response to microorganisms in the gut in genetically susceptible individuals underlie the development of IBD.[3–5] The current treatment paradigm is based on the goal of altering the dysregulated immune response and decreasing inflammation in the gut by targeting various proteins in the inflammatory cascade. Although the available drugs have the potential

Disclosures: None (A.S. Browne). Summit Therapeutics-consultant, Seres Health-site investigator (C.R. Kelly).
Department of Medicine, Alpert Medical School of Brown University, 146 West River Street, Providence, RI 02904, USA
* Corresponding author.
E-mail address: colleen_r_kelly@brown.edu

Gastroenterol Clin N Am 46 (2017) 825–837
http://dx.doi.org/10.1016/j.gtc.2017.08.005
0889-8553/17/© 2017 Elsevier Inc. All rights reserved.

to significantly improve patient symptoms, they are limited by their cost, side effects, and inconsistent efficacy.

THE MICROBIOME IN INFLAMMATORY BOWEL DISEASE

The gut microbiome has become an exciting new frontier for medical research not only because of the role that it may play in gastrointestinal disease but also for its potential activity in nongastrointestinal systemic disease, the obesity epidemic, mental health, and colon cancer.[6] This development has coincided with increased public interest in complementary and alternative medicine treatment options, including prebiotics and probiotics, as shown by a global probiotic market size in excess of $36 billion in 2015 that continues to grow.[7] Advances in DNA sequencing technology have allowed researchers to begin to characterize the exceedingly complex nature of the intestinal microbiome in both healthy and diseased patients. Patients with IBD have qualitative and quantitative differences in the bacterial species that make up their microbiomes compared with healthy individuals.[8,9] Certain bacteria, like *Fusobacterium*, *Escherichia*, and the Proteobacteria, are increased and other bacteria, like *Bacteroides*, *Bifidobacterium*, and *Clostridium* groups IV and XIVA, are decreased in patients with IBD and mouse models of colitis.[9,10] There is some evidence suggesting that variability in expression of NOD2, the first identified CD susceptibility gene encoding antimicrobial defensins, alters the bacterial milieu of the microbiome.[9,10] At this point, it is unclear whether the dysbiosis seen in IBD is a cause or consequence of chronic inflammation.[10] Most of the studies involving the composition of the microbiome so far have investigated its bacterial composition, although, as technology improves, studies are beginning assess the fungal and viral, especially bacteriophage, composition of the microbiome as well.[10]

At present, the most effective therapy available involving manipulation of the gut microbiome is fecal microbiota transplant (FMT) to treat recurrent *Clostridium difficile* infection (CDI). In FMT, stool from a healthy screened donor is administered to a recipient with the goal of restoring gut microbial diversity toward that of a healthy person. The first fecal transplants were performed in China in the fourth century to treat food poisoning and severe diarrhea.[11] The first known data on the use of FMT in the United States were published in 1958 by Eiseman and colleagues[12] in Denver, who administered fecal enemas to 4 patients with antibiotic-resistant pseudomembranous enterocolitis. The first case report of successfully treating CDI with FMT was published in 1983, with several subsequent case reports and retrospective case series reporting that FMT seemed to be an effective treatment in recurrent CDI.[13–15] The first randomized controlled trial to assess FMT for the treatment of recurrent CDI was published by van Nood and colleagues[16] in January 2013. Their study was stopped early after interim analysis showed a cure rate of 81% with a single nasoduodenal infusion compared with 31% of patients who received vancomycin alone and 23% who received vancomycin plus a bowel lavage. The overall cure rate after 1 to 2 FMTs was a remarkable 94%. Subsequent clinical trials of FMT for severe or recurrent CDI have shown cure rates as high as 100%, with a mean cure rate of 87% to 90%.[17] In the spring of 2013, the US Food and Drug Administration (FDA) announced that it was classifying stool used in FMT as a biologic drug, and therefore only physicians with an approved investigational new drug application could use FMT to treat patients. Later that summer, in response to outcry from patients and providers, the FDA changed their position to one of enforcement and discretion, stating that physicians could perform FMT specifically for cases of CDI not responding to standard therapies provided patients were given informed consent indicating that FMT is an experimental therapy.[18]

OBSERVATIONAL STUDIES

Before the landmark van Nood and colleagues[16] study, researchers had started to explore whether FMT could be an effective treatment of patients with IBD. The earliest case report of FMT as a treatment of UC was published in 1989 by Bennet and Brinkman.[19] Since then at least 18 case reports and case series containing between 1 and 16 adult and pediatric patients with either UC or CD have been published concerning the efficacy of FMT in inducing remission.[19–36]

There have been 2 systematic reviews specifically of FMT in IBD; the first was published in 2012 and the most recent was published in 2014.[37,38] Another systematic review published in 2014 discussed FMT as a therapy in gastrointestinal and nongastrointestinal disorders.[39] The systematic review and meta-analysis by Colman and Rubin[38] included 18 studies (9 prospective cohort studies, 5 case series, 3 case reports, and 1 randomized controlled trial by Moayyedi and colleagues[40]) that were conducted between 1989 and 2014, of which 11 were in patients with UC, 4 were in patients with CD, 2 included patients with IBD unspecified colitis, and 1 study that included more than 1 IBD subtype. These studies yielded 122 adult and pediatric patients, of whom 79 had UC, 39 had CD, and 4 had IBD unclassified. The analysis showed that 45% of patients overall achieved clinical remission after FMT. The meta-analysis of the 9 cohort studies alone revealed that 36.2% of patients achieved clinical remission from FMT with moderate heterogeneity ($I^2 = 37\%$). In the studies that included only patients with UC, 22% of patients achieved clinical remission with FMT and this was a statistically homogenous data set ($I^2 = 0\%$). In the studies that included only patients with CD, 60.5% of patients achieved clinical remission with FMT, but only 4 studies were included in the pooled analysis demonstrating moderate heterogeneity ($I^2 = 37\%$) and this was largely driven by 2 studies with larger sample sizes. The sources of stool in these studies varied from first-degree relatives to healthy anonymous donors, and protocols for administration of FMT differed (eg, enema, nasointestinal tube, endoscopic) as well as the number of FMTs (single or multiple). No study reported any serious adverse events, but some patients did experience fevers, chills, abdominal pain, bloating, nausea, vomiting, and diarrhea.

RANDOMIZED CONTROLLED TRIALS

To date, there have been no published randomized controlled trials studying FMT in CD. Three randomized controlled trials have been published on the use of FMT in UC (**Table 1**). The first 2, by Moayyedi and colleagues[40] and by Rossen and colleagues,[41] were published in 2015. The most recent study was published by Paramsothy and colleagues[42] in early 2017. Each study investigated the outcomes of FMT in patients with mild to moderate UC, but the studies differed in route and frequency of FMT delivery, the source of stool for FMT, and the type of placebo.

The study by Moayyedi and colleagues[40] in Canada was a double-blind randomized controlled trial of FMT versus placebo in adult patients 18 years of age or older with active UC. Each patient had a baseline Mayo score, Inflammatory Bowel Disease Questionnaire score, and a EuroQol score calculated before the study and underwent baseline flexible sigmoidoscopy.[43–45] Patients were then randomly assigned to receive FMT or placebo (brown water) via a 50-mL retention enema once per week for 6 weeks. Stool samples were collected each week and disease activity scores were repeated at week 7 as well as a follow-up flexible sigmoidoscopy. Stool was obtained from 6 healthy volunteers who were all screened according to previously published protocols.[46] The FMT preparation consisted of 50 g of donor stool mixed with 300 mL of commercial bottled drinking water. Patients did not undergo a bowel lavage

Table 1
Summary of 3 randomized controlled trials of fecal microbiota transplant in ulcerative colitis

Study	Mechanism of FMT	Frequency of FMT	Stool Source	FMT Preparation	Placebo Type	Bowel Lavage Before FMT	Medications Allowed During Study	Primary End Point Achieved
Moayyedi et al,[40] 2015	Retention enema	Once per week for 6 wk	6 Healthy donors (volunteer)	50 g of donor stool with 300 mL of commercial bottled drinking water	Water	No	Glucocorticoids Mesalamine Immunomodulators Anti-TNFs[a]	Yes
Rossen et al,[41] 2015	Nasoduodenal infusion	Two infusions 3 wk apart	15 healthy donors (patient directed or volunteer)	120 g of donor stool with 500 mL of normal saline	Autologous stool	Yes	Glucocorticoids Mesalamine Immunomodulators[b]	No
Paramsothy et al,[42] 2017	Colonoscopy, then enema	5 d/wk for 8 wk	Mixture of stool from 3–7 healthy donors organized into stool donor batches	37.5 g of stool with isotonic saline and then filtered to make a 150-mL infusion	Isotonic saline with brown food color and stool odor	Yes	Glucocorticoids Mesalamine Immunomodulators[c]	Yes

Abbreviation: TNF, tumor necrosis factor.

[a] On a stable dose for at least 12 weeks (4 weeks for steroids) and they still had active disease.

[b] Stable doses of mesalamine, thiopurines, and corticosteroids less than or equal to 10 mg daily permitted throughout the study; patients excluded if they were on anti-TNFs or methotrexate within 8 weeks or cyclosporine within 4 weeks.

[c] Oral mesalamine as long as the dose was stable for greater than or equal to 4 weeks, and thiopurines or methotrexate as long as the patients had been on these for at least 90 and the dose was stable for at least 4 weeks. Prednisone at a dose of less than or equal to 20 mg daily permitted as long as the dose had been stable for at least 2 weeks, with a mandatory steroid taper of up to 2.5 mg/wk with the goal of being steroid free by week 8. Anti-TNF agents and calcineurin inhibitors were not allowed during the study and in the preceding 12 weeks. Rectal corticosteroids and mesalamine were also not allowed during the study and within 2 weeks before enrollment, and antibiotics and probiotics were not allowed within 4 weeks of enrollment.

before FMT. Patients enrolled in this study could continue their current treatment of UC throughout the study, including glucocorticoids, mesalamine, immunomodulators like azathioprine, and tumor necrosis factor (TNF) antagonists (anti-TNF) if they had been on a stable dose for at least 12 weeks (4 weeks for steroids) and they still had active disease. The primary outcome of the Moayyedi and colleagues[40] study was clinical remission of UC at week 7 defined as a Mayo score less than 3 and endoscopic Mayo score of 0 indicating complete mucosal healing.

The study was stopped early about half way through recruitment by the Data Monitoring and Safety Committee (DSMC) for futility because they determined that the trial was unlikely to achieve its primary end point, although the patients who were already enrolled were allowed to complete the trial. Overall, 70 patients completed the trial, 36 in the FMT arm and 34 in the placebo arm (2 dropped out from the FMT arm and 3 from the placebo arm). The primary outcome was achieved by 9 of 38 (24%) patients in the FMT arm compared with 2 of 37 (5%) in the placebo arm ($P = .03$). No patients achieved an endoscopic Mayo score of 0 at the end of the trial. There were no significant differences between the two groups with regard to the various quality of life scores obtained. Serious adverse events occurred in 3 patients in the FMT group and 2 patients in the placebo group.

There were some intriguing findings in the Moayyedi and colleagues[40] study with regard to the source of the stool and the microbiome analysis. A particularly interesting finding in this study, was that one donor (donor B) was able to induce remission 39% of the time, compared with 10% in patients who received stool from one of the other donors. Although this did not reach statistical significance, it raised the question as to whether donor factors are important in FMT for IBD. Taxonomic profiles from donors included significant enrichment in the family Lachnospiraceae and the genera *Ruminococcus*, similar profiles to another donor associated with successful FMT in this trial. There was a trend toward responders who received stool from donor B to have microbiota compositions that were more similar to donor B's composition than to nonresponders but this did not reach statistical significance. A statistically significant difference in microbiota composition was found between the FMT group compared with the placebo group at week 6 versus baseline. In addition, after serial FMT, the microbiota composition of the FMT group was similar to their respective donors' microbiota composition compared with a control stool sample, and this reached statistical significance.

These results suggest that the microbiota composition of the donor stool potentially plays a critical role in terms of treatment success. There were 2 other intriguing observations from this study. The first is there was a trend for patients on immunosuppressive therapy to respond better than those not on therapy; however, this was not statistically significant. The second is that patients with a recent diagnosis of UC (defined as 1 year or less) were significantly more likely to respond to FMT compared with those patients with more long-standing disease, implying that early FMT shortly after a new diagnosis of UC may have greater benefit.

The study by Rossen and colleagues[41] in Amsterdam was also a double-blind randomized controlled trial of FMT versus placebo in adult patients with mild to moderately active UC. Each patient had a baseline Simple Clinical Colitis Activity Index (SCCAI) score and endoscopic Mayo score calculated and a baseline flexible sigmoidoscopy. Patients were then randomly assigned to receive 2 duodenal infusions of FMT or 2 duodenal infusions of placebo (autologous stool) administered via a nasoduodenal tube; the second infusion was administered 3 weeks after the first. Clinical and endoscopic follow-up was performed at week 6 and week 12 and stool samples were collected at baseline and at weeks 6 and 12. Stool was obtained from 15 healthy donors (1 partner, 1 friend, and 13 volunteers) who were all heavily screened according to prior protocols. The FMT preparation consisted of a median of 120 g of donor stool that was mixed with normal saline to create a 500-mL fecal suspension that was divided into multiple nontransparent syringes. Unlike the patients in the Moayyedi and colleagues[40] study, patients in this study did undergo a bowel lavage before naso-duodenal infusion (2 L of polyethylene glycol solution and 2 L of clear fluids). Patients could continue taking stable doses of mesalamine, thiopurines, and corticosteroids ($\leq$10 mg daily) throughout the study; however, unlike in the Moayyedi and colleagues[40] study, patients in this study were excluded if they had been treated with anti-TNFs or methotrexate within 8 weeks or cyclosporine within 4 weeks. The primary outcome of the study was clinical remission defined as an SCCAI score less than or equal to 2 along with a greater than or equal to 1-point improvement on the Mayo endoscopic score at 12 weeks compared with baseline.

This study was also stopped early by the DSMC for futility. In the end, 37 patients completed clinical and endoscopic follow-up and were included in the per-protocol analysis, and 48 patients were included in the intention-to-treat analysis. At week 6, 6 of 23 (26.1%) patients in the FMT group and 8 of 25 (32.0%) patients in the placebo group achieved clinical remission (P = .76). At week 12, 7 of 23 (30.4%) patients in the FMT group and 8 of 25 (32.0%) patients in the placebo group achieved clinical remission (P = 1.0). Rates of endoscopic response were also similar in both groups. Most patients in the study experienced mild adverse events such as transient dyspepsia and increase in stool frequency but there was no significant difference in these events between the two groups. Serious adverse events occurred in 2 patients in the FMT arm and 2 patients in the placebo arm.

The microbiota diversity index among responders in both the FMT and placebo groups increased significantly, whereas the microbiota diversity in nonresponders did not change over time. The microbiota composition in patients who responded to FMT shifted from similarity to the nonresponders at baseline to the donors at week 12. In the FMT group, the shift mainly consisted of an increase in Clostridium clusters and a decrease in Bacteroidetes. Patients in the autologous placebo FMT group who responded also had a shift in their microbiota composition compared with nonresponders; however, this shift was mostly associated with an increase in bacilli, Proteobacteria, and Bacteriodetes.

The most recent study, conducted in Australia by Paramsothy and colleagues,[42] was published earlier this year, and was a double-blind randomized controlled trial of FMT versus placebo in adult patients with mild to moderately active UC. Each patient had a clinical and endoscopic Mayo score calculated before study entry. Patients were then randomized to receive FMT or placebo, initially delivered via colonoscopy into the terminal ileum or cecum after a bowel prep and then via patient-administered enemas 5 d/wk for 8 weeks. Unlike the previous 2 studies, the stool that was used was a mixture of stool from 3 to 7 healthy donors that was organized into specific stool donor batches. Patients in the FMT arm received stool from the same donor batch throughout the study. A total of 37.5 g of stool was added to isotonic saline and then filtered to make a 150-mL infusion; the placebo arm got a 150-mL infusion of isotonic saline with brown food color and stool odorant.

Patients were allowed to remain on stable doses of oral mesalamine and thiopurines or methotrexate as long as they had been on these medications for at least 90 days and the dose was stable for at least 4 weeks. Patients were also permitted to be on prednisone at a dose of less than or equal to 20 mg daily as long as the dose had been stable for at least 2 weeks; however, enrolled patients had to undergo a mandatory steroid taper of up to 2.5 mg/wk with the goal of being steroid free by week 8. Anti-TNF agents and calcineurin inhibitors were not allowed during the study and in the preceding 12 weeks before the start of the study. Rectal corticosteroids and mesalamine were also not allowed during the study and within 2 weeks before enrolling; antibiotics and probiotics were not allowed within 4 weeks of enrollment. The primary outcome was steroid-free clinical remission and endoscopic response or remission at week 8, which was defined as a total Mayo score of 2 or less, all Mayo subscores of 1 or less, and a decrease of at least 1 point in the endoscopy score from baseline.

The investigators enrolled 41 patients in the FMT arm, of whom 32 completed the study, and 40 in the placebo arm, of whom 29 completed the study. In addition, after the study was completed, patients in the placebo arm were offered 8 weeks of open-label FMT that followed the same study protocol of 5 enemas per week for 8 weeks minus the initial colonoscopy with FMT. Thirty-seven patients elected to enroll in the open-label FMT arm, of whom 25 completed the 8-week study period. Eighty-one patients received at least 1 study infusion and were included in the modified intention-to-treat analysis. After 8 weeks, 11 of 41 (27%) patients in the FMT group and 3 of 40 (8%) patients in the placebo group achieved the primary end point in the modified intention-to-treat analysis ($P = .02$). In the per-protocol analysis, 11 of 32 (34%) of patients in the FMT arm and 3 of 29 (10%) patients in the placebo arm achieved the primary end point ($P = .02$). The primary end point remained significant on logistical regression analysis with regard to disease extent, disease severity, and medication use. Six serious adverse events occurred during the study: 2 in the FMT arm, 1 in the placebo arm, and 3 in the open-label FMT arm.

The microbiota composition of stool samples from patients, individual donors, and from the FMT batches was assessed. Unlike in the Moayyedi and colleagues[40] study, no donor batch or individual donor was responsible for significant differences in achieving the primary outcome. The diversity of the microbiota composition was significantly higher in the batches of donor stool compared with that of individual donors. The diversity of the microbiota composition was also significantly higher in batches and in individual donors compared with baseline patient samples. The diversity of the microbiota composition increased significantly compared with baseline in all patients in the FMT arm at 4 weeks and at 8 weeks, and this persisted 8 weeks after treatment. The types of bacterial species in the microbiota composition of the patients in the FMT arm shifted toward the types of bacterial species in the donor batch independent of clinical outcome. The researchers identified 87 taxa in the closed-label part of the study and 46 taxa in the open-label part of the study that were significantly associated with the primary outcome. One curious finding was that certain bacterial species were associated with achieving clinical remission in the closed FMT arm and different bacterial species were associated with achieving clinical remission in the open FMT arm. In addition, 2 bacterial species were associated with not achieving clinical remission in both the closed-label and open-label arms of the study.

These 3 studies are the first randomized controlled trials published on the use of FMT in UC. Two of the 3 studies achieved their primary end points even though 1 of them was stopped early. They each differed with regard to the mechanism and frequency of FMT delivery, the source of stool for FMT, the type of placebo, the types of medications patients were allowed to be on during the study, and whether there was a bowel lavage before FMT (see **Table 1**). Each of these differences individually, let alone collectively, could potentially play a significant role with regard to the efficacy of FMT at achieving clinical remission. The study by Paramsothy and colleagues[42] is intriguing not only because of the drastically increased frequency of FMT compared with the other 2 studies but also because of the way in which the donor stool was assembled into batches from multiple donors, which greatly increased the microbial diversity of the transplanted stool. These 3 studies provide the foundation for future studies to help address some key questions: what is the optimal mechanism and frequency for FMT? What is the optimal duration of treatment? Are there differences in achieving clinical remission when FMT is initiated early in the course of disease versus later? What is the optimal source of donor stool (individual donors vs pooled donors)? Are there specific bacterial species that consistently confer a significantly better chance of achieving clinical remission? Do the medications that patients are on during FMT enhance or hinder the ability to achieve stool engraftment and clinical remission?

SAFETY

There is a limited amount of data with regard to the safety of FMT, and almost all of these data come from the use of FMT for treatment of CDI, not for treatment of IBD. Most published findings are related to short-term adverse events because there are very few data on the long-term safety of FMT. Some studies have reported minor adverse events after FMT, such as transient fever and chills, borborygmus, bloating, abdominal pain, nausea, vomiting, diarrhea, and constipation.[17,38,41,42] There have been reports of serious adverse events after FMT, such as norovirus; *Escherichia coli* bacteremia; peritonitis in a patient on peritoneal dialysis, with resultant death; pneumonia in a patient with chronic obstructive pulmonary disease, resulting in death; and aspiration during a colonoscopy, resulting in death.[47–50] There were 5 serious adverse events in the Moayyedi and colleagues[40] study, 4 in the Rossen and colleagues[41] study, and 6 in the Paramsothy and colleagues[42] study (**Table 2**).

Table 2
Serious adverse events in the 3 randomized controlled trials of fecal microbiota transplant in ulcerative colitis

Study	Arm	Event	Outcome
Moayyedi et al,[40] 2015 (5 patients)	Placebo	Worsening colitis	Colectomy
	Placebo	Patchy inflammation and rectal abscess formation	Resolved with antibiotics
	FMT (2 patients)	Patchy inflammation and rectal abscess formation	Resolved with antibiotics
	FMT	Abdominal pain	Diagnosed with CDI
Rossen et al,[41] 2015 (4 patients)	Placebo	CMV infection	Resolved with IV ganciclovir
	Unclear	Possible small bowel perforation	Diagnosed with severe small bowel CD and improved with antibiotics
	Unclear	Abdominal pain that required admission	Resolved spontaneously
	Unclear	Cervical carcinoma	Surgery
Paramsothy et al,[42] 2017 (6 patients)	Placebo	Clinical deterioration	Hospital admission
	FMT	Clinical and endoscopic deterioration	Colectomy
	FMT	Clinical deterioration	Admitted for IV steroids
	Open label FMT (3 patients)	Clinical deterioration	Admission for IV steroids and anti-TNF

Abbreviations: CMV, cytomegalovirus; IV, intravenous.

There have been reports of UC flares and a new diagnosis of CD in patients after FMT.[50–53] In a multicenter retrospective review of FMT for CDI in immunocompromised patients published in 2014, Kelly and colleagues[50] reported that 14% of patients with IBD experienced an IBD flare after their FMT (3 were treated with steroids and 1 required a colectomy within 1 month after FMT); however, those 3 patients did have resolution of their CDI from the FMT. In this study, which showed that FMT in immunocompromised patients with CDI seemed to be a safe and effective treatment, patients with IBD did not experience a higher rate of adverse events compared with other immunocompromised patients.

In 2016, Fischer and colleagues[54] published a multicenter retrospective review of outcomes in patients with IBD who underwent FMT for recurrent or refractory CDI. A total of 67 adult patients from 8 different academic centers were reviewed between 2010 and 2015 (35 had CD, 31 had UC, and 1 had indeterminate colitis). All patients underwent FMT via sigmoidoscopy or colonoscopy and the source of the stool was either a patient-directed donor or an unrelated healthy volunteer. The primary outcome was CDI recurrence at 3 months. The initial FMT was successful in 53 patients (79%); however, the overall success rate to clear CDI after repeat FMT was 90%, which was similar to the CDI cure rates seen in patients without IBD.

The secondary outcomes assessed were IBD activity and severity 3 months after FMT and the safety of FMT in patients with IBD. At the time of FMT, 64% of the patients were on an immunosuppressive agent for IBD. Three months after FMT, the IBD clinical course was improved in 31 (46%), unchanged in 24 (36%), and worse in 12 (18%) patients. Disease activity scores before and after FMT were only available for 30 patients. In 23 patients there was a significant decrease in the Harvey-Bradshaw index score from a median of 7 before FMT to 2 after FMT ($P = .0042$). In 7 patients, there was a nonsignificant decrease in the Ulcerative Colitis Clinical Score from a median of 3.5 before FMT to 1.5 after FMT ($P = .22$). Of the 12 patients who got worse, 3 had extensive colitis at the time of FMT and were admitted for an IBD flare within 2 weeks after FMT. One patient with CD on adalimumab who was in clinical and endoscopic remission at the time of FMT was admitted with a CD flare 1 week after FMT and was found to have cytomegalovirus-positive cells on colonic biopsies. Two patients with severe colonic CD had surgery within 30 days of FMT, 1 patient with severe UC had a colectomy 8 weeks after FMT, and another patient with treatment-refractory UC had a colectomy more than 100 days after FMT. It is difficult to say whether some of these serious adverse events were from the FMT alone or were in part caused by the presence of CDI in patients with IBD with colonic involvement. It has been shown that a single CDI in an patient with IBD increases the risk of needing a colectomy 20-fold compared with a CDI in a patient without IBD.[55]

THE FUTURE OF FECAL MICROBIOTA TRANSPLANT IN INFLAMMATORY BOWEL DISEASE

With the current evidence from published case reports, case series, systematic reviews, and the 3 randomized controlled trials of FMT in UC, there is insufficient evidence to recommend FMT as a treatment modality for IBD at this time. Nevertheless, results from these early clinical studies are exciting. There are currently at least 38 trials registered on clinicaltrials.gov that are studying FMT as a treatment modality in pediatric and adult patients with IBD.[56] These studies are investigating patients with mild, moderate, and severe disease who receive FMT from different donor sources via various mechanisms (nasoenteral tube, colonoscopy, retention enema, frozen capsules) for different frequencies and durations. It is hoped that the numerous ongoing trials investigating FMT in IBD will help to clarify the efficacy of this modality as a treatment option. Patients with IBD are open to the possibility of FMT as part of their treatment regimens. In a study by Kahn and colleagues[57] that assessed the perceptions of 95 patients with UC regarding FMT as a potential treatment, 46% were willing to undergo FMT, 43% were unsure, and 11% were unwilling to undergo FMT. The percentage of patients willing to undergo FMT increased as the patient-reported severity of their UC increased; however, more than one-third of patients in remission were willing to undergo the procedure. Top factors influencing their decisions included proof of efficacy, safety, and whether other therapies had failed.

Further investigations into the bacterial, fungal, and viral compositions of both the healthy microbiome and the IBD microbiome should help to expand knowledge of the pathogenesis of IBD and also help to better characterize potential targets for therapy. Advances in DNA sequencing technology may lead to a future in which FMT is delivered as a defined microbial consortium instead of as a whole-stool transplant. Perhaps it will be possible, based on taxonomic profiling, to replete specific microbiological deficiencies in individual patients in an attempt to reverse the dysbiosis in IBD. It is likely that FMT will need to be administered on a maintenance schedule in these patients, who have been shown to return to baseline pre-FMT diversity within 6 months.[58] Encapsulated formulations would be ideal if ongoing therapy is determined to be necessary. Although not ready for general use, microbiota-based therapeutics are emerging and will change the way clinicians care for patients with IBD in the future.

REFERENCES

1. Colombel JF, Mahadevan U. Inflammatory bowel disease 2017: innovations and changing paradigms. Gastroenterology 2017;152:309–12.
2. Kaplan GG, Ng SC. Understanding and preventing the global increase of inflammatory bowel disease. Gastroenterology 2017;152:313–21.e2.
3. Baumgart DC, Sandborn WJ. Crohn's disease. Lancet 2012;380:1590–605.
4. Feuerstein JD, Cheifetz AS. Ulcerative colitis: epidemiology, diagnosis, and management. Mayo Clin Proc 2014;89:1553–63.
5. Knights D, Lassen KG, Xavier RJ. Advances in inflammatory bowel disease pathogenesis: linking host genetics and the microbiome. Gut 2013;62:1505–10.
6. Marchesi JR, Adams DH, Fava F, et al. The gut microbiota and host health: a new clinical frontier. Gut 2016;65:330–9.
7. Probiotics market size to exceed USD 64 billion by 2023: Global Market Insights Inc. 2016. Available at: http://www.prnewswire.com/news-releases/probiotics-market-size-to-exceed-usd-64-billion-by-2023-global-market-insights-inc-578769201.html. Accessed May 30, 2017.
8. De Cruz P, Prideaux L, Wagner J, et al. Characterization of the gastrointestinal microbiota in health and inflammatory bowel disease. Inflamm Bowel Dis 2012;18:372–90.
9. Kostic AD, Xavier RJ, Gevers D. The microbiome in inflammatory bowel disease: current status and the future ahead. Gastroenterology 2014;146:1489–99.
10. Sartor RB, Wu GD. Roles for intestinal bacteria, viruses, and fungi in pathogenesis of inflammatory bowel diseases and therapeutic approaches. Gastroenterology 2017;152:327–39.e4.
11. Zhang F, Luo W, Shi Y, et al. Should we standardize the 1,700-year-old fecal microbiota transplantation? Am J Gastroenterol 2012;107:1755 [author reply: 1755–6].

12. Eiseman B, Silen W, Bascom GS, et al. Fecal enema as an adjunct in the treatment of pseudomembranous enterocolitis. Surgery 1958;44:854–9.
13. Schwan A, Sjolin S, Trottestam U, et al. Relapsing *Clostridium difficile* enterocolitis cured by rectal infusion of homologous faeces. Lancet 1983;2:845.
14. Kassam Z, Lee CH, Yuan Y, et al. Fecal microbiota transplantation for *Clostridium difficile* infection: systematic review and meta-analysis. Am J Gastroenterol 2013; 108:500–8.
15. Cammarota G, Ianiro G, Gasbarrini A. Fecal microbiota transplantation for the treatment of *Clostridium difficile* infection: a systematic review. J Clin Gastroenterol 2014;48:693–702.
16. van Nood E, Vrieze A, Nieuwdorp M, et al. Duodenal infusion of donor feces for recurrent *Clostridium difficile*. N Engl J Med 2013;368:407–15.
17. Kelly CR, Kahn S, Kashyap P, et al. Update on fecal microbiota transplantation 2015: indications, methodologies, mechanisms, and outlook. Gastroenterology 2015;149:223–37.
18. US Food and Drug Administration. Guidance for industry: enforcement policy regarding investigational new drug requirements for use of fecal microbiota for transplantation to treat *Clostridium difficile* infection not responsive to standard therapies. 2013. Available at: https://www.fda.gov/downloads/BiologicsBloodVaccines/GuidanceComplianceRegulatoryInformation/Guidances/Vaccines/UCM361393.pdf. Accessed June 1, 2017.
19. Bennet JD, Brinkman M. Treatment of ulcerative colitis by implantation of normal colonic flora. Lancet 1989;1:164.
20. Borody TJ, George L, Andrews P, et al. Bowel-flora alteration: a potential cure for inflammatory bowel disease and irritable bowel syndrome? Med J Aust 1989;150:604.
21. Borody TJ, Leis S, McGrath K. Treatment of chronic constipation and colitis using human probiotic infusions. Presented at: Probiotics, Prebiotics and New Foods Conference; September 2-4, 2001; Rome, Italy.
22. Borody TJ, Warren EF, Leis S, et al. Treatment of ulcerative colitis using fecal bacteriotherapy. J Clin Gastroenterol 2003;37:42–7.
23. Borody T, Torres M, Campbell J, et al. Reversal of inflammatory bowel disease (IBD) with recurrent faecal microbiota transplants (FMT). Am J Gastroenterol 2011;106:S366.
24. Borody TJ, Campbell J, Torres M, et al. Reversal of idiopathic thrombocytopenic purpura (ITP) with fecal microbiota transplantation (FMT). Am J Gastroenterol 2011;106:S352.
25. Vermeire S, Joossens M, Verbeke K, et al. Pilot study on the safety and efficacy of faecal microbiota transplantation in refractory Crohn's disease. Gastroenterology 2012;142:S360.
26. Kunde S, Pham A, Bonczyk S, et al. Safety, tolerability, and clinical response after fecal transplantation in children and young adults with ulcerative colitis. J Pediatr Gastroenterol Nutr 2013;56:597–601.
27. Kellermayer R, Mir SA, Luna RA, et al. Complex bacteriotherapy in pediatric gastrointestinal disorders. J Pediatr Gastroenterol Nutr 2013;57:e66.
28. Kump PK, Grochenig HP, Lackner S, et al. Alteration of intestinal dysbiosis by fecal microbiota transplantation does not induce remission in patients with chronic active ulcerative colitis. Inflamm Bowel Dis 2013;19:2155–65.
29. Angelberger S, Reinisch W, Makristathis A, et al. Temporal bacterial community dynamics vary among ulcerative colitis patients after fecal microbiota transplantation. Am J Gastroenterol 2013;108:1620–30.

30. Kao D, Madsen K. Fecal microbiota transplantation (FMT) in the treatment of inflammatory bowel disease (IBD): a case report. Am J Gastroenterol 2013;108: S415–6.
31. Landy J, Al-Hassi HO, Mann ER, et al. A prospective controlled pilot study of fecal microbiota transplantation for chronic refractory pouchitis. Gastroenterology 2013;144:S897.
32. Zhang FM, Wang HG, Wang M, et al. Standard fecal microbiota transplantation through mid-gut is an effective therapy of refractory Crohn's disease. J Gastroenterol Hepatol 2013;28:9.
33. Suskind D, Wahbeh G, Vendetoulli H, et al. Fecal microbial transplant in pediatric Crohn's disease. Gastroenterology 2014;146:S834.
34. Damman C, Brittnacher M, Hayden H, et al. Single colonoscopically administered fecal microbiota transplant for ulcerative colitis-a pilot study to determine therapeutic benefit and graft stability. Gastroenterology 2014;146:S460.
35. Vaughn BP, Gevers D, Ting A, et al. Fecal microbiota transplantation induces early improvement in symptoms in patients with active Crohn's disease. Gastroenterology 2014;146:S591–2.
36. Suskind DL, Brittnacher MJ, Wahbeh G, et al. Fecal microbial transplant effect on clinical outcomes and fecal microbiome in active Crohn's disease. Inflamm Bowel Dis 2015;21:556–63.
37. Anderson JL, Edney RJ, Whelan K. Systematic review: faecal microbiota transplantation in the management of inflammatory bowel disease. Aliment Pharmacol Ther 2012;36:503–16.
38. Colman RJ, Rubin DT. Fecal microbiota transplantation as therapy for inflammatory bowel disease: a systematic review and meta-analysis. J Crohns Colitis 2014;8:1569–81.
39. Sha S, Liang J, Chen M, et al. Systematic review: faecal microbiota transplantation therapy for digestive and nondigestive disorders in adults and children. Aliment Pharmacol Ther 2014;39:1003–32.
40. Moayyedi P, Surette MG, Kim PT, et al. Fecal microbiota transplantation induces remission in patients with active ulcerative colitis in a randomized controlled trial. Gastroenterology 2015;149:102–9.e6.
41. Rossen NG, Fuentes S, van der Spek MJ, et al. Findings from a randomized controlled trial of fecal transplantation for patients with ulcerative colitis. Gastroenterology 2015;149:110–8.e4.
42. Paramsothy S, Kamm MA, Kaakoush NO, et al. Multidonor intensive faecal microbiota transplantation for active ulcerative colitis: a randomised placebo-controlled trial. Lancet 2017;389(10075):1218–28.
43. Irvine EJ, Feagan B, Rochon J, et al. Quality of life: a valid and reliable measure of therapeutic efficacy in the treatment of inflammatory bowel disease. Canadian Crohn's Relapse Prevention Trial Study Group. Gastroenterology 1994;106: 287–96.
44. Konig HH, Ulshofer A, Gregor M, et al. Validation of the EuroQol questionnaire in patients with inflammatory bowel disease. Eur J Gastroenterol Hepatol 2002;14: 1205–15.
45. D'Haens G, Sandborn WJ, Feagan BG, et al. A review of activity indices and efficacy end points for clinical trials of medical therapy in adults with ulcerative colitis. Gastroenterology 2007;132:763–86.
46. Bakken JS, Borody T, Brandt LJ, et al. Treating *Clostridium difficile* infection with fecal microbiota transplantation. Clin Gastroenterol Hepatol 2011;9:1044–9.

47. Schwartz M, Gluck M, Koon S. Norovirus gastroenteritis after fecal microbiota transplantation for treatment of *Clostridium difficile* infection despite asymptomatic donors and lack of sick contacts. Am J Gastroenterol 2013;108:1367.

48. Quera R, Espinoza R, Estay C, et al. Bacteremia as an adverse event of fecal microbiota transplantation in a patient with Crohn's disease and recurrent *Clostridium difficile* infection. J Crohns Colitis 2014;8:252–3.

49. Aas J, Gessert CE, Bakken JS. Recurrent *Clostridium difficile* colitis: case series involving 18 patients treated with donor stool administered via a nasogastric tube. Clin Infect Dis 2003;36:580–5.

50. Kelly CR, Ihunnah C, Fischer M, et al. Fecal microbiota transplant for treatment of *Clostridium difficile* infection in immunocompromised patients. Am J Gastroenterol 2014;109:1065–71.

51. De Leon LM, Watson JB, Kelly CR. Transient flare of ulcerative colitis after fecal microbiota transplantation for recurrent *Clostridium difficile* infection. Clin Gastroenterol Hepatol 2013;11:1036–8.

52. Kelly CR, Ziud H, Kahn S. New diagnosis of Crohn's colitis 6 weeks after fecal microbiota transplantation (ABSTR). Inflamm Bowel Dis 2014;20:S21.

53. Hohmann EL, Ananthakrishnan AN, Deshpande V. Case records of the Massachusetts General Hospital. Case 25-2014. A 37-year-old man with ulcerative colitis and bloody diarrhea. N Engl J Med 2014;371:668–75.

54. Fischer M, Kao D, Kelly C, et al. Fecal microbiota transplantation is safe and efficacious for recurrent or refractory *Clostridium difficile* infection in patients with inflammatory bowel disease. Inflamm Bowel Dis 2016;22:2402–9.

55. Razik R, Rumman A, Bahreini Z, et al. Recurrence of *Clostridium difficile* infection in patients with inflammatory bowel disease: The RECIDIVISM Study. Am J Gastroenterol 2016;111:1141–6.

56. ClinicalTrials.gov. Clinical trials for fecal transplant and inflammatory bowel disease. Available at: https://clinicaltrials.gov/ct2/results?term=fecal+transplant+and+inflammatory+bowel+disease&pg=4. Accessed May 30, 2017.

57. Kahn SA, Vachon A, Rodriquez D, et al. Patient perceptions of fecal microbiota transplantation for ulcerative colitis. Inflamm Bowel Dis 2013;19:1506–13.

58. Hourigan SK, Chen LA, Grigoryan Z, et al. Microbiome changes associated with sustained eradication of *Clostridium difficile* after single faecal microbiota transplantation in children with and without inflammatory bowel disease. Aliment Pharmacol Ther 2015;42:741–52.

The Brain-Gut Axis and Stress in Inflammatory Bowel Disease

Charles N. Bernstein, MD

KEYWORDS

• Stress • Depression • Anxiety • Brain-gut axis • Vagus nerve • Gut microbiota

KEY POINTS

- The brain gut axis serves as a circuit that incorporates the human experience, the state of mind, the gut microbiome, and the immune response that ultimately drives the phenotypic expression of inflammatory bowel disease (IBD).
- There are several biological pathways through which stress can play a deleterious role in IBD, including through increasing intestinal permeability and thereby facilitating intestinal translocation of bacteria, which in turn can stimulate innate and adaptive immune responses.
- Increased perceived stress is associated with increased symptoms in persons with IBD; the relationship though between stress and symptoms is bidirectional.
- Although attention to stress and psychiatric comorbidity is important in the management of IBD, there are few clinical trials to direct management based on strong evidence.

THE BIOLOGY OF THE BRAIN-GUT AXIS AND STRESS IN INFLAMMATORY BOWEL DISEASE

A biopsychosocial understanding of illness describes clinical outcome and disease exacerbation as influencing and strongly influenced by both biological and psychosocial factors.[1] The brain and the gut communicate through the autonomic nervous system and the circumventricular organs both in physiologic and pathologic conditions.[1] This brain-gut axis serves as a circuit that incorporates the human experience, the state of mind, the gut microbiome, and the immune response that ultimately drives

Disclosure: Dr C.N. Bernstein is supported in part by the Bingham Chair in Gastroenterology. He has served on advisory boards for Abbvie Canada, Ferring Canada, Janssen Canada, Shire Canada, Takeda Canada, Pfizer Canada, and Cubist Pharmaceuticals and has consulted for Mylan Pharmaceuticals. He has received educational grants from Abbvie Canada, Shire Canada, Takeda Canada, and Janssen Canada. He has been on the speaker's panel for Abbvie Canada, Ferring Canada, and Shire Canada.
Department of Internal Medicine, University of Manitoba IBD Clinical and Research Centre, Max Rady College of Medicine, 804-715 McDermot Avenue, Winnipeg, MB R3E3P4, Canada
E-mail address: charles.bernstein@umanitoba.ca

the phenotypic expression of inflammatory bowel disease (IBD).[1] It is through this circuit that stress impacts gastrointestinal symptoms in health and IBD. Stress is conceptualized as the feeling of being challenged by a threatening event or an evolving situation.[2] Persistent stress may precipitate the development of major depression or chronic anxiety. Depression may affect more than 25% and anxiety more than 30% of persons with IBD, 2 to 3 times higher than in the general population.[3]

Stress may play a deleterious role in IBD through 8 main pathways (as reviewed in Ref.[1]). These pathways include the following: (a) activation of mast cells and the sympathetic nervous system, (b) vagus nerve inhibition on inflammatory pathways, (c) the prefrontal cortex and amygdala control over the hypothalamic pituitary axis (HPA), (d) the hypothalamic-corticotropin releasing factor (CRF)-ergic system, (e) the peripheral CRF-ergic system, (f) the effect of early life events on colitis (the HPA axis is programmed by early life events, and neonatal inflammatory stimuli exert long-term changes in HPA activity), (g) the impact of depression on exacerbating colitis possibly through shared proinflammatory cytokines, and (h) the intestinal microbiota-brain axis.

The vagus nerve is thought to have anti-inflammatory effects, and stress decreases vagus nerve efferent outflow[4] and increases sympathetic outflow and adrenomedullary activity, leading to increased norepinephrine and epinephrine levels.[4] Decreased vagus nerve outflow and increased sympathetic tone can lead to inhibition of immune cell functions and ultimately intestinal inflammation.[1] Furthermore, chronic stress can lead to an adaptation of the hypothalamic CRFergic system.[5] In rats, stress and CRF increase colonic permeability.[6] Stress-increased intestinal permeability allows bacteria to cross the epithelial barrier to activate the mucosal immune response[7] and to translocate to secondary lymphoid organs[8] to stimulate the innate immune system.

The neurohormonal control of intestinal immune response has been studied over decades. However, it has only been in the past 10 to 15 years that the gut microbiome has emerged as a likely critical compartment in the evolution of IBD. Stress-mediated changes may shift the microbial colonization patterns on the mucosal surface and alter the susceptibility of the host to infection. In turn, these changes in host-microbe interactions may also influence neural activity in stress-responsive brain areas.[9] Commensal microbiota can affect the postnatal development of brain systems involved in the endocrine response to stress.[10] Rat models of maternal separation, an important neonatal stress model, are associated with important changes in the HPA axis as well as in intestinal immunologic and microbial responses.[1] Altering the microbiota can also impact behavior and brain structures. Germ-free mice have been shown to reduce anxiety-like behavior in comparison to specific pathogen-free mice. This reduced anxiety-like behavior is accompanied by changes in plasticity-related genes in the hippocampus and amygdala.[11] Altering the gut microbiota in mice with a combination of antibiotics was associated with a change in gut bacteria, also an altered brain-derived neurotropic factor in the hippocampus and amygdala, and an increase in mouse exploratory behavior.[12] Behavioral traits of the donor mice were transferred to adult germ-free mice of a different strain by transplanting gut microbiota.[12]

The mechanisms by which the gut microbiota impact the gut-brain axis are being investigated. Candidates include the gamma-aminobutyric acid (GABA) and serotonin signaling pathways, which are implicated in the neurobiology of depression and anxiety.[13] GABA, a major inhibitory neurotransmitter, is a metabolite of certain gut microbes,[14,15] and increased serotonin turnover is observed in germ-free mice.[16] Neurotransmitters with well-known immune effects, including catecholamines, acetylcholine, and serotonin, are metabolites of gut microbiota.[17–19]

HUMAN STUDIES

People with chronic disease may have higher levels of distress, health anxiety, and perceived stress, and it has been shown that persons with IBD have higher lifetime rates of panic, generalized anxiety, and obsessive-compulsive disorders as well as major depression compared with control populations.[3] Compared with community controls, the 12-month prevalence of major depression in a population-based cohort of subjects with IBD was 9.1% versus 5.5% (odds ratio [OR], 1.72; 95% confidence interval [CI], 1.07 to 2.76).[3] The lifetime prevalence of major depression in the subjects with IBD was 27.2% versus 12.3% (OR, 2.20; 95% CI, 1.64–2.95). About one-half of those with a mood disorder experienced a first episode of depression more than 2 years before the onset of IBD.[3] Therefore, although it is expected that people with chronic disease like IBD may develop psychiatric comorbidity as a response to having a chronic disease, these data suggest that psychiatric comorbidity may even predispose to IBD. Whether antedating the disease or emerging after diagnosis, a great deal of the functional impairment and disability associated with health conditions such as IBD is related to the presence of anxiety or depression.[20–22] Further psychiatric comorbidity in IBD is an independent predictor of health care utilization and in turn a driver of health care costs.[23,24]

The Manitoba IBD Cohort Study is a prospective longitudinal population-based study following a cohort of IBD patients every 6 months with surveys and annually with interviews over 12 years. In this study, psychological factors had a greater contribution to health perception for the IBD cohort compared with a control population. However, those with inactive disease were quite similar to those in the non-IBD controls.[25] It is not having the disease per se that relates to psychological difficulties, but rather that disease activity is pivotal. In a sample of patients with IBD seen in a gastroenterology clinic, it was found that disease severity and psychological symptoms contributed independently to impaired quality of life.[26] In another gastroenterology clinic study, better psychological adjustment was associated with greater bowel and systemic health, increased engagement in activities and symptom tolerance, less pain, less perceived stress, and fewer gastroenterologist visits in a clinic sample of persons with IBD.[27] Hence, improving disease activity can improve psychological health and improving psychological health may improve disease activity.

In a study assessing potential triggers of symptomatic flares of IBD, nearly 600 subjects drawn from the population-based University of Manitoba IBD Research Registry completed surveys on health issues every 3 months for 1 year.[28] In any 3-month period, approximately 50% experienced some type of stress, and most reported stresses were everyday life stresses: family stress was the most commonly reported, followed by work or school, and financial stress. In terms of the association between variables experienced in one 3-month period and a symptomatic flare in the next 3-month period, only the psychological factors, including occurrence of a major life event, high perceived stress (as measured by the Cohen's Perceived Stress Scale, CPSS), and high negative mood during a previous 3-month period, were significantly associated with the subsequent occurrence of a flare.[28] On multivariate logistic regression analyses of these variables, only high perceived stress (OR 2.40; 95% CI, 1.35–4.26) was associated with an increased risk of flare. There are variable physiologic effects of acute and chronic stress, but perceived stress is how the individual appraises the demands created by stress in general and their resources to cope with the stress. To determine if increased perceived stress was driving a symptomatic flare or an actual flare of inflammatory disease, the Manitoba group undertook a second cohort study. They enrolled nearly 480 persons who completed similar questionnaires every 3 months for 6 months. At the time of returning surveys, the participants also submitted a stool sample to be tested for fecal calprotectin as a measure of intestinal inflammation. Perceived stress was associated with symptomatic activity for both Crohn disease and ulcerative colitis (1.07 per 1-point increase on the CPSS, 95% CI 1.03–1.10).[29] However, there was no significant association between perceived stress and intestinal inflammation for either Crohn disease or ulcerative colitis. Active symptoms were associated with intestinal inflammation in ulcerative colitis (OR 3.94, 95% CI 1.65–9.43), but not in Crohn disease (OR 0.98, 95% CI 0.51–1.88). The investigators concluded that despite a strong relationship between perceived stress and gastrointestinal symptoms, perceived stress was unrelated to concurrent intestinal inflammation. However, it is important to note that fecal calprotectin has limited sensitivity in small bowel Crohn disease compared with colonic inflammation. Furthermore, some symptoms in Crohn disease may be related to fibrotic stricturing disease or secondary to previous intestinal resections and not necessarily inflammatory disease. Whether stress can drive symptoms generated from these scenarios is unknown, but considering that the physiologic effects of stress may impact gut motility, it is plausible that it can.

In a follow-up to this Manitoba study, Sexton and colleagues[30] reported changes in symptoms and stress over time. Both symptom activity and perceived stress were remarkably stable from baseline to 6 months later in both Crohn disease and ulcerative colitis. Although it had been reported that baseline perceived stress predicted symptoms at 3 months,[28,29] this analysis showed that month 0 symptom activity predicted change in perceived stress from 0 to 3 months for both Crohn disease and ulcerative colitis. Hence, in this prospective study, there was a bidirectional relationship between perceived stress and IBD symptoms. This finding raises the possibility that stress and symptoms each maintain one another at higher levels over time. Whether high levels of stress trigger symptom exacerbations, or whether prolonged symptom activity promotes elevated stress, the presence of either seems to promote elevations in the other.

In this same study, participants rated their sources of stress on a Likert scale.[31] The group that reported persistently active symptoms over the 6 months of the study had higher general stress at both baseline and 3 months later than the persistently inactive group but also higher mean ratings of most sources of stress. IBD was rated as a highly frequent source of stress by 20% to 30% of the persistently active group compared with 1% to 2% of the persistently inactive group. It is noteworthy that despite reporting ongoing symptoms a maximum of 30% considered their IBD to be a source of stress. Furthermore, among asymptomatic persons at most 2% viewed their IBD as a source of stress. In sync with the data that those with inactive IBD have similar psychological health as the general population,[25] these data suggest that when the patient is well, IBD is not a source of stress even though it is a disease that can flare and become symptomatic. Finances, work, and family were rated as high-frequency stresses in the persistently active group at a similar level to IBD stress.[31] The authors of this study concluded that persons with active symptoms may benefit from targeted stress interventions.

A range of prospective studies with few exceptions have also reported that higher levels of perceived stress experience a greater likelihood of symptom reoccurrence.[32–35] Two other studies have also reported on the disconnection between active symptoms and intestinal inflammation in IBD.[36,37] In the Levenstein study,[33] persons with ulcerative colitis who were asymptomatic yet had increased levels of histologic inflammation reported higher chronic perceived stress than those asymptomatic participants without inflammation, standing out as one study showing some relationship between perceived stress and inflammation.

TREATMENT OF MENTAL HEALTH IN INFLAMMATORY BOWEL DISEASE

As reviewed herein, there is convincing literature that stress and psychiatric comorbidity impact adversely on persons with IBD. The presence of psychiatric comorbidity worsens outcomes in IBD through either reduced adherence to treatment, additional morbidity, or biological mechanisms.[38] Furthermore, undertreatment of depression or anxiety in the context of IBD complicates disease management, adversely impacting patient outcomes and health, and increasing the resource burden to the health care system. Unfortunately, there has been little research on intervening on psychiatric comorbidity in IBD. A systematic review suggested a beneficial effect of antidepressants in patients with IBD.[39] However, a recent systematic review assessing treatment of depression and anxiety in IBD populations turned up only one controlled trial.[40] Even though experts recommend cognitive behavioral therapy for treatment of pain and psychiatric comorbidity in IBD[38] when it has been studied in a randomized controlled trial in persons with IBD, it did not positively impact anxiety, depression, or coping at 1 year.[41] Hence, more studies are needed to explore optimal interventions of depression and anxiety in IBD and to determine how management of psychiatric comorbidity will ultimately impact the gastrointestinal manifestations of the IBD. On a practical basis, stress is an everyday occurrence and not only do persons with IBD experience stress but also there is ample evidence that stress adversely impacts IBD symptoms. Hence, it is imperative that clinicians discuss and manage stress

---

Box 1
Highlights of brain-gut axis and stress in inflammatory bowel disease

1. The vagus nerve has an anti-inflammatory role; enhanced cholinergic activity is anti-inflammatory, whereas sympathetic activity is proinflammatory.

2. Stress increases intestinal permeability, which can allow bacteria to cross the epithelial barrier to activate the mucosal immune response and ultimately the innate immune system.

3. In mouse models, behavioral traits of donor mice can be transferred to adult germ-free mice of a different strain by transplanting gut microbiota, underscoring that the gut microbiota can impact mental processes.

4. Persons with IBD have a 2 -to 3-fold elevated rate of depression and anxiety than the general population. These conditions may antedate the diagnosis of IBD by years and hence are not only sequelae of having a chronic disease.

5. Psychiatric comorbidity in IBD negatively impacts clinical outcomes and increases rates of disability, health care utilization, and ultimately, health care costs.

6. High perceived stress is a predictor of increased symptoms in persons with IBD. The relationship between stress and symptoms is bidirectional.

7. There are limited data suggesting that stress exacerbates frank intestinal inflammation; however, this requires further study.

8. In persons with active symptoms, only up to 30% may rate their IBD as being stressful, whereas in asymptomatic patients as little as 2% rate their IBD as being stressful. Persons with IBD suffer from the usual life stressors as the general population does: finances, work, and family being the leading stressors reported.

9. There are few controlled studies exploring the management of psychiatric comorbidity in IBD or the impact of psychotropic drugs on IBD outcomes.

10. Clinicians must engage patients with IBD on issues of mental health because they impact greatly on symptoms, and improving mental health may improve outcomes in terms of both the IBD and general well-being.

and mental health with their patients with IBD. It is also imperative that researchers explore optimal ways to manage stress and mental health in IBD (**Box 1**).

REFERENCES

1. Bonaz B, Bernstein CN. Brain-gut interactions in inflammatory bowel disease. Gastroenterology 2013;144:36–49.
2. Selye H. Confusion and controversy in the stress field. J Human Stress 1975;1: 37–44.
3. Walker JR, Ediger J, Graff LA, et al. The Manitoba IBD Cohort Study: a population-based study of the prevalence of lifetime and 12-month anxiety and mood disorders. Am J Gastroenterol 2008;103:1989–97.
4. Taché Y, Bonaz B. Corticotropin-releasing factor receptors and stress-related alterations of gut motor function. J Clin Invest 2007;117:33–40.
5. Bonaz B, Rivest S. Effect of a chronic stress on CRF neuronal activity and expression of its type 1 receptor in the rat brain. Am J Physiol 1998;275:R1438–49.
6. Santos J, Saunders PR, Hanssen NP, et al. Corticotropin-releasing hormone mimics stress-induced colonic epithelial pathophysiology in the rat. Am J Physiol 1999;277:G391–9.
7. Kiliaan AJ, Saunders PR, Bijlsma PB, et al. Stress stimulates transepithelial macromolecular uptake in rat jejunum. Am J Physiol 1998;275:G1037–44.
8. Bailey MT, Engler H, Sheridan JF. Stress induces the translocation of cutaneous and gastrointestinal microflora to secondary lymphoid organs of C57BL/6 mice. J Neuroimmunol 2006;171:29–37.
9. Lyte M, Vulchanova L, Brown DR. Stress at the intestinal surface: catecholamines and mucosa-bacteria interactions. Cell Tissue Res 2011;343:23–32.
10. Sudo N, Chida Y, Aiba Y, et al. Postnatal microbial colonization programs the hypothalamic-pituitary-adrenal system for stress response in mice. J Physiol 2004;558:263–75.
11. Neufeld KM, Kang N, Bienenstock J, et al. Reduced anxiety-like behavior and central neurochemical change in germ-free mice. Neurogastroenterol Motil 2011;23:255–64.
12. Bercik P, Denou E, Collins J, et al. The intestinal microbiota affect central levels of brain-derived neurotrophic factor and behavior in mice. Gastroenterology 2011; 141:599–609.
13. Foster JA, McVey Neufeld KA. Gut-brain axis: how the microbiome influences anxiety and depression. Trends Neurosci 2013;36(5):305–12.
14. Barrett E, Ross RP, O'Toole PW, et al. Gamma-aminobutyric acid production by culturable bacteria from the human intestine. J Appl Microbiol 2012;113(2): 411–7.
15. Higuchi T, Hayashi H, Abe K. Exchange of glutamate and gamma aminobutyrate in a Lactobacillus strain. J Bacteriol 1997;179(10):3362–4.
16. Diaz Heijtz R, Wang S, Anuar F, et al. Normal gut microbiota modulates brain development and behavior. Proc Natl Acad Sci U S A 2011;108(7):3047–52.
17. Komatsuzaki N, Nakamura T, Kimura T, et al. Characterization of glutamate decarboxylase from a high gamma-aminobutyric acid (GABA)-producer, Lactobacillus paracasei. Biosci Biotechnol Biochem 2008;72(2):278–85.
18. Tsavkelova EA, Botvinko IV, Kudrin VS, et al. Detection of neurotransmitter amines in microorganisms with the use of high-performance liquid chromatography. Dokl Biochem 2000;372(1–6):115–7.

19. Girvin GT, Stevenson JW. Cell free choline acetylase from Lactobacillus plantarum. Can J Biochem Physiol 1954;32(2):131–46.
20. Walker JR, Graff LA, Dutz JP, et al. Psychiatric disorders in patients with immune-mediated inflammatory diseases: prevalence, association with disease activity, and overall patient wellbeing. J Rheumatol 2011;88:31–5.
21. Kessler RC, Ormel J, Demler O, et al. Comorbid mental disorders account for the role impairment of commonly occurring chronic physical disorders: results from the National Comorbidity Survey. J Occup Environ Med 2003;45:1257–66.
22. Buist-Bouwman MA, de Graaf R, Volleburgh WA, et al. Comorbidity of physical and mental disorders and the effect on work-loss days. Acta Psychiatr Scand 2005;111:436–43.
23. Click B, Ramos Rivers C, Koutroubakis IE, et al. Demographic and clinical predictors of high healthcare use in patients with inflammatory bowel disease. Inflamm Bowel Dis 2016;22:1442–9.
24. Limsrivilai J, Stidham PW, Govani SM, et al. Factors that predict high health care utilization and costs for patients with inflammatory bowel diseases. Clin Gastroenterol Hepatol 2017;15:385–92.
25. Graff LA, Walker JR, Clara I, et al. Stress coping, distress, and health perceptions in inflammatory bowel disease and community controls. Am J Gastroenterol 2009; 104:2959–69.
26. Guthrie E, Jackson J, Shaffer J, et al. Psychological disorder and severity of inflammatory bowel disease predict health-related quality of life in ulcerative colitis and Crohn's disease. Am J Gastroenterol 2002;97:1994–9.
27. Kiebles JL, Doerfler B, Keefer L. Preliminary evidence supporting a framework of psychological adjustment to inflammatory bowel disease. Inflamm Bowel Dis 2010;16:1685–95.
28. Bernstein CN, Singh S, Graff LA, et al. A prospective population based study of symptomatic triggers of flares in IBD. Am J Gastroenterol 2010;105:1994–2002.
29. Targownik LE, Sexton KA, Bernstein MT, et al. The relationship among perceived stress, symptoms, and inflammation in persons with inflammatory bowel disease. Am J Gastroenterol 2015;110(7):1001–12.
30. Sexton KA, Walker JR, Graff LA, et al. Evidence of bidirectional associations between perceived stress and symptom activity: a prospective longitudinal investigation in inflammatory bowel disease. Inflamm Bowel Dis 2017;23(3):473–83.
31. Bernstein MT, Targownik LE, Sexton KA, et al. Assessing the relationship between sources of stress and symptom changes among persons with IBD over time: a prospective study. Can J Gastroenterol Hepatol 2016;2016:1681507.
32. Duff y LC, Zielezny MA, Marshall JR, et al. Lag time between stress events and risk of recurrent episodes of inflammatory bowel disease. Epidemiology 1991; 2:141–5.
33. Levenstein S, Prantera C, Varvo V, et al. Stress and exacerbation in ulcerative colitis: a prospective study of patients enrolled in remission. Am J Gastroenterol 2000;95:1213–20.
34. Bitton A, Sewitch MJ, Peppercorn MA, et al. Psychosocial determinants of relapse in ulcerative colitis: a longitudinal study. Am J Gastroenterol 2003;98:2203–8.
35. Langhorst J, Hofstetter A, Wolfe F, et al. Short-term stress, but not mucosal healing nor depression was predictive for the risk of relapse in patients with ulcerative colitis: a prospective 12-month follow-up study. Inflamm Bowel Dis 2013;19:2380–6.

36. Falvey JD, Hoskin T, Meijer B, et al. Disease activity assessment in IBD: clinical indices and biomarkers fail to predict endoscopic remission. Inflamm Bowel Dis 2015;21(4):824–31.

37. Gracie DJ, Williams CJM, Sood R, et al. Poor correlation between clinical disease activity and mucosal inflammation, and the role of psychological comorbidity, in inflammatory bowel disease. Am J Gastroenterol 2016;111:541–51.

38. Regueiro M, Greer JB, Szigethy E. Etiology and treatment of pain and psychosocial issues in patients with inflammatory bowel diseases. Gastroenterology 2017; 152:430–9.

39. Mikocka-Walus AA, Turnbull DA, Moulding NT, et al. Antidepressants and inflammatory bowel disease: a systematic review. Clin Pract Epidemiol Ment Health 2006;2:24.

40. Fiest K, Bernstein CN, Walker JR, et al. Systematic review of interventions for depression and anxiety in persons with inflammatory bowel disease. BMC Res Notes 2016;9(1):404.

41. Mikocka-Walus A, Bampton P, Hetzel D, et al. Cognitive behavioural therapy has no effect on disease activity but improves quality of life in subgroups of patients with inflammatory bowel disease: a pilot randomized controlled trial. BMC Gastroenterol 2015;15:54.

Psychological Considerations and Interventions in Inflammatory Bowel Disease Patient Care

Tiffany H. Taft, PsyD[a],*, Sarah Ballou, PhD[b], Alyse Bedell, MS[a],
Devin Lincenberg, PsyD[c]

KEYWORDS

- Inflammatory bowel disease • Psychology • Mental health • Psychotherapy
- Behavioral interventions

KEY POINTS

- Psychological health is an important yet neglected aspect of inflammatory bowel disease (IBD) patient care, with challenges in identifying proper treatments and mental health resources.
- Psychological distress typically occurs due to disease impact, treatment concerns, intimacy concerns, and stigma. Left untreated, psychological distress has direct negative impacts on patient outcomes.
- Several evidence-based treatments are available for most causes of psychological distress in patients with IBD, the most widely accepted being rooted in cognitive behavioral theory.
- Patients want their gastroenterologist to discuss psychological issues during routine visits, and many are open to or desire referral to qualified mental health providers for concurrent treatment.

INTRODUCTION

Psychosocial challenges for patients with inflammatory bowel disease (IBD) are critical considerations when managing care. These constructs have garnered much needed attention in recent years. However, psychological research represents only

Disclosures: T.H. Taft has an ongoing speaker relationship with Janssen pharmaceuticals for patient education programs. All other authors have nothing to disclose.
Funding: Funded by NIH (1T32DK101363).
[a] Division of Gastroenterology, Northwestern University Feinberg School of Medicine, 676 North Saint Clair Street #1400, Chicago, IL 60611, USA; [b] Department of Medicine, Beth Israel Deaconess Medical Center, 330 Brookline Avenue, Boston, MA 02215, USA; [c] Oak Park Behavioral Medicine LLC, 101 N. Marion Street #313, Oak Park, IL 60301, USA
* Corresponding author. 676 North Saint Clair Street #1400, Chicago, IL 60611.
E-mail address: ttaft@northwestern.edu

http://dx.doi.org/10.1016/j.gtc.2017.08.007
0889-8553/17/© 2017 Elsevier Inc. All rights reserved.
gastro.theclinics.com

approximately 2% of all published IBD-related inquiry (74 of 4470 articles indexed on PubMed in 2016) and translation of research findings to clinical practice is challenging. Considerable evidence shows IBD impacts health-related quality of life,[1] causes psychological distress,[2] and psychological and behavioral interventions can mitigate some negative impacts to patient outcomes.[3,4]

Anxiety and depression are the most commonly researched psychological comorbidities in IBD. A 2016 systematic review reports the prevalence of clinical anxiety *disorders* is 21% in patients with IBD, whereas the prevalence of anxiety *symptoms* (eg, subclinical scores on standardized anxiety measures) is 35%; rates of depression are somewhat lower, with 15% having a depressive disorder and 22% reporting depressive symptoms.[2] Detailed reviews of anxiety and depression in IBD are conducted elsewhere. Rather, we aim to review potential psychosocial challenges for patients with IBD within these 2 overarching, often-used terms and provide recommendations for appropriate interventions to mitigate negative impacts on patient care and outcomes.

PSYCHOLOGICAL CONSIDERATIONS IN INFLAMMATORY BOWEL DISEASE

We know approximately one-third of patients with IBD experience anxiety and depression, but what is driving these symptoms? The 1991 study by Drossman and colleagues[5] outlines 4 main areas of patient concerns: disease impact, treatment, intimacy, and stigma. Subsequent research on IBD psychosocial issues generally tracks these domains, with additional nuance emerging as investigation in this area evolves.[6] Evidence-based psychological treatments exist for most IBD mental health concerns. Of available psychotherapies, cognitive behavioral therapy (CBT), originally developed to treat depression,[7] shows consistent efficacy when applied to a wide range of psychiatric and medical conditions, including IBD, and may be effective in mitigating several of the psychological issues outlined in this review.

What Is Cognitive Behavioral Therapy?

In CBT, patients are taught to understand the relationship among situations, thoughts, behaviors, physical reactions, and emotions. Patients learn to change thoughts (through cognitive reframing), behaviors (through scheduled or prescribed changes in activity or responses), and levels of physiologic arousal (through relaxation exercises) to reduce emotional distress. In behavioral medicine settings, the CBT model is used to help patients cope with distress related specifically to a medical condition. In IBD, CBT has not been shown to consistently alter disease outcomes, but is effective in improving quality of life, coping skills, medical adherence, and underlying symptoms of anxiety or depression.[8] As such, as we outline psychological distress in patients with IBD, potential CBT-based interventions are proposed in **Box 1**.

INFLAMMATORY BOWEL DISEASE IMPACT
Disordered Eating

Food is a fundamentally important aspect of life that can pose particular challenges for patients with IBD. Most patients hold strong beliefs about how food impacts their illness, but many do not receive adequate help.[9,10] Many patients with IBD determine what foods are "safe" versus "unsafe" based on subjective experience.[11,12] Some turn to one of many popular exclusion diets. Following long-term dietary regimens can produce maladaptive attitudes, including anxiety, toward food.[13] Although clinical eating disorder pathology (ie, anorexia nervosa) is possible, the more common risk in IBD is development of *disordered eating (DE)*, or dysfunctional eating behaviors,

---

Box 1
Evidence-based behavioral interventions for inflammatory bowel disease (IBD) mental health concerns

Disordered Eating
- Traditional cognitive behavioral therapy (CBT) for disordered eating
- Enhanced CBT (CBT-E) if clinical eating disorder present
- Intensive outpatient or inpatient eating disorder center

Insomnia
- CBT for insomnia (CBT-I)
- Medical hypnotherapy
- Sleep Healthy Using the Internet (SHUTi) http://www.myshuti.com

Fatigue
- Traditional CBT
- Behavioral self-management

Posttraumatic Stress Disorder
- Cognitive processing therapy
- Prolonged exposure therapy
- Select psychotropic medications
- http://www.ptsd.va.gov/professional/treatment/overview

Treatment Concerns
- Traditional CBT
- Behavioral self-management

Intimacy Concerns
- CBT for sexual dysfunction
- Medical hypnotherapy
- Pelvic floor physical therapy
- Education about IBD and pregnancy

Stigma
- Individual or group CBT
- Educational programs for family, friends, significant others

---

such as skipping meals, binge eating, restricting, and fasting.[14] We recommend The Food-Related Quality of Life Questionnaire to assess IBD patient eating concerns.

People with gastrointestinal illness, including IBD, are at higher risk for developing DE, which is associated with increased psychological distress and symptom severity,[15] and is independent of remission status.[16] Patients may limit social interactions to mitigate food anxiety, which in turn increases psychological distress, creating a vicious cycle.[16,17] Depending on how restrictive the diet is, nutritional deficiencies may develop from DE, further complicating treatment. Overnutrition is also a growing problem in IBD, with rates of overweight and obesity similar to the general population,[18,19] especially in patients with mild disease or in remission. Patients with IBD are susceptible to DE habits, which may increase caloric intake, including binges or emotional eating associated with anxiety or depression.

Insomnia and Fatigue

Sleep is important in IBD management, as insomnia is known to impact both physical and psychological well-being. A large body of research demonstrates sleep problems are associated with poorer outcomes in anxiety and depression[20] and insomnia predicts future mental health problems in individuals without current psychological distress.[21] Fatigue is one of the most burdensome IBD symptoms[22] and is highly prevalent, with 44% to 86% of patients with active disease and 22% to 41% with inactive disease reporting clinically significant levels of fatigue.[22–24] Being female, and having psychological distress, disease-related worry, low quality of life, disability, and poor sleep quality are all associated with greater fatigue. Two measures of IBD fatigue include the Inflammatory Bowel Disease Fatigue Scale and the Multidimensional Fatigue Inventory.

Posttraumatic Stress Disorder

To date, no study evaluates posttraumatic stress disorder (PTSD) in IBD. However, based on the nature of IBD, it is plausible PTSD may be present in a subset of patients. PTSD symptoms may increase over time or be intermittent throughout the course of illness and include intrusive thoughts, nightmares, or flashbacks[25]; avoidance of thoughts or feelings related to the trauma; social withdrawal; and emotional numbing.[25] There are multiple risk factors for PTSD, including heightened psychological distress following diagnosis, female sex,[26] lower socioeconomic status,[27] more severe disease,[28] uncontrolled pain, younger age at diagnosis,[28,29] type of surgery, subjective intensity of symptoms,[30] and at least 1 disease recurrence.

Compared with trauma associated with combat or natural disasters, the PTSD-stressor in IBD comes from an internal event (ie, the disease), and as such the patients with IBD cannot flee the actual threat. Avoidance behaviors may manifest in treatment nonadherence[31–33] or missed follow-up care,[34] as these may be triggers of intrusive symptoms. Conversely, PTSD may drive health-related anxiety resulting in excessive health care utilization and costs[35] due to somatic symptoms or pain perception[36] not associated with IBD disease activity. PTSD also is associated with enhanced cellular immune response[37] and alterations to the hypothalamic-pituitary-adrenal axis,[38] thereby complicating its relationship with IBD disease course. Rapid assessment tools exist to screen patients with IBD for PTSD, including the Primary Care PTSD Screen and PTSD Checklist–Civilian Version.

INFLAMMATORY BOWEL DISEASE TREATMENT CONCERNS

A recent paradigm shift in IBD treatment outlines top-down (ie, biologic medication first) versus traditional bottom-up approaches[39]; 24% of patients with IBD were current or past users of biologic medications in 2014,[40] with increasing trends of use.[41] Starting a biologic medication may cause distress in some patients. Escalation in therapy may serve as a sign of worsening disease.[42] Some patients may be afraid of potential side effects of biologic therapies, and others may be more tolerable of risk than their physician.[43] Injection anxiety is an underdeveloped area of research in IBD, but is associated with lower medication adherence in other illness groups.[44,45] If anxiety poses a barrier to initiating or adhering to a biologic, or other IBD medications, traditional CBT or behavioral self-management (outlined later in this article) are effective treatments.

INTIMACY CONCERNS
Body Image

Up to two-thirds of patients with IBD report some body image dissatisfaction,[46,47] with higher rates in women (75% vs 50% of men). Dissatisfaction is related to weight loss, hair loss, weight gain from corticosteroids, extraintestinal dermatologic manifestations, increased disease activity, high symptom burden, longer duration of steroid use, other extraintestinal symptoms including fistulas, and surgical history.[47,48] Negative body image is logically associated with decreased quality of life and increased psychological distress[46,49]; however, it is infrequently discussed during routine medical visits. The 9-item Body Image Scale is recommended for assessment.

Sexuality

Up to 31% of men and 80% of women with IBD report low or no interest in sex.[50,51] Depressed mood is the strongest predictor of sexual dysfunction across genders. Patients with prior surgical resection report lower libido and less frequent sexual activity compared with nonoperated patients.[52] Permanent ostomy also impairs sexual functioning in both men and women, with an increased rate of anorgasmia in female patients with ostomy. Longer disease duration is associated with fewer sexual problems, possibly due to increased coping skills over time.[50] Twenty-five percent of women report pain during intercourse, which is not associated with disease type or activity, use of steroids, or presence of perianal disease and may be related to pelvic floor dysfunction. Unfortunately, many providers do not inquire about sexual functioning during regular visits.[53] In a survey of 64 women with IBD, only 12 (18.8%) had discussed sexuality/sexual functioning with their gastroenterologist, and of those who did, 100% were patient-generated conversations. Several validated assessment tools exist, including the Sexual Functions Questionnaire, International Index of Erectile Function, and Female Sexual Function Index.

Childbearing Concerns

Many women with IBD report a higher rate of voluntary childlessness[54,55]: 18% in Crohn's Disease (CD) and 14% in Ulcerative Colitis (UC) compared with 6.2% in the general population. Primary motivators include worry about IBD heritability, risk of congenital abnormalities, and medication teratogenicity. Common pregnancy concerns, which are associated with poor understanding of actual risks of pregnancy with IBD,[56] include infertility, effects of medications on the fetus, vaginal delivery versus cesarean delivery, and breastfeeding.[57] However, only 28% of women with IBD demonstrate "good" to "very good" knowledge in these areas.[58]

STIGMA

Although stigmatization is widely studied in human immunodeficiency virus/AIDS and mental illness, research into IBD-related stigma is relatively new. A 2016 comprehensive review of IBD stigma finds patients with IBD perceive that others hold stigmatizing views toward them and the disease; some patients internalize these negative beliefs, whereas others resist them, and stigmatizing attitudes and behaviors exist among those without IBD.[59,60] Like stigma toward other diseases, IBD stigma is associated with poorer outcomes[61] and may cause or exacerbate feelings of depression or anxiety. Clinicians should be mindful of potential stigma being experienced by their patients and inquire about its impacts on social experiences and interpersonal relationships.

INTEGRATING MENTAL HEALTH INTO INFLAMMATORY BOWEL DISEASE PATIENT CARE

This review, as several others, demonstrates patients with IBD have mental health needs that, if unchecked, can have direct and indirect impacts on patient outcomes. Yet, integration of behavioral medicine services into gastroenterology practice is limited, mostly to tertiary, university-based centers in major metropolitan areas. How, then, can the vast majority of gastroenterologists ensure effective management of the mental health issues of their patients?

Psychological distress over the disease course of IBD is consistent and can be independent from disease activity,[62] so merely treating IBD symptoms is insufficient in its alleviation. Newly diagnosed patients have the greatest need for psychotherapy,[63] and early intervention, before the patient is significantly distressed, leads to better outcomes.[64] Unfortunately, several barriers exist, including social stigma, financial burdens, and a lack of mental health professionals trained in working with patients with IBD,[65] preventing timely referral to a mental health specialist; only 15% of patients with IBD report referral for mental health treatment, whereas half would desire such referral.[65]

Two 2017 studies found most patients and providers do not discuss how IBD may affect quality of life, emotional functioning, and overall mental health during routine visits,[65] both in the United States and Europe[42]; 75% of patients would like their providers to address these impacts. Gastroenterologists may feel compelled to try to treat mental health themselves, feel unsure of how to broach the topic of mental health, not detect psychological distress,[66] or prioritize other disease management issues due to appointment time constraints.[67]

In the era of the rapid medical encounter, it is vital for the practicing gastroenterologist to efficiently recognize potential psychosocial issues that may impact patient outcomes and establish a referral process for reliable and reputable mental health treatments. **Box 2** provides recommendations for streamlining referrals to mental health services. In addition to CBT approaches previously described, additional psychological interventions are available and may be efficacious for some patients with IBD.

Behavioral Self-Management

For patients who do not exhibit psychological distress and/or who are not interested in traditional psychotherapy, behavioral or self-management therapy may be effective.[68,69] In this treatment, the goal is to target negative health behaviors (eg, poor medication compliance, dietary nonadherence) to improve overall physical health. This therapy is informed by the CBT model but does not incorporate the cognitive component of traditional CBT, which evaluates negative or distressing thought patterns.

Box 2
Integrating mental health services into IBD patient care

Know Your Resources
- Generate a referral list of qualified mental health professionals in your area that are easily accessible in clinic. See the Resources section for directory recommendations.
- Seek clinicians with specialization in clinical health psychology or behavioral medicine and who primarily use a CBT treatment approach.

Therapists Directories
- *Psychology today* therapist finder: https://therapists.psychologytoday.com
- Directory of Cognitive Behavioral Therapists: http://www.abct.org
- Society of Behavioral Medicine: www.sbm.org
- Gut-Directed Hypnotherapy Providers: http://www.ibshypnosis.com

Have the Discussion
- Establish a solid therapeutic alliance with open communication with each patient.
- Discuss social and emotional aspects of IBD early, even in the absence of overt distress.
- Ask patients about stress, mood, anxiety, and intimacy regularly to ensure early intervention.

Integration of Care
- Communicate with mental health providers working with your patients with IBD to ensure continuity of care.
- Ask patients about their experience with mental health treatment once referred.

Medical Hypnotherapy

Medical hypnotherapy is an effective intervention for many diseases and disorders. Gut-directed hypnotherapy is a variation of medical hypnotherapy that focuses hypnotic suggestions on the health of the gastrointestinal tract.[4,70,71] This treatment typically involves 7 to 12 weekly sessions in which patients learn to achieve a deep hypnotic state and are then led through a series of scripted, gut-focused imageries with suggestions. Patients practice these exercises at home using audio recordings. Recent pediatric research suggests self-directed hypnotherapy is as effective in treating functional abdominal pain and irritable bowel syndrome as treatment with a clinician,[72] which would make this treatment more accessible.

In IBD, a handful of studies (limited by small sample sizes) evaluate the efficacy of gut-directed hypnotherapy. Findings show reduced rectal mucosal inflammatory responses (interleukin (IL)-6, IL-13, tumor necrosis factor-α, substance P, histamine) in patients after 1 session,[73] prolonged clinical remission by approximately 2.5 months in patients with quiescent UC compared with controls after 7 sessions of hypnotherapy,[74] and maintained remission in one-quarter of patients with active IBD at 5-year follow-up after 12 sessions.[75]

Telemental Health

Telemental health interventions are a promising alternative for patients with IBD needing behavioral intervention. Four studies on Web-based interventions exist for IBD.[76] The existing literature is promising, suggesting improved outcomes in IBD with use of these interventions.[77,78] Web-based psychological interventions are effective in treating depression and anxiety,[79–81] insomnia,[82] and irritable bowel syndrome.[83,84] These strategies may bridge the treatment gap that currently exists for integrated behavioral medicine practice in gastroenterology.

SUMMARY

Psychological considerations are vital for proper IBD management, as patients with IBD experience a complex interplay between their physical and emotional health. Although there is a dearth of gastrointestinal psychologists at present, identifying mental health clinicians with chronic illness experience trained in evidenced-based interventions such as CBT should be a priority. Patients express desires for, at a minimum, conversations about IBD's impact on quality of life and emotional well-being, yet these needs remain unmet in most. Although these topics may be difficult or potentially time-consuming, if left unchecked psychological distress can hamper disease and symptom management. As IBD treatment continues to evolve, giving appropriate credence to the psychology of the patient with IBD will lead to improved patient satisfaction and care.

REFERENCES

1. Sainsbury A, Heatley RV. Review article: psychosocial factors in the quality of life of patients with inflammatory bowel disease. Aliment Pharmacol Ther 2005;21: 499–508.
2. Neuendorf R, Harding A, Stello N, et al. Depression and anxiety in patients with inflammatory bowel disease: a systematic review. J Psychosom Res 2016;87:70–80.
3. Fiest KM, Bernstein CN, Walker JR, et al. Systematic review of interventions for depression and anxiety in persons with inflammatory bowel disease. BMC Res Notes 2016;9:404.

4. Peters SL, Muir JG, Gibson PR. Review article: gut-directed hypnotherapy in the management of irritable bowel syndrome and inflammatory bowel disease. Aliment Pharmacol Ther 2015;41:1104–15.

5. Drossman DA, Leserman J, Li ZM, et al. The rating form of IBD patient concerns: a new measure of health status. Psychosom Med 1991;53:701–12.

6. Casati J, Toner BB, de Rooy EC, et al. Concerns of patients with inflammatory bowel disease: a review of emerging themes. Dig Dis Sci 2000;45:26–31.

7. Beck AT. The past and future of cognitive therapy. J Psychother Pract Res 1997;6: 276–84.

8. Knowles SR, Monshat K, Castle DJ. The efficacy and methodological challenges of psychotherapy for adults with inflammatory bowel disease: a review. Inflamm Bowel Dis 2013;19:2704–15.

9. Prince A, Whelan K, Moosa A, et al. Nutritional problems in inflammatory bowel disease: the patient perspective. J Crohns Colitis 2011;5:443–50.

10. Tinsley A, Ehrlich OG, Hwang C, et al. Knowledge, attitudes, and beliefs regarding the role of nutrition in IBD among patients and providers. Inflamm Bowel Dis 2016;22:2474–81.

11. Triggs CM, Munday K, Hu R, et al. Dietary factors in chronic inflammation: food tolerances and intolerances of a New Zealand Caucasian Crohn's disease population. Mutat Res 2010;690:123–38.

12. Limdi JK, Aggarwal D, McLaughlin JT. Dietary practices and beliefs in patients with inflammatory bowel disease. Inflamm Bowel Dis 2016;22:164–70.

13. Quick VM, Byrd-Bredbenner C, Neumark-Sztainer D. Chronic illness and disordered eating: a discussion of the literature. Adv Nutr 2013;4:277–86.

14. Grilo C. Eating and weight disorders. New York: Psychology Press; 2006.

15. Satherley R, Howard R, Higgs S. Disordered eating practices in gastrointestinal disorders. Appetite 2015;84:240–50.

16. Hughes L, Lindsay JO, Lomer MC, et al. Psychosocial impact of food and nutrition in people with inflammatory bowel disease: a qualitative study. Gut 2013;62:A168.

17. Daniel JM. Young adults' perceptions of living with chronic inflammatory bowel disease. Gastroenterol Nurs 2002;25:83–94.

18. Nic Suibhne T, Raftery TC, McMahon O, et al. High prevalence of overweight and obesity in adults with Crohn's disease: associations with disease and lifestyle factors. J Crohns Colitis 2013;7:e241–8.

19. Steed H, Walsh S, Reynolds N. A brief report of the epidemiology of obesity in the inflammatory bowel disease population of Tayside, Scotland. Obes Facts 2009;2: 370–2.

20. Ranjbaran Z, Keefer L, Farhadi A, et al. Impact of sleep disturbances in inflammatory bowel disease. J Gastroenterol Hepatol 2007;22:1748–53.

21. Johnson EO, Roth T, Breslau N. The association of insomnia with anxiety disorders and depression: exploration of the direction of risk. J Psychiatr Res 2006; 40:700–8.

22. Graff LA, Vincent N, Walker JR, et al. A population-based study of fatigue and sleep difficulties in inflammatory bowel disease. Inflamm Bowel Dis 2011;17: 1882–9.

23. Jelsness-Jorgensen LP, Bernklev T, Henriksen M, et al. Chronic fatigue is associated with increased disease-related worries and concerns in inflammatory bowel disease. World J Gastroenterol 2012;18:445–52.

24. Gracie DJ, Ford AC. Letter: causes of fatigue in inflammatory bowel disease remain uncertain. Aliment Pharmacol Ther 2017;45:762–3.

25. Tedstone JE, Tarrier N. Posttraumatic stress disorder following medical illness and treatment. Clin Psychol Rev 2003;23:409–48.
26. Hilerio CM, Martinez J, Zorrilla CD, et al. Posttraumatic stress disorder symptoms and adherence among women living with HIV. Ethn Dis 2005;15:S5-47-50.
27. Cordova MJ, Andrykowski MA, Kenady DE, et al. Frequency and correlates of posttraumatic-stress-disorder-like symptoms after treatment for breast cancer. J Consult Clin Psychol 1995;63:981–6.
28. Epping-Jordan JE, Compas BE, Osowiecki DM, et al. Psychological adjustment in breast cancer: processes of emotional distress. Health Psychol 1999;18: 315–26.
29. Bennett P, Conway M, Clatworthy J, et al. Predicting post-traumatic symptoms in cardiac patients. Heart Lung 2001;30:458–65.
30. Bruggimann L, Annoni JM, Staub F, et al. Chronic posttraumatic stress symptoms after nonsevere stroke. Neurology 2006;66:513–6.
31. Boarts JM, Sledjeski EM, Bogart LM, et al. The differential impact of PTSD and depression on HIV disease markers and adherence to HAART in people living with HIV. AIDS Behav 2006;10:253–61.
32. Shemesh E, Rudnick A, Kaluski E, et al. A prospective study of posttraumatic stress symptoms and nonadherence in survivors of a myocardial infarction (MI). Gen Hosp Psychiatry 2001;23:215–22.
33. Kronish IM, Edmondson D, Goldfinger JZ, et al. Posttraumatic stress disorder and adherence to medications in survivors of strokes and transient ischemic attacks. Stroke 2012;43:2192–7.
34. Alonzo AA. Acute myocardial infarction and posttraumatic stress disorder: the consequences of cumulative adversity. J Cardiovasc Nurs 1999;13:33–45.
35. Marciniak MD, Lage MJ, Dunayevich E, et al. The cost of treating anxiety: the medical and demographic correlates that impact total medical costs. Depress Anxiety 2005;21:178–84.
36. Sherman JJ, Turk DC, Okifuji A. Prevalence and impact of posttraumatic stress disorder-like symptoms on patients with fibromyalgia syndrome. Clin J Pain 2000;16:127–34.
37. Altemus M, Dhabhar FS, Yang R. Immune function in PTSD. Ann N Y Acad Sci 2006;1071:167–83.
38. de Kloet CS, Vermetten E, Geuze E, et al. Assessment of HPA-axis function in posttraumatic stress disorder: pharmacological and non-pharmacological challenge tests, a review. J Psychiatr Res 2006;40:550–67.
39. Devlin SM, Panaccione R. Evolving inflammatory bowel disease treatment paradigms: top-down versus step-up. Med Clin North Am 2010;94:1–18.
40. Vester-Andersen MK, Prosberg MV, Jess T, et al. Disease course and surgery rates in inflammatory bowel disease: a population-based, 7-year follow-up study in the era of immunomodulating therapy. Am J Gastroenterol 2014;109:705–14.
41. Duricova D. What can we learn from epidemiological studies in inflammatory bowel disease? Dig Dis 2017;35:69–73.
42. Rubin DT, Dubinsky MC, Martino S, et al. Communication between physicians and patients with ulcerative colitis: reflections and insights from a qualitative study of in-office patient-physician visits. Inflamm Bowel Dis 2017;23:494–501.
43. Johnson FR, Hauber B, Ozdemir S, et al. Are gastroenterologists less tolerant of treatment risks than patients? Benefit-risk preferences in Crohn's disease management. J Manag Care Pharm 2010;16:616–28.

44. Turner AP, Williams RM, Sloan AP, et al. Injection anxiety remains a long-term barrier to medication adherence in multiple sclerosis. Rehabil Psychol 2009;54:116–21.

45. Mann DM, Ponieman D, Leventhal H, et al. Predictors of adherence to diabetes medications: the role of disease and medication beliefs. J Behav Med 2009;32:278–84.

46. McDermott E, Mullen G, Moloney J, et al. Body image dissatisfaction: clinical features, and psychosocial disability in inflammatory bowel disease. Inflamm Bowel Dis 2015;21:353–60.

47. Muller KR, Prosser R, Bampton P, et al. Female gender and surgery impair relationships, body image, and sexuality in inflammatory bowel disease: patient perceptions. Inflamm Bowel Dis 2010;16:657–63.

48. Trindade IA, Ferreira C, Pinto-Gouveia J. The effects of body image impairment on the quality of life of non-operated Portuguese female IBD patients. Qual Life Res 2017;26:429–36.

49. Dunker MS, Stiggelbout AM, van Hogezand RA, et al. Cosmesis and body image after laparoscopic-assisted and open ileocolic resection for Crohn's disease. Surg Endosc 1998;12:1334–40.

50. Timmer A, Bauer A, Kemptner D, et al. Determinants of male sexual function in inflammatory bowel disease: a survey-based cross-sectional analysis in 280 men. Inflamm Bowel Dis 2007;13:1236–43.

51. Timmer A, Kemptner D, Bauer A, et al. Determinants of female sexual function in inflammatory bowel disease: a survey based cross-sectional analysis. BMC Gastroenterol 2008;8:45.

52. Bel LG, Vollebregt AM, Van der Meulen-de Jong AE, et al. Sexual dysfunctions in men and women with inflammatory bowel disease: the influence of IBD-related clinical factors and depression on sexual function. J Sex Med 2015;12:1557–67.

53. Borum ML, Igiehon E, Shafa S. Physicians may inadequately address sexuality in women with inflammatory bowel disease. Inflamm Bowel Dis 2010;16:181.

54. Mountifield R, Bampton P, Prosser R, et al. Fear and fertility in inflammatory bowel disease: a mismatch of perception and reality affects family planning decisions. Inflamm Bowel Dis 2009;15:720–5.

55. Marri SR, Ahn C, Buchman AL. Voluntary childlessness is increased in women with inflammatory bowel disease. Inflamm Bowel Dis 2007;13:591–9.

56. Selinger CP, Eaden J, Selby W, et al. Inflammatory bowel disease and pregnancy: lack of knowledge is associated with negative views. J Crohns Colitis 2013;7:e206–13.

57. Nguyen GC, Seow CH, Maxwell C, et al. The Toronto consensus statements for the management of inflammatory bowel disease in pregnancy. Gastroenterology 2016;150:734–57.e1.

58. Selinger CP, Eaden J, Selby W, et al. Patients' knowledge of pregnancy-related issues in inflammatory bowel disease and validation of a novel assessment tool ('CCPKnow'). Aliment Pharmacol Ther 2012;36:57–63.

59. Taft TH, Keefer L. A systematic review of disease-related stigmatization in patients living with inflammatory bowel disease. Clin Exp Gastroenterol 2016;9:49–58.

60. Taft TH, Bedell A, Naftaly J, et al. Stigmatization toward irritable bowel syndrome and inflammatory bowel disease in an online cohort. Neurogastroenterol Motil 2017;29:e12921. http://dx.doi.org/10.1111/nmo.12921.

61. Taft TH, Keefer L, Leonhard C, et al. Impact of perceived stigma on inflammatory bowel disease patient outcomes. Inflamm Bowel Dis 2009;15:1224–32.

62. Lix LM, Graff LA, Walker JR, et al. Longitudinal study of quality of life and psychological functioning for active, fluctuating, and inactive disease patterns in inflammatory bowel disease. Inflamm Bowel Dis 2008;14:1575–84.

63. Miehsler W, Weichselberger M, Offerlbauer-Ernst A, et al. Which patients with IBD need psychological interventions? A controlled study. Inflamm Bowel Dis 2008; 14:1273–80.

64. Evers AW, Kraaimaat FW, van Riel PL, et al. Tailored cognitive-behavioral therapy in early rheumatoid arthritis for patients at risk: a randomized controlled trial. Pain 2002;100:141–53.

65. Quinton S, Bedell A, Craven M, et al. Disparities in the integration of mental health treatment in inflammatory bowel disease (IBD) patient care. Gastroentrol 2017;5: S746–7.

66. Keefer L, Sayuk G, Bratten J, et al. Multicenter study of gastroenterologists' ability to identify anxiety and depression in a new patient encounter and its impact on diagnosis. J Clin Gastroenterol 2008;42:667–71.

67. Spiegel BM, Gralnek IM, Bolus R, et al. Clinical determinants of health-related quality of life in patients with irritable bowel syndrome. Arch Intern Med 2004; 164:1773–80.

68. Keefer L, Doerfler B, Artz C. Optimizing management of Crohn's disease within a project management framework: results of a pilot study. Inflamm Bowel Dis 2012; 18:254–60.

69. Keefer L, Kiebles JL, Kwiatek MA, et al. The potential role of a self-management intervention for ulcerative colitis: a brief report from the ulcerative colitis hypnotherapy trial. Biol Res Nurs 2012;14:71–7.

70. Riehl ME, Keefer L. Hypnotherapy for esophageal disorders. Am J Clin Hypn 2015;58:22–33.

71. Whorwell PJ. Review article: the history of hypnotherapy and its role in the irritable bowel syndrome. Aliment Pharmacol Ther 2005;22:1061–7.

72. Rutten JM, Vlieger AM, Frankenhuis C, et al. Home-based hypnotherapy self-exercises vs individual hypnotherapy with a therapist for treatment of pediatric irritable bowel syndrome, functional abdominal pain, or functional abdominal pain syndrome: a randomized clinical trial. JAMA Pediatr 2017;171(5):470–7.

73. Mawdsley JE, Jenkins DG, Macey MG, et al. The effect of hypnosis on systemic and rectal mucosal measures of inflammation in ulcerative colitis. Am J Gastroenterol 2008;103:1460–9.

74. Keefer L, Taft TH, Kiebles JL, et al. Gut-directed hypnotherapy significantly augments clinical remission in quiescent ulcerative colitis. Aliment Pharmacol Ther 2013;38:761–71.

75. Miller V, Whorwell PJ. Treatment of inflammatory bowel disease: a role for hypnotherapy? Int J Clin Exp Hypn 2008;56:306–17.

76. Stiles-Shields C, Keefer L. Web-based interventions for ulcerative colitis and Crohn's disease: systematic review and future directions. Clin Exp Gastroenterol 2015;8:149–57.

77. Cross RK, Cheevers N, Rustgi A, et al. Randomized, controlled trial of home telemanagement in patients with ulcerative colitis (UC HAT). Inflamm Bowel Dis 2012; 18:1018–25.

78. Cross RK, Finkelstein J. Feasibility and acceptance of a home telemanagement system in patients with inflammatory bowel disease: a 6-month pilot study. Dig Dis Sci 2007;52:357–64.

79. Godleski L, Darkins A, Peters J. Outcomes of 98,609 U.S. Department of Veterans Affairs patients enrolled in telemental health services, 2006-2010. Psychiatr Serv 2012;63:383-5.
80. Backhaus A, Agha Z, Maglione ML, et al. Videoconferencing psychotherapy: a systematic review. Psychol Serv 2012;9:111-31.
81. Steel K, Cox D, Garry H. Therapeutic videoconferencing interventions for the treatment of long-term conditions. J Telemed Telecare 2011;17:109-17.
82. van der Zweerde T, Lancee J, Slottje P, et al. Cost-effectiveness of i-sleep, a guided online CBT intervention, for patients with insomnia in general practice: protocol of a pragmatic randomized controlled trial. BMC Psychiatry 2016;16:85.
83. Ljotsson B, Falk L, Vesterlund AW, et al. Internet-delivered exposure and mindfulness based therapy for irritable bowel syndrome–a randomized controlled trial. Behav Res Ther 2010;48:531-9.
84. Ljotsson B, Hedman E, Andersson E, et al. Internet-delivered exposure-based treatment vs. stress management for irritable bowel syndrome: a randomized trial. Am J Gastroenterol 2011;106:1481-91.

Mindfulness-Based Interventions in Inflammatory Bowel Disease

Megan M. Hood, PhD[a],*, Sharon Jedel, PsyD[b]

KEYWORDS

• IBD • Mindfulness • Crohn's disease • Ulcerative colitis • Yoga

KEY POINTS

• Mindfulness-based interventions may provide a viable treatment for improving health and well-being in patients with IBD.

• A small number of studies have assessed interventions that include mindfulness, with fairly strong support for their effects on quality of life and anxiety/depression, but mixed or low support in other psychosocial areas.

• There has been limited support thus far for the effects of mindfulness interventions on disease-related and physiologic outcomes.

INTRODUCTION

Inflammatory bowel diseases (IBD), including Crohn's disease (CD) and ulcerative colitis (UC), are chronic relapsing disorders associated with disabling physical and psychological symptoms, particularly during periodic flare-ups. Given that there is no cure for IBD, psychosocial interventions are increasingly recommended as a component of a multidisciplinary treatment approach. These interventions aim to help individuals with IBD cope more effectively with the distressing and unpredictable symptoms of the disease, decrease symptoms of depression and/or anxiety, and improve quality of life. Additionally, psychosocial interventions focus on stress management and, as such, have the potential to prevent stress-triggered disease flare-ups and to improve quality of life.

Mindfulness-based interventions are increasingly being used to reduce stress, foster more adaptive coping, and improve overall functioning in medical populations,

Disclosures: The authors report no conflicts of interest or funding sources for this article.
[a] Department of Behavioral Sciences, Rush University Medical Center, 1645 West Jackson, Suite 400, Chicago, IL 60612, USA; [b] Division of Digestive Diseases and Nutrition, Department of Internal Medicine, Rush University Medical Center, 1725 West Harrison Street, Suite 207, Chicago, IL 60612, USA
* Corresponding author.
E-mail address: Megan_Hood@rush.edu

including in patients with such conditions as chronic pain, cancer, cardiovascular disease risk factors, and functional gastrointestinal disorders, such as irritable bowel syndrome.[1–3] These interventions focus on increasing mindfulness, defined as intentionally focusing one's attention on the present moment in a nonjudgmental way.[4] Possible mechanisms by which mindfulness can improve physical and mental health include changing pain perceptions and tolerance; reducing psychological symptoms, such as stress, anxiety, and depression; improving health behaviors (eg, adherence, diet, exercise); or even by directly affecting biologic pathways, such as the autonomic nervous system and the immune system.[5]

Mindfulness-based interventions are derived from Buddhist traditions designed to reduce suffering and improve well-being.[2] Traditional mindfulness practices have been adapted in Western treatments to form well-studied programs, including mindfulness-based stress reduction (MBSR)[4] and mindfulness-based cognitive therapy (MBCT).[6] Mindfulness is also a key component of other complementary and meditation-focused interventions, such as yoga.

Mindfulness-based interventions have strong empirical support for the reduction of stress and psychological concerns,[7–10] but have been used minimally for patients with IBD thus far. This article summarizes and discusses interventions with mindfulness components that have been used for patients with IBD and suggests future directions.

METHODS
Search Strategy and Study Selection

An electronic search of the literature was conducted using PubMed, Psychinfo, and Cochrane databases from 1960 through December 2016. Search terms included combinations of "mindfulness" and "meditation" with "inflammatory bowel," "ulcerative colitis," and "Crohns" and article reference searches. "Yoga" was later added as a search term for comprehensiveness when studies that included mindful yoga were retrieved from the previously mentioned searches. Studies were included in this review if they were English-language articles that described original data collection of studies testing interventions that reported including mindfulness-based treatment components for patients with IBD. Articles were excluded if they did not describe original data collection (eg, reviews, commentaries). Eighty articles were found in the initial search. After eliminating duplicates and those that did not meet review criteria, eight articles were included (**Table 1**). In total, 444 participants were included in this review, with study samples ranging from 29 to 100 participants per study. Participants were more often female (64%), and spanned a broad age range (19–85 years) (gender/age data were unavailable for four participants). Samples were predominantly comprised of patients with UC (67%), with fewer patients with CD (32%). One additional patient had indeterminate colitis and another had lymphocytic pancolitis. Although it was unclear in a few studies whether patients were symptomatic (flaring), most participants seemed to be in remission, which should be considered when generalizing these results to other patients with IBD. Despite only including a small number of studies, these programs were tested in several geographic regions (Wales, Germany, United States, Australia, Scotland, and India), suggesting an international interest in mindfulness interventions for patients with IBD.

RESULTS AND DISCUSSION

Study methodology details and outcomes for the articles included in this review are described in **Table 1**. Of the reviewed articles, four included interventions with mindfulness as the primary focus MBSR,[11] MBCT,[12] mindfulness-based intervention for

Table 1
Methods and results of reviewed studies

Authors, Year (Location)	Patients	Treatment	Control	Randomized?	Retention	Outcomes	Results
Berrill et al,[14] 2014, (Wales)	66 IBD pts (73% UC, 27% CD) in clinical remission, subgrouped into those with IBS-type symptoms (n = 38) and/or high perceived stress levels (n = 48)	MCT plus standard medical therapy (n = 33)	Standard medical therapy (n = 33)	Yes; patients with IBS-type symptoms were stratified according to type of IBD (UC or CD) and severity of IBS; patients with high perceived stress were stratified by type of IBD	MCT: 8 did not attend intervention, 6 dropped out during intervention, 27 completed 4-mo assessment Control: 32 completed 4-mo assessment	Primary: quality of life (IBDQ) at 4 mo, also assessed at baseline 8 and 12 mo Secondary: changes in disease activity (relapse rate, fecal calprotectin, need for escalation in IBD medications), perceived stress (PSQ), and coping (WCC) at baseline, 4, 8, and 12 mo	IBDQ (4 mo) MCT: increase Control: no change Between group differences Complete case: $P = .08$ Per protocol: $P = .04$ IBDQ (4, 8, 12 mo) Repeated measures = ns IBDQ in IBS-type subgroup (4 mo) MCT > control: $P = .02$ IBDQ in perceived stress subgroup (4 mo) MCT > control: $P = .095$ 4, 8, 12 mo Relapse rates: ns Medication escalations: ns PSQ: ns Coping-Wishful Thinking: ns Coping-Positive Thinking: ns Coping-Avoidance: ns Coping-Seek Advice: ns (4), $P = .08$ (8), $P = .009$ (12), MCT > control Coping-Self-Blame: ns

(continued on next page)

Table 1
(continued)

Authors, Year (Location)	Patients	Treatment	Control	Randomized?	Retention	Outcomes	Results
Elsenbruch et al,[16] 2005; Langhorst et al,[17] 2007 (Germany)	60 patients with UC in remission or with low disease activity (n = 30 in Elsenbruch et al[16]), 10 healthy control subjects	Mind-body intervention[16] (n = 15; cohort 1) aka comprehensive lifestyle modification program[17] (n = 30, cohorts 1 and 2)	Waitlist control/ usual care (n = 30; 15 per cohort)	57 randomized, 3 chose group based on scheduling conflicts. Two control pts crossed over into the intervention group to take open spaces from withdrawals and were not included in analyses	Two intervention group pts dropped out before starting the intervention, 2 control dropped out	Quality of life[16,17] (German versions of SF-36 and IBDQ), perceived stress[16] (German version of PSS), psychological distress[17] (BSI, German version), health behavior questionnaire,[17] clinical disease activity[17] (CAI), self-assessed disease status,[17] cortisol,[16] prolactin,[16] growth hormone,[16] leukocytes and lymphocyte subsets,[16] TNF-α[16] at baseline and 10 wk at baseline, 3 mo,[16,17] and 12 mo[17]	Baseline to 3 and 12 mo (within CLMP) CAI: ns Self-assessed disease activity: ns Relaxation practice: P<.0001 Diet: ns Exercise: ns Baseline to 3 mo (between groups, cohort 1 only) Perceived Stress: ns Cortisol: ns Prolactin: ns Growth hormone: ns Baseline to 3 mo (between groups, both cohorts) SF-36 Physical: P = .02, CLMP > control IBDQ scales: ns BSI-18-Anxiety: P = .03, CLMP > control Baseline to 12-mo (between groups) SF-36 scales: ns IBDQ scales: ns BSI-18-Anxiety: ns UC (cohort 1) vs health controls Basal leukocytes, granulocytes, monocytes: all P<.05, UC > control TNF-α: P = .09, UC < control Circulating lymphocyte subsets: ns

Study	Population	Intervention	Control	Randomized	Dropouts/Completion	Outcomes	Results
Gerbarg et al,[15] 2015, (United States)	29 IBD pts (18 CD, 9 UC, 1 indeterminate colitis, 1 lymphocytic pancolitis)	BBMW (n = 16)	Active time control 9-h ES (6 h in Day 1, two additional 90-min sessions, plus 6 weekly educational lectures on IBD quality of life issues; n = 13)	Yes	2 (1 BBMW, 1 ES) dropouts during groups, 15 BBMW and 12 ES completed 6-wk follow-up, 14 BBMW and 11 ES completed 26-wk follow-up	Anxiety (BAI), depression (BDI), general distress (BSI-18), quality of life (IBDQ), perceived disability (PDS), perceived stress (PSQ), digestive disease acceptance (DDAQ), illness perception (BIPQ), FCP, C-reactive protein (CRP), body temperature, blood pressure, pulse, at baseline, 6, and 26 wk	Baseline to 6 and to 26 wk (within BBMW) BSI-18: $P = .02$ BAI: $P = .02$ IBDQ: $P = .01$ DDAQ: ns BIPQ: ns FCP: ns Temperature: $P = .02$ (BL to 6 wk only) Blood pressure: ns Pulse: ns Baseline to 26 wk (within BBMW) PDS: $P = .001$ PSQ: $P = .01$ BDI: $P = .01$ CRP: $P = .01$ Baseline to 6 wk (between groups) BSI-18: $P = .02$, BBMW > control IBDQ: $P = .08$, BBMW > control Baseline to 26 wk (between groups) BSI-18: $P = .01$, BBMW > control IBDQ: $P = .04$, BBMW > control PDS: $P = .05$, BBMW > control PSQ: $P = .01$, BBMW > control

(continued on next page)

Table 1
(continued)

Authors, Year (Location)	Patients	Treatment	Control	Randomized?	Retention	Outcomes	Results
Jedel et al,[11] 2014 (United States)	55 pts with inactive UC	8-wk MBSR (n = 27)	8-wk time/attention control mind/body medicine lectures/videos focused on stress education with no UC or coping training, articles for homework (n = 26)	Yes	2 (1 in MBSR, 1 in control) dropped before intervention; 2 (1 in MBSR, 1 in control) dropped during the course	Primary: flare rate (UCDAI) at 8 wk and at flare time or 12 mo if no flare Secondary: inflammation and disease activity (calprotectin, cytokines, CRP, time to flare up, severity of flare up), quality of life (IBDQ), markers of stress (serum ACTH), perceived stress (PSQ), depression (BDI), trait anxiety (STAI-trait), mindfulness (MAAS), perceived health competence (PHCS)	Flare rate: ns Calprotectin: ns Cytokines: IL-6 and IL-8 = ns, IL-10: inc in MBSR flared pts but dec in control flared pts CRP: $P = .05$, MBSR flared pts < control flared pts IBDQ Total: $P = .001$, MBSR flared > control flared IBDQ-Bowel: $P = .01$, MBSR flared > control flared IBDQ-Emotion: $P = .01$, MBSR flared > control flared IBDQ-Bowel: $P = .02$, MBSR > control (last visit) IBDQ-Systemic: $P = .03$, MBSR > control (last visit) Flare-free survival time: ns Severity of flare: ns Serum ACTH: $P = .007$, MBSR flared < control flared Cortisol: ns Perceived stress: $P = .04$, MBSR flared < control flared at last visit Depression, mindfulness, perceived health competence, anxiety: ns

Study	Participants	Intervention	Control	Randomization	Dropout/follow-up	Outcomes measured	Results
Neilson et al,[13] 2016 (Melbourne)	60 pts (44 CD), 24 with active disease (12 CD, 12 UC)	MI-IBD (n = 33; 23 CD, 10 UC, 14 with active disease)	Medical treatment as usual (n = 27; 21 CD, 6 UC, 10 with active disease)	No; participants self-selected groups	N = 7 lost to follow-up at Week 8 (n = 5 intervention, n = 2 control); n = 8 lost to follow-up at 32 wk (n = 5 intervention, n = 3 control), n = 27 completed the intervention (attended at least 6 sessions)	Quality of life (WHOQoL-BREF), depression, and anxiety (HADS), mindfulness (FFMQ), at baseline, 8, and 32 wk	BL to 8 wk and to 32 wk between group differences (MI-IBD > control) Anxiety: $P<.05$ (BL to 8 wk only) Depression: $P<.05$ QoL Physical Health: $P<.01$ (BL to 8 wk only) QoL Psychological Health: $P<.01$ (BL to 8 wk only) QoL Social Wellbeing: ns QoL Environment: ns FFMQ Observing: $P<.001$ FFMQ Describing: $P<.01$ FFMQ Nonreactivity: $P<.01$ FFMQ Activing with Awareness: ns FFMQ Nonjudgment: ns FFMQ Total: $P<.001$
Schoultz et al,[12] 2015 (Scotland)	44 IBD pts (22 CD, 22 UC) at two study locations	MBCT (n = 22; 9 CD, 13 UC)	Wait-list control (n = 22; 12 CD, 10 UC) including Crohn's and Colitis UK educational leaflet	Yes; stratified by disease type (UC vs CD) and sex	1 MBCT drop out before start of treatment, 19 (10 in control, 9 in MBCT) dropped out before MBCT completion, post-MBCT and 6-mo follow-up data on 12 in control and 12 in MBCT	Recruitment/dropout rate, depression rate (BDI-II), anxiety (STAI), disease activity (CDAI or SCCAI), dispositional mindfulness (MAAS), quality of life (IBDQ) at baseline, 8 wk, and 6 mo	15% recruitment rate, 44% dropout rate BL to 8 wk and 6 mo (repeated measures group × time interaction, MBCT > control) Depression: $P = .03$ State Anxiety: $P = .08$ Trait Anxiety: $P = .048$ Dispositional Mindfulness: $P = .03$ Disease activity: ns (UC or CD) IBDQ: ns

(continued on next page)

Table 1
(continued)

Authors, Year (Location)	Patients	Treatment	Control	Randomized?	Retention	Outcomes	Results
Sharma et al,[18] 2015 (India)	100 pts with IBD in remission (UC = 60, CD = 40)	Yoga plus standard medical therapy (n = 50; 20 CD, 30 UC)	Standard medical therapy (n = 50; 20 CD, 30 UC)	Yes; stratified by UC/CD diagnosis	6 drop outs in yoga group, 7 drop outs in control group (at 2 mo)	Heart rate variability (HR, LST, DBT, VM, BP, HGT, CPT); ECP and sIL-2R for immune markers, anxiety (STAI), symptom diary, at 1 and 2 mo	UC and CD within and between groups: Parasympathetic, Sympathetic Activity measures: ns LF power reduction: $P = .05$, yoga > control Rise in diastolic BP in response to HGT: $P = .05$, yoga > control Immune markers: ns Symptoms: ns Fewer arthralgia symptoms: $P < .05$ (BL to 2 mo, yoga group only) State anxiety: $P = .01$, UC group only Trait anxiety: $P = .001$, UC group only

Abbreviations: ACTH, adrenocorticotropic hormone; BAI, Beck Anxiety Inventory; BBMW, body-mind workshop; BDI, Beck Depression Inventory; BIPQ, brief illness perception questionnaire; BL, baseline; BP, blood pressure; BSI-18, Brief Symptoms Inventory; CAI, clinical activity index; CDAI, Crohn's Disease Activity Index; CLMP, comprehensive lifestyle modification program; CPT, cold presser test; CRP, C-reactive protein; DBT, deep breathing test; DDAQ, digestive disease acceptance questionnaire; ECP, serum eosinophilic cationic protein; ES, educational seminar; FCP, fecal calprotectin; FFMQ, five facet mindfulness questionnaire; HADS, Hospital Anxiety and Depression Scale; HGT, isometric hand grip test; HR, heart rate; IBDQ, inflammatory bowel disease questionnaire; IBS, irritable bowel syndrome; LF, low frequency; LST, response to lying to standing test; MAAS, mindful attention awareness scale; MCT, multiconvergent therapy; MI-IBD, mindfulness-based intervention for IBD; PDS, perceived disability scale; PHCS, perceived health competence scale; PNAS, positive and negative affect schedule; PSQ, perceived stress questionnaire; PSS, perceived stress scale; SCCAI, simple clinical colitis activity index; SF-36, 36 item Short Form Survey; sIL-2R, soluble interleukin-2 receptor; STAI, state trait anxiety inventory; TNF, tumor necrosis factor; UCDAI, May UC activity index; VM, Valsalva maneuver; WCC, ways of coping checklist; WHOQoL-BREF, World Health Organization Quality of Life BREF.

IBD (MI-IBD),[13] and multiconvergent therapy (MCT),[14] all of which were fairly recently published and used interventions that had at least some empirical support in other populations. Other interventions included mindfulness training as a component of a broader intervention, including a body-mind workshop (BBMW),[15] a mind-body medicine and comprehensive lifestyle modification program,[16,17] and a yoga intervention.[18] Other than MBSR, which was tested in Jedel and colleagues[11] and Neilson and colleagues,[13] each other intervention that was identified has only been tested in one study (Elsenbruch[16] and Langhorst[17] reported on different time points of the same study), making it difficult to generalize results to other samples. It is unclear whether any of the interventions were adapted specifically for patients with IBD, other than MI-IBD, which was adapted from standard MBSR for patients with IBD[13] (adaptations described later). All but one intervention[13] used randomization, although one[16] also included a few participants who chose their group assignment. Waitlist or usual care groups were the most common control group used, although two interventions[11,15] used active control groups (weekly educational sessions of the same duration as the intervention). These two interventions found fairly different psychosocial outcome effects, suggesting that additional research is needed to better understand how, and whether, mindfulness interventions improve outcomes above and beyond attention- and group-based effects. Retention rates seemed to be similar in intervention and control groups, suggesting fairly good acceptance of the interventions by participants. The interventions were facilitated by instructors with specialized training in the intervention. The studies included instructors with various qualifications, including physicians,[11,15] a psychiatrist,[13] psychologists,[11,13] a psychotherapist,[14] and a yoga instructor.[18] In one study,[15] the intervention was administered by the physician who originally developed it.

Interventions

Mindfulness-based stress reduction
MBSR, an empirically validated curriculum for teaching mindfulness, was developed by Kabat-Zinn[4] as a complement to standard medical treatment and as an approach for coping more effectively with pain and chronic illness through the use of mindfulness and self-compassion, and has been used with IBD patients.[11] The intervention was comprised of 8 weekly sessions, spanning 2 to 2.5 hours in length, and an optional half-day retreat. Sessions included instruction and practice in formal guided meditations (eg, sitting mediation, body scan, and yoga) and informal practices (eg, awareness of personal reactions to daily events). The goal of these practices was to facilitate mindfulness in daily life. Weekly homework assignments (45 min/d, 6 d/wk) were designed to reinforce techniques and strategies introduced in class. Participants were encouraged to continue their meditation practice on completion of the 8-week intervention and through the end of the study (12-month follow-up).

Mindfulness-based intervention for inflammatory bowel disease
MI-IBD was adapted from MBSR and tailored to patients with IBD.[13] The program was comprised of eight weekly 2.5-hour group sessions, one 7-hour weekend session, and weekly homework assignments. The standard components from MBSR included guided meditations, exploring a variety of exercises designed to enhance mindfulness in daily life, and group discussions to allow participants to discuss challenges and learn from each other's and facilitators' experiences. The class was tailored to patients with IBD with the inclusion of the following IBD-specific components: discussions about the brain-gut axis and the impact of mindfulness meditation on bowel symptoms and living with IBD; input from the class facilitators about their clinical

experiences of working with patients with bowel symptoms in hospital settings and relating such experiences to IBD; and guided meditations that focused on physical sensations, emotions, and thoughts associated with IBD symptoms (written communication, March 2017).

Mindfulness-based cognitive therapy

MBCT is an evidence-based, structured psychological group program that teaches participants to develop better awareness and understanding of their individual responses to stress (psychological or physical) and learn alternative ways for responding to stress.[12] Mindfulness is the core skill that is taught in this 8-week program. In this study, the MBCT curriculum was based on the standardized MBCT manual.[6] Sessions were approximately 2 hours each and included instruction in meditation, cognitive behavioral exercises, and informal practices and discussions with personal reflections of daily life events. Weekly homework assignments (up to 45 min/d, 6 d/wk) reinforced the content from group sessions.

Multiconvergent therapy

MCT is a therapeutic intervention that combines mindfulness meditation and components of cognitive behavioral therapy. In this study[14], the intervention was standardized and followed a session plan that included instruction in the biopsychosocial model of treatment and the stress response, learning how to identify stressors and coping mechanisms, use of mindfulness meditation and breathing exercises, and efforts to prevent relapse of gains from MCT skills. Six face-to-face sessions (40 minutes each) occurred over 16 weeks.

Body-mind workshop

BBMW was described as a program that includes physical movement, breathing techniques, and meditation.[15] The program was developed by Richard P. Brown, MD, based on his study of martial arts, aikido, Zen, yoga, and qigong. In this study, Dr Brown administered the workshop, which occurred over 2 consecutive days for a total of 9 hours. Subjects were taught four breathing techniques, qigong movements coordinated with breathing, and a type of meditation called Open Focus Attention Training. Weekly follow-up sessions of 90 minutes each were offered for 6 weeks and then monthly from Week 7 through Week 26. Dr Brown administered the class and conducted all follow-up sessions. Weekly homework assignments reinforced the content from group sessions.

Mind-body intervention program and comprehensive lifestyle modification program

This intervention was based on multiple components of the mind-body program from the Mind/Body Medical Institutes at Harvard Medical University[19] and MBSR,[4] and was geared toward improving psychological and physical well-being.[16,17] The intervention included instruction in stress management, mindfulness meditation, cognitive behavioral techniques, and effective coping skills. Participants were also encouraged to consume a Mediterranean diet and participate in light to moderate exercise. The intervention followed a structured format of 6-hour instruction 1 day per week for 10 weeks. Elsenbruch and coworkers[16] reported the pre-post intervention results of the first cohort (n = 30; 15 in the intervention and 15 in the control groups) and Langhorst and coworkers[17] described the long-term (up to 12 months) results in the total sample (n = 30 in the intervention group and n = 26 in the control group).

Yoga

The yoga intervention was comprised of various yoga postures, a controlled breathing technique called pranayama, and meditation.[18] A certified yoga instructor administered the intervention for 1 h/d over 1 week. For the next 7 weeks, participants were instructed to continue with the intervention at home on a daily basis and were provided with audio recordings and instruction manuals to assist with their home practice. Compliance was monitored by a symptom diary, which participants brought to follow-up visits. During follow-up visits (at 1 and 2 months), a yoga session was offered to participants.

Outcomes

Psychological outcomes

Quality of life Quality of life was the most commonly assessed outcome, typically assessed with the disease-specific Inflammatory Bowel Disease Questionnaire[20] and/or the more generic Short Form-36,[21] or in one study[13] the World Health Organization-Quality of Life BREF.[22] Most studies that assessed quality of life found significantly greater improvements, or trends toward greater improvements, over control groups in many quality-of-life areas from prestudy to poststudy,[13–17] with some improvements occurring over long-term follow-up,[11,15] and others failing to remain significantly different.[13,14,17] The MCT study showed particularly good improvements in quality of life in the subgroup of patients with irritable bowel syndrome–type symptoms.[14] Only the MBCT study[12] found no differences in quality of life. Langhorst and colleagues[17] found that greater use of relaxation strategies at posttreatment was associated with greater improvements in quality-of-life scores. Jedel and coworkers[11] found that when comparing MBSR participants who flared during the study with those in the control group who flared, IBD-specific quality of life was significantly better in MBSR participants than control subjects at the time of the flare, suggesting a possible protective role of MBSR on the impact of flares on quality of life. When both an IBD-specific quality-of-life scale and a generic quality-of-life scale were used in the same study,[16,17] significant improvements seemed to be found more commonly in generic quality-of-life areas than IBD-specific quality-of-life areas.

Perceived stress Perceived stress was assessed in four studies, and measured with the Perceived Stress Questionnaire[23] and/or the Perceived Stress Scale.[24] Interestingly, no studies found significant improvements in perceived stress from pretreatment to posttreatment,[11,14–16] although a few found significant improvements in long-term follow-up, ranging from 26 weeks to 12 months.[11,15]

Anxiety and depression Anxiety and depression were assessed with the Hospital Anxiety and Depression Scale,[25] the Beck Depression Inventory,[26,27] the Beck Anxiety Inventory,[28] and/or the State-Trait Anxiety Inventory.[29] Most studies found greater improvements in anxiety[12,13,15] and depression[12,13] in interventions over control subjects from pretreatment to posttreatment, including long-term improvements in anxiety[15] and depression[13,15] at follow-up of 26 to 32 weeks. Only Jedel and coworkers[11] found no changes in anxiety or depression, potentially because of low baseline levels of anxiety and depression. In the yoga study,[18] patients with UC, but not patients with CD, experienced significant reductions in anxiety.

Mindfulness Mindfulness was only assessed in three studies, using either the Mindful Attention Awareness Scale[30] or the Five Facet Mindfulness Questionnaire.[31] The MBI-IBD[13] and MBCT[12] studies found significantly greater improvements in mindfulness areas in the intervention over the control groups at posttreatment and at follow-up of 6 months to 32 weeks. In contrast, the MBSR study[11] found no changes in mindfulness.

Other psychosocial measures A few other psychosocial variables were assessed in one to two studies each. Psychological distress and self-efficacy improved more in the intervention than control groups at posttreatment[15,17] and at follow-up in one study.[15] Greater improvements in perceived disability[15] were found at long-term follow-up. Langhorst and coworkers[17] found that within their intervention group, frequency of relaxation exercises increased, whereas diet and exercise variables did not change. No changes were found in digestive disease acceptance,[15] illness perception,[15] or perceived health competence.[11] Coping styles generally did not change[14] following the intervention.

Summary Mindfulness interventions seem to improve general and IBD-specific quality of life, anxiety, depression, and self-reported mindfulness during the course of the treatment and in some cases in the long term. Surprisingly, given that mindfulness interventions have been commonly associated with perceived stress improvements in other studies, perceived stress did not seem to be reduced in the studies in this review. A possible reason for this lack of effect may be that most participants were in remission at the time of the study and rates of stress and psychological concerns tend to be higher during flares. This may have contributed to rates of perceived stress being in the average range at baseline in many studies, leading to a floor effect. Evidence is preliminary and mixed in terms of the effects of mindfulness interventions on other psychosocial functioning areas.

Possible psychosocial mechanisms of change were rarely statistically tested in these studies. There are early data to suggest that subgroups of patients with IBD, such as those with irritable bowel syndrome–type symptoms, may in particular benefit from mindfulness interventions and that MBSR may even be protective against the effect of flares on quality of life. Although few studies reported on adherence to weekly homework assignments or associations with practice and outcomes, one study found that higher rates of relaxation practice at the end of the study was associated with better quality-of-life outcomes, preliminarily suggesting that greater use of the skills taught in the intervention may be associated with better outcomes. Only three studies assessed mindfulness, the primary proposed mechanism of change of mindfulness-based interventions. Two of these three studies reported improvements in mindfulness and in anxiety and depression, providing some preliminary support for the association between improvements in mindfulness and psychological concerns.

Physiologic outcomes
Disease activity Disease activity was assessed in all studies. A variety of measures were used, including the Crohn's Disease Activity Index,[32] the Ulcerative Colitis Disease Activity Index,[33] the Mayo Ulcerative Colitis Disease Activity Index,[34] a modified Simple Clinical Colitis Activity Index,[35] the Colitis Activity Index,[36] a modified Harvey Bradshaw index score,[37] and symptom diaries. None of the studies found significant differences in change in clinical disease activity,[11,12,14,16,17] time to flare up,[11] severity of flare up,[11,14] or rates of relapse[11,14] in intervention participants compared with control subjects. One study[13] did not report on disease activity outcomes, but rather measured disease activity only at baseline. No significant differences in need for IBD medication escalations were found between patients in the intervention group compared with control subjects at 4, 8, or 12 months in Berrill and colleagues.[14] In two studies,[17,18] patients also self-assessed their clinical symptoms. In the Sharma and colleagues[18] study, fewer IBD participants in the yoga group reported arthralgia compared with control subjects and control participants reported significantly more intestinal colicky pain compared with yoga participants following the intervention,

whereas no differences were found in Langhorst and colleagues[17] in self-reported UC symptoms between the intervention and control groups at 3 or 12 months.

Serum C-reactive protein Serum C-reactive protein was measured in two studies.[11,15] Gerbarg and colleagues[15] found that median C-reactive protein values demonstrated significant improvement in the BBMW group at 26 weeks, compared with baseline measurements. Jedel and colleagues[11] found significantly better last visit C-reactive protein levels among flared subjects in MBSR compared with control subjects who flared, and a significantly better change in C-reactive protein levels over the 12-month time period in MBSR versus control groups among subjects who did not flare.

Fecal calprotectin No significant changes were found in the four studies that assessed fecal calprotectin.[10,11,14,15]

Cytokines Jedel and colleagues[11] measured interleukin (IL)-6, IL-8, and IL-10. No significant differences in IL-6 and IL-8 were found between MBSR and control groups or between those who flared and those who did not at 3, 6, or 12 months. However, there was a significant difference in IL-10 between MBSR patients who flared and control group patients who flared at the 12-month follow-up. No significant differences were found in sIL-2R between intervention participants and control subjects in the yoga study.[18]

Other physiologic outcomes Several other physiologic measures were assessed in various studies. In the MBSR study, a significant improvement in serum adrenocorticotropic hormone levels was found over time between flared subjects in the MBSR group compared with flared subjects in the control group.[11] In the yoga study, CD intervention patients exhibited a greater rise in diastolic blood pressure in response to the handgrip test compared with control subjects.[18] Patients with IBD in the yoga group also demonstrated a significantly reduced low-frequency power, a measure of sympathetic activity, compared with control subjects.[18] No significant between- or within-group differences were found in blood pressure,[15,18] body temperature,[15] pulse,[15] heart rate,[18] heart rate variability,[18] deep breathing and the Valsalva maneuver,[18] the isometric handgrip and cold pressor tests,[18] serum eosinophilic cationic protein,[18] circulating lymphocytes and lymphocyte subsets,[18] tumor necrosis factor-α,[16] prolactin,[16] growth hormones,[16] urine catecholamines,[16] and plasma cortisol.[11,16]

Summary Mindfulness interventions do not seem to impact disease activity and other disease-related factors in patients with UC or CD. These findings are consistent with data from other psychosocial interventions,[38,39] which did not demonstrate a positive impact on IBD clinical course. There is limited, preliminary evidence that mindfulness interventions may have a positive impact on some inflammatory markers. This is consistent with data from other studies that found that MBSR modulated proinflammatory cytokine profiles to anti-inflammatory pattern in patients with breast or prostate cancer[40] and human immunodeficiency virus.[41] Mindfulness interventions did not typically impact other physiologic variables that were assessed. However, many of the studies did not include such assessments. Based on these studies, it is difficult to determine whether IBD interventions are effective for altering IBD disease course and other physiologic factors. It is possible that longer, more sustained interventions that are tailored to a subset of patients, would be beneficial. More studies are necessary to better understand how mindfulness interventions could affect IBD course and markers of mucosal or systemic inflammation.

DIRECTIONS FOR FUTURE RESEARCH

Given the results of this review, we suggest that future research consider the following:

- Measurement of psychosocial functioning: To better understand the mechanisms by which mindfulness-based interventions affect psychosocial outcomes, studies should consider assessing and testing the effects of mindfulness, homework completion/practice, or other proposed mechanisms during the course of the intervention. Given the heterogeneity of the types of mindfulness interventions that are being studied, use of the same measures of commonly assessed constructs (eg, quality of life, perceived stress, anxiety/depression) may allow for more accurate comparisons across studies.
- Methodologic vigor: Intervention testing is affected by several methodologic issues, highlighting the importance of the use of high-quality intervention testing strategies, such as randomization, intervention fidelity monitoring, and blinding. Although control group selection depends on the study research question, additional studies that use active controls will allow for a better understanding of how mindfulness-based interventions compare with attention alone and other psychosocial interventions that have been used with patients with IBD.[42]
- Further testing of empirically supported mindfulness interventions: It is promising that some of the most widely supported mindfulness-based interventions (eg, MBSR and MBCT) have been preliminarily tested in the IBD population. These studies are recent, suggesting that this may be a new direction in the field. Few studies have been reported so far with each intervention, suggesting that additional studies of these interventions with patients with IBD are needed to develop a better understanding of the possible role of mindfulness interventions in the treatment of patients with IBD in different samples.
- IBD adaptations: Considering adaptations for the IBD population may be beneficial. Although few studies reported on whether their interventions were adapted in some way, it is possible that mindfulness-based treatments may be challenging for some patients with IBD, particularly those with active disease. Procedural adaptations, such as taking frequent breaks or including IBD-relevant imagery/terminology in meditations, and including discussions of the relationships between the mindfulness skills being discussed and IBD, may be beneficial.
- IBD subsample testing: Early data suggest that certain types of IBD participants may benefit more than others from mindfulness-based interventions. Additional studies testing the effects of these interventions based on participant and disease factors (eg, active vs inactive disease, elevated baseline stress or anxiety/depression, interest in mindfulness-based interventions) would allow for better matching of psychosocial interventions with participants who are more likely to benefit from the treatment.

REFERENCES

1. Aucoin M, Lalonde-Parsi MJ, Cooley K. Mindfulness-based therapies in the treatment of functional gastrointestinal disorders: a meta-analysis. Evid Based Complement Alternat Med 2014;2014:140724.
2. Baer R. Mindfulness based treatment approaches. Burlington (MA): Elsevier; 2006.
3. Loucks EB, Schuman-Olivier Z, Britton WB, et al. Mindfulness and cardiovascular disease risk: state of the evidence, plausible mechanisms, and theoretical framework. Curr Cardiol Rep 2015;17(12):112.

4. Kabat-Zinn J. Full catastrophe living: using the wisdom of your body and mind to face stress, pain and illness. New York: Delacorte Press; 1990.
5. Ludwig DS, Kabat-Zinn J. Mindfulness in medicine. JAMA 2008;300(11):1350–2.
6. Segal Z, Williams M, Teasdale J. Mindfulness-based cognitive therapy for depression: a new approach to preventing relapse. Guilford Press; 2002.
7. Grossman P, Niemann L, Schmidt S, et al. Mindfulness-based stress reduction and health bene fits: a meta-analysis. J Psychosom Res 2004;57:35–43.
8. Fjorback LO, Arendt M, Ornbol E, et al. Mindfulness-based stress reduction and mindfulness-based cognitive therapy: a systematic review of randomized controlled trials. Acta Psychiatr Scand 2011;124:102–19.
9. Gotink RA, Chu P, Busschbach V, et al. Standardised mindfulness-based interventions in healthcare: an overview of systematic reviews and meta-analyses of RCTs. PLoS One 2015;10:e0124344.
10. Huang HP, He M, Wang H, et al. A meta-analysis of the benefits of mindfulness-based stress reduction (MBSR) on psychological function among breast cancer (BC) survivors. Breast Cancer 2016;23(4):568–76.
11. Jedel S, Hoffman A, Merriman P, et al. A randomized controlled trial of mindfulness-based stress reduction to prevent flare-up in patients with inactive ulcerate colitis. Digestion 2014;89(2):142–55.
12. Schoultz M, Atherton I, Watson A. Mindfulness-based cognitive therapy for inflammatory bowel disease patients: findings from an exploratory pilot randomised controlled trial. Trials 2015;16:379.
13. Neilson K, Ftanou M, Monshat K, et al. A controlled study of a group mindfulness intervention for individuals living with inflammatory bowel disease. Inflamm Bowel Dis 2016;22(3):694–701.
14. Berrill JW, Sadlier M, Hood K, et al. Mindfulness-based therapy for inflammatory bowel disease patients with functional abdominal symptoms or high perceived stress levels. J Crohns Colitis 2014;8(9):945–55.
15. Gerbarg PL, Jacob VE, Stevens L, et al. The effect of breathing, movement, and meditation on psychological and physical symptoms and inflammatory biomarkers in inflammatory bowel disease: a randomized controlled trial. Inflamm Bowel Dis 2015;21(12):2886–96.
16. Elsenbruch S, Langhorst J, Popkirowa K, et al. Effects of mind-body therapy on quality of life and neuroendocrine and cellular immune functions in patients with ulcerative colitis. Psychother Psychosom 2005;74(5):277–87.
17. Langhorst J, Mueller T, Luedtke R, et al. Effects of a comprehensive lifestyle modification program on quality-of-life in patients with ulcerative colitis: a twelve-month follow-up. Scand J Gastroenterol 2007;42(6):734–45.
18. Sharma P, Poojary G, Dwivedi SN, et al. Effect of yoga-based intervention in patients with inflammatory bowel disease. Int J Yoga Therap 2015;25(1):101–12.
19. Benson H, Stuart EM. The wellness book: the comprehensive guide to maintaining health and treating stress-related illness. New York: Simon & Schuster; 1992.
20. Guyatt G, Mitchell A, Irvine EJ, et al. A new measure of health status for clinical trials in inflammatory bowel disease. Gastroenterology 1989;96(3):804–10.
21. Ware JE, Snow KK, Kosinski M. SF-36 health survey manual and interpretation guide. Boston: New England Medical Center, The Health Institute; 1993.
22. The World Health Organization Quality of Life Assessment (WHOQOL). Development and general psychometric properties. Soc Sci Med 1998;46:1569–85.
23. Levenstein S, Prantera C, Varvo V, et al. Development of the perceived stress questionnaire: a new tool for psychosomatic research. J Psychosom Res 1993; 37(1):19–32.

24. Cohen S, Kamarck T, Mermelstein R. A global measure of perceived stress. J Health Soc Behav 1983;24:386–96.
25. Zigmond AS, Snaith RP. The Hospital Anxiety and Depression Scale. Acta Psychiatr Scand 1983;67(6):361–70.
26. Beck AT, Ward CH, Mendelson M, et al. An inventory for measuring depression. Arch Gen Psychiatry 1961;4:561–71.
27. Beck AT, Steer RA, GKB. Manual for the Beck Depression Inventory-II. San Antonio (TX): Psychological Corporation; 1996.
28. Beck AT, Epstein N, Brown GK, et al. An inventory for measuring clinical anxiety: psychometric properties. J Consult Clin Psychol 1988;56:893–7.
29. Spielberger CD. Manual for the State-Trait Anxiety Inventory. Palo Alto (CA): STAI(Consulting Psychologists Press); 1983.
30. Brown KW, Ryan RM. The benefits of being present: mindfulness and its role in psychological well-being. J Pers Soc Psychol 2003;84:822–48.
31. Baer RA, Smith GT, Hopkins J, et al. Using self-report assessment methods to explore facets of mindfulness. Assessment 2006;13:27–45.
32. Best WR, Becktel JM, Singleton JW, et al. Development of a Crohn's disease activity index. National Cooperative Crohn's Disease Study. Gastroenterology 1976; 70:439–44.
33. Sutherland LR, Martin F, Greer S, et al. 5-Aminosalicylic acid enema in the treatment of distal ulcerative colitis, proctosigmoiditis, and proctitis. Gastroenterology 1987;92(6):1894–8.
34. Schroeder KW, Tremaine WJ, Ilstrup DM. Coated oral 5-aminosalcylic acid therapy for mildly to moderately active ulcerative colitis. N Engl J Med 1987;317: 1625–9.
35. Walmsley RS, Ayres RC, Pounder RE, et al. A simple clinical colitis activity index. Gut 1998;43(1):29–32.
36. Rachmilewitz D. Coated mesalazine (5-aminosalicylic acid) versus sulphasalazine in the treatment of active ulcerative colitis: a randomised trial. BMJ 1989; 298:82–6.
37. Harvey RF, Bradshaw JM. A simple index of Crohn's-disease activity. Lancet 1980;1(8167):514.
38. von Wietersheim J, Kessler H. Psychotherapy with chronic inflammatory bowel disease patients: a review. Inflamm Bowel Dis 2006;12(12):1175–84.
39. Mikocka-Walus A, Bampton P, Hetzel D, et al. Cognitive-behavioural therapy for inflammatory bowel disease: 24-month data from a randomised controlled trial. Int J Behav Med 2017;24(1):127–35.
40. Carlson LE, Speca M, Patel KD, et al. Mindfulness-based stress reduction in relation to quality of life, mood, symptoms of stress, and immune parameters in breast and prostate cancer. Psychosom Med 2003;65:571–8.
41. Robinson FP, Mathews HL, Witek-Janusek L. Psycho-endocrine-immune response to mindfulness-based stress reduction in individuals infected with the human immunodeficiency virus: a quasiexperimental study. J Altern Complement Med 2003;9:683–94.
42. Ballou S, Keefer L. Psychological interventions for irritable bowel syndrome and inflammatory bowel diseases. Clin Transl Gastroenterol 2017;8(1):e214.

Massage Acupuncture, Moxibustion, and Other Forms of Complementary and Alternative Medicine in Inflammatory Bowel Disease

 CrossMark

Daniel J. Stein, MD

KEYWORDS

- Crohn disease • Ulcerative colitis • Massage • Acupuncture • Moxibustion
- Complementary and alternative therapy

KEY POINTS

- Complementary and alternative medicine (CAM) therapy is frequently used by patients with inflammatory bowel disease (IBD).
- Massage therapy, acupuncture, and moxibustion therapy are some of the most commonly used CAMs by IBD patients who use CAM.
- Massage therapy, although it may provide benefit in other medical conditions, is poorly studied in the IBD patient population.
- Acupuncture and moxibustion therapy when used alone or in combination have shown to improve inflammation and symptoms in animal and human studies.
- Current clinical trials of acupuncture and moxibustion, although encouraging, are insufficient to recommend these therapies as alternatives to conventional IBD therapies.

MASSAGE, ACUPUNCTURE, MOXIBUSTION, AND OTHER FORMS OF COMPLEMENTARY AND ALTERNATIVE MEDICINE IN INFLAMMATORY BOWEL DISEASE

Complementary and alternative medicine (CAM) comprises an assorted group of nonconventional medical and health care systems, practices, and products. Complementary medicine is defined as use of nonconventional treatments together with conventional medicines. In contrast, alternative therapy is defined as nonconventional treatments used instead of conventional medicines. CAM can include herbal therapy,

Disclosure Statement: The author has received speaker honorariums for Abbvie, Takeda, and Janssen pharmaceutical companies.
Division of Gastroenterology and Hepatology, Medical College of Wisconsin, 9200 West Wisconsin Avenue, Milwaukee, WI 53226, USA
E-mail address: dstein@mcw.edu

probiotics and prebiotics, dietary supplements, dietary practices, mind-body practices, and spiritual healing. Many of these practices have been used for many years and have more recently gained traction in westernized medicine.

CAMs are used frequently by inflammatory bowel disease (IBD) patients.[1,2] Patients often do not reveal the use of CAM to their treating physicians and, even more concerning, they may be less compliant with their conventional therapy because of CAM usage.[3–5] On the physician side of the problem, physician understanding of what and how CAM works is often extremely limited. Physicians may be quick to discount or disregard a patient's use of CAM as inconsequential, an attitude that can strain the physician-patient relationship.

Some of the most commonly CAMs used by IBD patients center around mind-body techniques such as massage, acupuncture, and moxibustion.[1,6–8] Because acupuncture and moxibustion are relatively new to western society, most physicians are unaware of what exactly is involved with these therapies. Given that these therapies are being used with increasing frequency within the IBD patient population, this review is undertaken with the purpose of familiarizing physicians with massage, acupuncture, and moxibustion. It is hoped that gaining a better understanding of these therapies will assist in avoiding any additional strain on the physician-patient relationship.

Massage Therapy

Massage therapy involves applying pressure on the joints and muscles of the body in a variety of ways. Pressure is most commonly applied with the hands, but knees, feet, and elbows are sometimes used. A massage can be applied with a device that may or may not vibrate. Commonly, the patient is in the prone or supine position on a specially designed massage table. Massage is possibly among the oldest CAMs, with evidence of it being used in ancient Greece, China, Italy, and Japan, and by Native Americans. Massage has been reported to benefit all sorts of medical conditions, but is it most commonly used for sports-related and muscle-related injuries.[9] Many studies have reported benefit in a variety of conditions, including pain, depression, and anxiety.[10] Massage therapy does require specific training and it is regulated in some form by 44 states, which does provide some consistency across providers, as well as safety assurances.

For these reasons, it is no surprise that a Swedish study reported that 20% of IBD subjects who use CAMs used massage.[11] Another study from Manitoba, Canada, reported that 30% of CAM-using IBD subjects used massage and another 14% used chiropracty.[6] Other trials have reported chiropractor use as high as 40% and massage use at 22% in subjects who used CAM. Despite the high level of utilization of this therapy among IBD subjects, clinical trials evaluating the efficacy of massage therapy in IBD subjects are lacking. This may be a result of the difficulty around appropriate trial design that has hampered massage therapy study in other disease states; in particular, developing a sham massage treatment is very difficult. Any sort of even light touch may be perceived has having a relaxing or calming effect on patients.

Acupuncture and Moxibustion

What is acupuncture?

Acupuncture consists of placing thin needles into the skin at specific locations (acupoints) with the hopes of providing a therapeutic benefit to the patient. There are several variations on this technique, sometime using small electrical currents or in conjunction with heat. This has perhaps been around even longer than massage therapy. It has been used by the Chinese for more than 4000 years and is central to Chinese traditional medicine.[12]

What is moxibustion?

Moxibustion, like acupuncture, is a traditional Chinese medicine therapy thought to be more than 4000 year old. It involves burning dried mugwort (moxa) cones that are placed on particular points on the body, depending on what ailment is being treated. Sometimes the skin is allowed to burn; however, in most cases the point is warmed and then removed the cone before the skin burns. Alternatively, the point is warmed by holding a burning moxa stick, which is similar in appearance to a cigar, near the area. Different herbs are also added to the burning moxa, depending on the desired effect; this is called herb-partitioned moxibustion. Frequently this technique is used in conjunction with acupuncture.[13]

ACUPUNCTURE AND MOXIBUSTION IN INFLAMMATORY BOWEL DISEASE

Animal Models of Complementary and Alternative Medicine in Inflammatory Bowel Disease: Acupuncture

Acupuncture and electroacupuncture have been studied in several different animal models of IBD. Albeit a heterogeneous group of studies, these therapies seem to have a modest effect on animal models of IBD. In mouse and rat models of IBD, they have been shown to decrease the levels of tumor necrosis factor (TNF) and TNF receptors, as well as interleukin (IL)-6, IL-8, and nuclear factor-kappa beta (NF-$\kappa\beta$).[14–17] As with many animal studies, the models of colitis vary between studies, making drawing generalized conclusions difficult.

Animal Models of Complementary and Alternative Medicine in Inflammatory Bowel Disease: Moxibustion

Moxibustion has also been studied in several animal models of IBD. It does seem to improve microscopic inflammation in rats and has been shown to decrease levels of TNF receptors, as well as TNF levels.[17–20] Moxibustion also seems to upregulate tight junction proteins and decrease epithelial cell apoptosis in animal models, which might explain the decrease in inflammation.[21,22] Again, similar to the acupuncture studies, because of the heterogeneity of the methods it is difficult to draw meaningful conclusions.

Human Studies in Crohn Disease: Acupuncture, Moxibustion, and Combination

Human studies looking at tight junction protein expression have discovered results similar to those found in the animal models. One study in Crohn subjects randomized to mesalamine therapy versus moxibustion combined with acupuncture. Similar results were seen in both treatment arms in regard to increased expression of tight junction proteins, suggesting moxibustion plus acupuncture was at least as effective as mesalamine therapy.[23] However, there was no placebo or sham arm of the trial.[23]

A randomized controlled trial in Crohn subjects compared moxibustion plus acupuncture to sham moxibustion plus sham acupuncture (burning bran and shallow placement of needles at nonacupoints). The trial showed improvement in Crohn disease activity index (CDAI) scores in the therapeutic arm.[24] Additionally, they showed reductions in IL-17 levels and an increase in T-regulatory cells compared with the sham group.[24] Another study looking at mild to moderate Crohn disease using a similar sham technique was able to show a significant improvement in CDAI, C-reactive protein, and hemoglobin levels, favoring the moxibustion plus acupuncture group; however, no difference was seen during endoscopic evaluation of the 2 groups.[25] One small study looking at acupuncture alone also showed a modest but significant decrease in the CDAI compared with a sham acupuncture group.[26] However, there was a robust placebo effect in the sham group and no difference was seen in C-reactive protein levels between the groups.[26]

Human Studies in Ulcerative Colitis: Acupuncture, Moxibustion, and Combination

A small trial in ulcerative colitis (UC) subjects comparing acupuncture and moxibustion to sham acupuncture showed a modest improvement in colitis activity index; however, again, there was a large placebo effect and no change in inflammatory markers.[27] A larger study in UC randomized subjects to herb-partitioned moxibustion to a sham (bran partitioned) moxibustion. The UC subjects in the herb-partitioned moxibustion group had significantly inhibited levels of both mRNA and protein IL-8 and Inter Cellular Adhesion Molecule-1 expression compared with the sham group. However, their clinical outcomes did not follow a commonly used disease activity index, which makes these results difficult to compare with other therapies.[28]

A meta-analysis of 43 studies comparing sulfasalazine therapy to moxibustion (with or without acupuncture) for IBD (Crohn disease and UC combined) therapy ultimately identified 10 reports of high enough quality to be analyzed in the meta-analysis. Methodology across the studies was poor, but there was little heterogeneity between the studies. Overall, there was a significant treatment effect favoring the moxibustion and acupuncture versus sulfasalazine therapy by a factor of approximately 5 times.[29] Another meta-analysis, looking only at UC subjects treated with moxibustion compared with mesalamine therapies, was able to identify 5 studies of sufficient quality to analyze. They found a more modest but still significant effect of moxibustion versus mesalamine therapy.[30]

SAFETY OF MASSAGE, ACUPUNCTURE, AND MOXIBUSTION

Across all studies there has been a favorable safety profile for massage, moxibustion, and acupuncture. Massage should be undertaken with great care in patients with underlying orthopedic injuries or in the setting of malignancy.[10] Mild superficial burns have been reported with moxibustion and local superficial hematomas have been reported with acupuncture.[25] Contamination of the acupuncture needles and subsequent local skin infections have also been reported.[12]

ISSUES FOR FUTURE STUDY

To date, studies of moxibustion or acupuncture have varied widely in clinical endpoints and few have been of high enough methodologic quality to enable the authors to make a meaningful recommendation about use with patients. Additionally, similar to the massage therapy trials, there is considerable debate about appropriate shams or placebos that could be applied to acupuncture and moxibustion trials. Burning bran still produces some heat to the skin and superficial needle injections still produce some degree of sensation. So, even if the heat or needle is not in the traditional location, the patient still perceives a sensation that they may interpret as positive or negative. Developing more rigorous study design and outcome measures will be essential to evaluate the role of these therapies going forward.

SUMMARY

Based on the current level of evidence, it remains difficult to make recommendations for or against massage, acupuncture, or moxibustion therapy in IBD patients. Although there is some evidence of upregulation of tight junction proteins and downregulation of inflammatory cytokines, these trials have not been conclusive. Additionally, although there have been several clinical trials showing favorable effects of acupuncture and moxibustion, they have, in general, been of low quality and of considerable heterogeneity to warrant incorporation into routine clinical practice. Nonetheless, these therapies seem safe and may have a modest clinical effect based on a few early clinical trials. Therefore, IBD patients who perceive benefit from massage, acupuncture, or moxibustion should continue, provided they are using them as a complement and not an alternative to their conventional therapy.

REFERENCES

1. Koning M, Ailabouni R, Gearry RB, et al. Use and predictors of oral complementary and alternative medicine by patients with inflammatory bowel disease: a population-based, case-control study. Inflamm Bowel Dis 2013;19(4):767–78.
2. Cheifetz AS, Gianotti R, Luber R, et al. Complementary and alternative medicines used by patients with inflammatory bowel diseases. Gastroenterology 2017; 152(2):415–29.e15.
3. Mountifield R, Andrews JM, Mikocka-Walus A, et al. Covert dose reduction is a distinct type of medication non-adherence observed across all care settings in inflammatory bowel disease. J Crohns Colitis 2014;8(12):1723–9.
4. Hung A, Kang N, Bollom A, et al. Complementary and alternative medicine use is prevalent among patients with gastrointestinal diseases. Dig Dis Sci 2015;60(7): 1883–8.
5. Nguyen GC, Croitoru K, Silverberg MS, et al. Use of complementary and alternative medicine for inflammatory bowel disease is associated with worse adherence to conventional therapy: the COMPLIANT study. Inflamm Bowel Dis 2016;22(6): 1412–7.
6. Rawsthorne P, Clara I, Graff LA, et al. The Manitoba Inflammatory Bowel Disease Cohort Study: a prospective longitudinal evaluation of the use of complementary and alternative medicine services and products. Gut 2012;61(4):521–7.
7. Abitbol V, Lahmek P, Buisson A, et al. Impact of complementary and alternative medicine on the quality of life in inflammatory bowel disease: results from a French national survey. Eur J Gastroenterol Hepatol 2014;26(3):288–94.
8. Weizman AV, Ahn E, Thanabalan R, et al. Characterisation of complementary and alternative medicine use and its impact on medication adherence in inflammatory bowel disease. Aliment Pharmacol Ther 2012;35(3):342–9.
9. Brummitt J. The role of massage in sports performance and rehabilitation: current evidence and future direction. N Am J Sports Phys Ther 2008;3(1):7–21.
10. Health, U.S.D.o.H.a.H.S.N.I.o. Massage therapy for health purposes. 2016. Available at: https://nccih.nih.gov/health/massage/massageintroduction.htm. Accessed September 12, 2017.
11. Oxelmark L, Lindberg A, Löfberg R, et al. Use of complementary and alternative medicine in Swedish patients with inflammatory bowel disease: a controlled study. Eur J Gastroenterol Hepatol 2016;28(11):1320–8.
12. Health, U.S.D.o.H.a.H.S.N.I.o. Acupuncture: in depth. 2016. Available at: https://nccih.nih.gov/health/acupuncture/introduction. Accessed September 12, 2017.
13. Health, U.S.D.o.H.a.H.S.N.I.o. Traditional chinese medicine: in depth. 2013. Available at: https://nccih.nih.gov/health/whatiscam/chinesemed.htm. Accessed September 12, 2017.
14. Ho TY, Lo HY, Chao DC, et al. Electroacupuncture improves trinitrobenzene sulfonic Acid-induced colitis, evaluated by transcriptomic study. Evid Based Complement Alternat Med 2014;2014:942196.

15. Wu HG, Liu HR, Tan LY, et al. Electroacupuncture and moxibustion promote neutrophil apoptosis and improve ulcerative colitis in rats. Dig Dis Sci 2007; 52(2):379–84.

16. Yan J, Liu HR, Tan LY, et al. Effects of electroacupuncture at Shangjuxu (ST 37) on interleukin-1beta and interleukin-4 in the ulcerative colitis model rats. J Tradit Chin Med 2009;29(1):60–3.

17. Wu HG, Zhou LB, Pan YY, et al. Study of the mechanisms of acupuncture and moxibustion treatment for ulcerative colitis rats in view of the gene expression of cytokines. World J Gastroenterol 1999;5(6):515–7.

18. Shi Y, Zhou EH, Wu HG, et al. Moxibustion treatment restoring the intestinal epithelium barrier in rats with Crohn's disease by down-regulating tumor necrosis factor alpha, tumor necrosis factor receptor 1, and tumor necrosis factor receptor 2. Chin J Integr Med 2011;17(3):212–7.

19. Shi Y, Qi L, Wang J, et al. Moxibustion activates mast cell degranulation at the ST25 in rats with colitis. World J Gastroenterol 2011;17(32):3733–8.

20. Wang XM, Lu Y, Wu LY, et al. Moxibustion inhibits interleukin-12 and tumor necrosis factor alpha and modulates intestinal flora in rat with ulcerative colitis. World J Gastroenterol 2012;18(46):6819–28.

21. Bao CH, Wu LY, Shi Y, et al. Moxibustion down-regulates colonic epithelial cell apoptosis and repairs tight junctions in rats with Crohn's disease. World J Gastroenterol 2011;17(45):4960–70.

22. Wu HG, Gong X, Yao LQ, et al. Mechanisms of acupuncture and moxibustion in regulation of epithelial cell apoptosis in rat ulcerative colitis. World J Gastroenterol 2004;10(5):682–8.

23. Shang HX, Wang AQ, Bao CH, et al. Moxibustion combined with acupuncture increases tight junction protein expression in Crohn's disease patients. World J Gastroenterol 2015;21(16):4986–96.

24. Zhao C, Bao C, Li J, et al. Moxibustion and Acupuncture Ameliorate Crohn's Disease by Regulating the Balance between Th17 and Treg Cells in the Intestinal Mucosa. Evid Based Complement Alternat Med 2015;2015:938054.

25. Bao CH, Zhao JM, Liu HR, et al. Randomized controlled trial: moxibustion and acupuncture for the treatment of Crohn's disease. World J Gastroenterol 2014; 20(31):11000–11.

26. Joos S, Brinkhaus B, Maluche C, et al. Acupuncture and moxibustion in the treatment of active Crohn's disease: a randomized controlled study. Digestion 2004; 69(3):131–9.

27. Joos S, Wildau N, Kohnen R, et al. Acupuncture and moxibustion in the treatment of ulcerative colitis: a randomized controlled study. Scand J Gastroenterol 2006; 41(9):1056–63.

28. Zhou EH, Liu HR, Wu HG, et al. Down-regulation of protein and mRNA expression of IL-8 and ICAM-1 in colon tissue of ulcerative colitis patients by partition-herb moxibustion. Dig Dis Sci 2009;54(10):2198–206.

29. Ji J, Lu Y, Liu H, et al. Acupuncture and moxibustion for inflammatory bowel diseases: a systematic review and meta-analysis of randomized controlled trials. Evid Based Complement Alternat Med 2013;2013:158352.

30. Lee DH, Kim JI, Lee MS, et al. Moxibustion for ulcerative colitis: a systematic review and meta-analysis. BMC Gastroenterol 2010;10:36.

Sleep and Circadian Hygiene and Inflammatory Bowel Disease

Garth R. Swanson, MD[a],*, Helen J. Burgess, PhD[b]

KEYWORDS

• Advance • Circadian • Delay • Light • Sleep

KEY POINTS

• Inflammatory bowel disease (IBD) is associated with sleep disturbance and possibly some circadian disruption.
• Sleep and circadian disruption can worsen IBD disease course.
• Possible approaches to reduce sleep and circadian disruption in patients are reviewed.
• Large placebo-controlled randomized trials in human patients are needed to fully understand the potential benefits and mechanisms of chronotherapeutic treatments for IBD.

INTRODUCTION

Inflammatory bowel disease (IBD) consists of 2 distinct phenotypic patterns: Crohn disease (CD) and ulcerative colitis (UC), that affects ~1.6 million Americans with as many as 70,000 new cases diagnosed each year.[1] IBD is typically diagnosed at a young age (20s to 30s), has a relapsing and remitting disease course, and has no known cure. This combination of factors leads to a significant health care cost and burden on society that continues to increase as IBD-related hospitalizations cost ~$4 billion annually in the United States.[2] Although a significant portion of patients with IBD will have an aggressive disease course with frequent disease flares, hospitalizations, and surgery, IBD has a highly heterogeneous disease course, and some patients will have mild disease that requires little if any medications.

Disclosure Statement: The authors have nothing to disclose.
H.J. Burgess and G.R. Swanson are supported by grants from the National Institutes of Health. The content is solely the responsibility of the authors and does not necessarily represent the official views of the National Institutes of Health.
[a] Department of Digestive Diseases, Rush University Medical Center, 1725 West Harrison Street, Suite 206, Chicago, IL 60612, USA; [b] Biological Rhythms Research Laboratory, Department of Behavioral Sciences, Rush University Medical Center, 1645 West Jackson Boulevard, Suite 425, Chicago, IL 60612, USA
* Corresponding author.
E-mail address: Garth_R_Swanson@rush.edu

Gastroenterol Clin N Am 46 (2017) 881–893
http://dx.doi.org/10.1016/j.gtc.2017.08.014
0889-8553/17/© 2017 Elsevier Inc. All rights reserved.

One group of factors that can have a crucial impact on IBD disease course is environmental stressors. The most well-studied environmental factor that is known to impact IBD course is cigarette smoking. Interestingly, cigarette smoking impacts UC and CD differently because it reduces disease flares in UC and induces disease flares and the risk of surgery in CD.[3] The focus of this review is on sleep and circadian disruption, which have recently received significant interest as important environmental factors that may attribute to disease flare in IBD. This is because both sleep and circadian alterations are capable of impacting key components in IBD disease flares, such as intestinal permeability, translocation of bacterial endotoxins and products, induction of intestinal dysbiosis, and increasing proinflammatory cytokines.[4,5] Here, the authors review the basics of sleep and circadian timing and common forms of circadian disruption that gastroenterologists may see in their clinical patients. A summary of the literature is also provided that examines sleep and circadian disruption in IBD (see **Table 1**). Then, the authors review a range of treatment approaches for circadian disruption, which may be applicable to some patients with IBD.

SLEEP AND CIRCADIAN TIMING
A Basic Overview

The neural circuitry underlying sleep and circadian timing is complex.[6] A key brain center that promotes sleep onset and the consolidation of sleep is the ventrolateral preoptic nucleus.[6] The activity of this brain region is influenced by sleep pressure, which builds up homeostatically as the duration of wakefulness increases. The circadian system interacts with this and other sleep/wake centers to promote the timing of sleep onset and the consolidation of sleep.[6] The central circadian pacemaker (suprachiasmatic nuclei, SCN) also generates and regulates circadian rhythms in the periphery, and those rhythms assist in transmitting the central circadian signal to other systems in the brain and body.[7] Indeed, the central circadian clock has a direct influence on peripheral inflammatory processes[8] and also influences peripheral clocks that exist in almost every cell, tissue, and organ in the body.[9] Both sleep and circadian timing are widely recognized as having a widespread and profound influence on mental and physical health.[10–12]

More than 70% of humans have an endogenous circadian clock with a period greater than 24 hours (on average ∼24.2 hours).[13,14] Thus, for most humans, the internal circadian clock takes more than 24 hours to complete one cycle, which results in an endogenous or intrinsic tendency to drift later ("phase delay") each day. This is most commonly seen in the later sleep times that many people adopt on the weekend or on work-free days.[15] To remain in synchrony or "entrained" to the external 24-hour day, and indeed to 9 to 5 society, the circadian clock needs to regularly, if not daily, shift earlier ("phase advance"). The strongest environmental influence on circadian timing is the light-dark (LD) cycle, which is captured by various photoreceptors in the retina and transmitted to the SCN.[16] Light in the evening typically phase delays circadian timing and thus exacerbates the intrinsic tendency to drift later, whereas light in the morning typically phase advances circadian timing and thus can correct for the intrinsic tendency to drift later.[7] The human circadian clock is particularly sensitive to short wavelength or blue light,[17] such as that seen during sunrise and sunset, and also emitted from many electronic devices, such as cell phones and tablets.

The peripheral circadian rhythm often measured to infer the timing of the central circadian clock in humans is the endogenous melatonin rhythm, because the secretion of melatonin from the pineal gland is controlled by the SCN.[18] Specifically, the most reliable marker of circadian timing is the dim light melatonin onset (DLMO),[19] which is the time when endogenous melatonin levels begin to increase in dim light ~2 to 3 hours before habitual bedtime.[20] Endogenous melatonin must be measured in dim light, because light suppresses melatonin.[21] The DLMO can be assessed either in the laboratory or at home from half-hourly or hourly saliva samples collected in the ~6 hours or so before habitual sleep onset time, which are later assayed for melatonin concentration.[22] A shift in the DLMO reflects a shift in the timing of the central circadian clock.

RISK FACTORS FOR SLEEP AND CIRCADIAN DISRUPTION

Sleep disturbance is increasingly prevalent in society. For example, up to 30% of Americans regularly sleep 6 hours or less per night,[23] and 10% to 15% of the adult population suffer from chronic insomnia.[24] Other sleep disorders such as sleep apnea and restless leg syndrome also affect significant proportions of the general population.[25,26] Sleep disturbance can also be a symptom of underlying circadian disruption, as seen in a variety of circadian rhythm sleep disorders.[27,28] Importantly, sleep disruption results in increases in inflammatory markers.[29,30] Sleep disruption also affects dietary intake, such as increasing the appetite for fats and sugars.[31,32] Indeed, sleep disruption may also alter gut microbiota,[33] although this has not been found consistently.[34] In this review, the authors focus on forms of circadian disruption that gastroenterologists are more likely to see in their clinical patients, namely shift work and social jet lag.

Shift Work

Approximately 15% of the general work force is engaged in some sort of "nonstandard" work hours.[35] There is a large variety of shift work schedules including permanent night shifts, evening shifts or morning shifts, and slow or fast rotating shifts that can rotate forward (such as morning, evening, to night shifts) or backwards (such as night to evening to morning shifts). Most of these if not all are associated with some degree of circadian misalignment. Shift work is also associated with reduced sleep duration and sleep quality, particularly during morning and night shifts.[36,37] Given the sleep and circadian disruption that occurs during shift work, it is not surprising that shift work is associated with worse physical and mental health outcomes, including depression, cardiometabolic health, and cancer.[36,37] One likely contributor to these negative health effects is an increase in systemic inflammation as observed in shift workers.[4,38,39] Shift workers also tend to eat less nutritious foods,[40] probably in part due to the associated sleep deprivation, which increases the appetite for fats and sugars as mentioned earlier, but also in part because of the limited availability of nutritious foods during odd work hours, such as the food typically available in vending machines.

Chronotype and Social Jet Lag

Chronotype, or diurnal preference, refers to people's self-reported actual or preferred timing in their behaviors, including sleep timing, and reflects either a tendency toward morningness, eveningness, or somewhere in the middle ("intermediate or neither types"). Chronotype or diurnal preference can be assessed via different questionnaires and correlates with the DLMO, such that morning types tend to have earlier DLMOs and evening types tend to have later DLMOs.[41] Chronotype tends to vary with age, such that younger people tend to have more eveningness, which shifts more toward morningness with increasing age. In general, evening types, or people who typically sleep later, tend to have increased rates of depression,[42] consume more alcohol, caffeine, and nicotine,[43] and have less healthy dietary habits.[44]

People with higher eveningness can fall into 1 of 2 groups. Some evening types have a lot of control over their sleep times and thus are able to regularly sleep and wake as late as they wish, such as students or self-employed workers. Then there are those that are forced to shift to earlier sleep times on some days of the week, in order to meet their social responsibilities such as work or childcare responsibilities. Such shifting of desired sleep times on work days is referred to as "social jet lag," which can be defined as a 2-hour or more difference between the timing of the midpoint of sleep on work days versus work-free days.[43] Thus, social jet lag is in many ways a milder form of the chronic circadian misalignment seen in night workers and is quite prevalent, with estimates suggesting it occurs in about 30% of the general population.[45] Social jet lag is also associated with a host of negative health effects, including increased rates of depression,[12] higher body mass index,[45] higher resting heart rate,[46] higher HbA1c,[47] and an increase in inflammatory markers such as C-reactive protein.[47] Social jet lag is also associated with the increased consumption of alcohol, nicotine, and caffeine,[43] which may reflect circadian misalignment, the associated sleep deprivation, or self-medication behaviors to treat the impaired sleep and alertness associated with social jet lag.

OBSERVATIONAL STUDIES IN SLEEP AND CIRCADIAN DISRUPTION IN INFLAMMATORY BOWEL DISEASE
Sleep and Inflammatory Bowel Disease

Several observational studies have found an increased prevalence of sleep and sleep disturbances in IBD (see **Table 1**). Most studies have used validated questionnaires to examine sleep quality, fatigue, or sleepiness, such as the Pittsburgh Sleep Quality Index (PSQI), the Patient-Reported Outcomes Measurement Information System (PROMIS), the Modified Fatigue Impact Scale (MFIS), or the Epworth Sleepiness Scale (ESS). However, one of the first studies to objectively measure sleep in IBD was by Keefer and colleagues,[48] who used polysomnography (PSG) in 16 inactive IBD subjects compared with 9 patients with IBS and 7 healthy controls. They found that IBD subjects had decreased total sleep time, an increase in stage 1 sleep, and overall arousal index compared with healthy controls. Using the PSQI in larger cohort studies to strengthen this evidence, Ranjbaran and colleagues[49] studied 199 subjects with inactive IBD finding high rates of poor sleep in CD (78%) and UC (39%), and poor sleep correlated with a worse IBD-specific quality-of-life score. Subsequently, a study by Graff and colleagues[50] in 318 IBD with active and inactive disease found that disease activity correlated with poor sleep quality (PSQI) and also fatigue (MFIS) and sleepiness (ESS). The largest study to date and some of the strongest evidence to support the impact of sleep in IBD was by Ananthakrishnan and colleagues,[51] who studied 3173 IBD patients with the PROMIS Sleep Disturbance questionnaire and found that disease activity, depression, female sex, smoking, and corticosteroid or narcotics use were all associated with sleep disturbance. Very interestingly, in this study, the investigators found that over a 6-month timeframe poor sleep was associated with an increased risk of flare in CD but not UC. This difference on the impact of sleep disturbance in CD and UC requires further study. The only study to examine mucosal inflammation and sleep[52] also found a strong association in 41 IBD patients between histologic inflammation and sleep disturbance as measured by PSQI. These preliminary studies on mucosal disease activity need to be further validated with additional markers of subclinical inflammation, such as stool calprotectin, intestinal permeability, and the intestinal microbiota. Finally, a recent study by Wilson and colleagues[53] found that IBD subjects had poor sleep as measured by PROMIS even when controlling for nocturnal symptoms, and another study by van Langenberg and colleagues[54]

Table 1
Observational studies in sleep and inflammatory bowel disease

Study, y	Subjects	Measure	Outcome	Main Finding
Keefer et al,[48] 2006	Inactive IBD, IBS, & healthy controls	PSG	↓ Sleep time, ↓ Sleep efficiency	Sleep worsened IBD-Q
Ranjbaran et al,[49] 2007	Inactive IBD, IBS, & healthy controls	PSQI	↑ Sleep latency, ↑ Sleep fragmentation	Sleep worsened IBD-Q
Burgess et al,[55] 2010	Inactive IBD	Actigraphy DLMO	↑ Sleep latency, ↓ Sleep efficiency	2/4 IBD patients had circadian disruption
Graff et al,[50] 2011	Active & inactive IBD	PSQI MFI ESS	↑ Stress, ↓ global sleep, & ↑ fatigue	↓ Sleep in active & inactive IBD
Ananthakrishnan et al,[51] 2013	Active & inactive IBD	PSQI PROMIS	↓ Sleep quality in active disease, depression, smokers, & steroid or narcotic use	Sleep disturbance associated with ↑ risk of flare in CD at 6 mo
Ali et al,[52] 2013	Active & inactive IBD	PSQI Colonoscopy	↓ Sleep in active disease	↓ Sleep associated with inflammation
Wilson et al,[53] 2015	Active & inactive IBD	PROMIS	Poor sleep present regardless of nocturnal symptoms	↑ CRP associated with poor sleep
van Langenberg et al,[54] 2015	CD	Actigraphy	↑ Sedentary, ↑ Sleep fragmentation	Poorer sleep quality and less physical activity

found that Crohn's patients had increased sleep fragmentation and less physical activity than healthy controls by wrist actigraphy. The results of these observational studies are summarized in **Table 1**. The consistent results from these studies strengthen the high prevalence of poor sleep in IBD and the association of poor sleep with disease activity. However, further prospective controlled studies are needed to determine if sleep disruption is a potential modifiable risk factor for a disease flare or if it is only a consequence of uncontrolled inflammation and disease activity.

Circadian and Inflammatory Bowel Disease

The number of studies examining circadian disruption in IBD is much smaller. In a small pilot study, the authors measured for the first time sleep and circadian rhythmicity in 4 patients with IBD that were asymptomatic at the time of assessment.[55] Three (1 UC, 2 CD) of the 4 patients took longer to fall asleep and had lower sleep efficiency than age- and sex-matched controls. Two patients (1 UC, 1 CD) displayed relatively early to normal DLMOs, occurring between 6:30 PM and 8:30 PM. However, one patient (CD) had a relatively late DLMO at about 11:00 PM, and the last patient (CD) had no circadian rhythmicity in their melatonin profile at all. These results highlight the possibility that some IBD patients, especially CD patients, may have circadian disruption, which could contribute to sleep disruption.

The strongest data on the impact of circadian disruption in IBD come from animal models. The effect of a continuous 12-hour phase shift in the LD cycle every 5 days for 3 months compared with a control group that stayed on a constant 12:12-hour LD cycle was examined in a dextran sodium sulfate (DSS) model. Preuss and colleagues[56] found that phase shifted animals developed more severe colitis that was associated with more significant weight loss and an overall higher mortality compared with those mice in a stable LD cycle. The severity of the colitis was confirmed by tissue histopathologic scoring and was also associated with an increase in neutrophil activation as evidenced by elevation in MPO activity. Subsequently, Tang and colleagues[57] repeated a similar experiment examining the effect of sleep deprivation in a DSS colitis model. In this study, the mice were placed in a rotating mechanical wheel to keep them awake either acutely for one 24-hour period or chronically for 6 hours every other day. The investigators found a worsening of the DSS colitis in the chronically sleep-deprived animals as manifested again by greater weight loss and MPO activity in the colon compared with the acutely sleep-deprived control animals. Finally, the proinflammatory milieu of the intestinal microbiota could be another factor that could impact IBD. A study by Voigt and colleagues[5] found that in a similar model of 12-hour LD phase shifts for 5 months significantly altered the intestinal microbiota in mice fed a high-fat diet, which included a significant decrease in Bacteroidetes and increase in proinflammatory Firmicutes. Similarly, the first human study data on the impact of an 8- to 10-hour jet lag on intestinal microbiota by Thaiss and colleagues[58] also found an increase in Firmicutes and an increased susceptibility of metabolic syndrome when human fecal transfer was done into a germ-free mouse model.

Overall, these studies highlight circadian disruption as a potential risk factor for disease course in IBD, but also reveal the lack of human studies and limitations of the available data. For instance, one prior epidemiologic study based in Denmark did not find an association between shift work and the risk of hospitalization in patients with IBD[59]; however, genetic studies examining one of the core clock genes, PER3, found a polymorphism of the PER 3 gene to be associated with an increased use of immunosuppressive drugs and structuring/fistulizing phenotype in CD.[60] Overall, these studies point to a possible association between circadian rhythms and IBD, but better studies are needed to examine the effect of shift work, chronotype, social jet lag, and sleep debt in IBD to make a more definitive evaluation of established risk factors for disease flare such as mucosal inflammation, intestinal permeability, and increased proinflammatory cytokines.

POSSIBLE TREATMENT APPROACHES FOR INFLAMMATORY BOWEL DISEASE PATIENTS WITH SLEEP AND CIRCADIAN DISRUPTION

Patients who regularly sleep less than 7 hours a night may benefit from some education about the importance of sleep to mental and physical health (**Table 2**). The American Academy of Sleep Medicine and Sleep Research Society recently released a consensus statement recommending adults obtain at least 7 hours of sleep per night.[61] As the consensus panel concluded after an extensive literature review, adults who regularly sleep less than 7 hours per night are at greater risk for adverse health outcomes, including impaired immune function, increased pain, depression, cardio-metabolic disease, and death.[61] Most people have fixed wake times because of social responsibilities such as work or child care, and thus, sleep extension is often achieved with earlier bedtimes. Earlier bedtimes not only increase the opportunity for sleep but, because of the associated reduction in evening light, also result in circadian phase advances,[62] which is usually an additional benefit to most people.

As the circadian system is relatively slow to shift, even with the addition of light treatment, sudden shifts in sleep timing are to be avoided. Instead, small progressive shifts in sleep timing of 30 minutes to 1 hour per day will permit the circadian clock to shift in synchrony with sleep, thereby reducing the likelihood of inadvertently creating some circadian misalignment.[63] Patients who voluntarily cut their sleep short each night may be encouraged to try to extend their sleep to 7 to 8 hours per night for 1 to 2 weeks to experience possible improvements in their health and well-being. For evening

Table 2
Potential treatments for patients with possible sleep/circadian disruption

Sleep/Circadian Disruption	Potential Treatment
Voluntary short sleeper	• Educate on importance of sleep to health • Suggest trial of obtaining 7–8 h/sleep for 1–2 wk to experience possible improvements in health
Evening chronotype (night owl) with or without social jet lag	• If desires earlier sleep times, suggest slowly shifting sleep times earlier by 30 min to 1 h/d • Educate on importance of a consistent sleep wake schedule, and avoidance of sleeping in on days off • Educate on importance of evening light avoidance • Educate on importance of morning light exposure via morning activities or a light device (light box or wearable light treatment) • Educate on importance of avoiding afternoon/evening caffeine
Shift work	• Consider switching to day or evening shifts if possible • If rotating shift work, consider avoiding night shifts especially if morning type (early bird), or avoiding early morning shifts especially if evening type (night owl) • If permanent night shifts (≥2 wk), consider shifting later by seeking evening/night light, avoiding morning light (sunglasses, to bed within 2 h of end of night shift), and sleeping late on days off (up until around noon)

chronotypes (late sleepers) who wish to shift their sleep timing earlier (phase advance), further manipulation of the LD cycle will be useful, because light is the strongest environmental influence on circadian timing. Avoidance or reduction of evening light will be of benefit,[64] which means earlier bedtimes, dimming ambient lighting, and if possible, reducing exposure to light-emitting electronic devices,[65] such as tablets and cell phones, either by reducing use or dimming the screens and increasing the distance between the device and eyes (such as a cell phone). In addition, the use of orange-colored "blue blocker" glasses in the evening, which filter out the short "blue" wavelengths of light the circadian system is most sensitive to, may contribute to phase advances.[64] Last, caffeine in the 3 hours before usual bedtime can not only disturb sleep[66] but may also phase delay the circadian clock,[67] and thus should be avoided.

Enhancing morning light exposure will also assist with phase advancing. For some patients, this could be achieved by encouraging outdoor morning activities in sunlight such as walking the dog or going for a morning jog. Avoiding the use of sunglasses in the morning will also help to increase morning light exposure. Otherwise, morning light exposure can be enhanced with a morning light treatment, either from a light box or from recently available wearable light devices, such as the Re-timer (re-timer.com) or Luminette (myluminette.com).[7,28] So-called dawn simulators have also been tested, but they appear to only be effective if they wake subjects up early, because only 1% to 2% of light passes through closed eyelids.[7] Nonetheless, they may be an option for patients with low motivation to engage in a morning light treatment.[7] In the authors' morning light treatment trials, they use a 1-hour light treatment duration for larger clinical effects, but a 30-minute duration could be used if patients do not have time in the morning for a full hour of treatment. The authors advise not initially starting a morning light treatment any earlier that 1 hour before the patient's average wake time, because starting the light treatment any earlier than that risks inadvertently phase delaying the clock.[7] Thereafter, the timing of morning light can be nudged earlier with wake time. Morning light is generally considered safe. For example, in the light treatment of winter depression, a daily light treatment in the fall and winter for 6 years did not lead to any ophthalmologic changes.[68] Nonetheless, morning light treatment does have some side effects, most commonly headaches, eyestrain, nausea, and agitation,[69] but these are typically minimal and spontaneously remit,[69,70] and patients rarely stop treatment because of side effects.[70] Morning light is usually not recommended to patients with existing eye disease, migraine headaches if light is a headache trigger, patients on medications that photosensitize to blue light, or in patients with a history of mania.[69,70] Notably, morning light exposure also has an immediate alerting and mood-enhancing effect.[71] Indeed, light treatment as a nonpharmacologic therapy is usually attractive to many patients. In general, once desired sleep times are met, patients should try wherever possible to reduce the variability in their sleep times, such as any social jet lag. Given the associations between social jet lag and worse health outcomes, as reviewed above, a regular bed and wake time, within about a 1-hour range, may well lead to some health benefits.

Shift workers should first consider if they can switch to day or evening shifts, which are associated with more sleep. Otherwise, encouraging morning types to avoid night shifts and evening types to avoid early morning shifts has been shown to result in an increase of about 30 minutes of sleep per night and an increase in overall well-being.[72] Because the central circadian clock is quite slow to shift, circadian adaptation to night shifts should only be attempted if there will be at least 2 weeks of night shifts.[73,74] This involves increasing late night light exposure (up until about 4 AM) with a light device if permitted in the workplace, avoiding morning light (sunglasses during commute home, and sleep in dark bedroom within 2 hours of end of night shift), and continuing to sleep late (eg, sleeping until noon) on days off.[73,74]

Melatonin and melatonin agonists can also be used to shift circadian timing in humans.[75] In addition, animal models of IBD suggest potential benefits of melatonin treatment because it prevents increased intestinal permeability and ameliorates proinflammatory cytokines such as tumor necrosis factor-α.[76,77] However, in humans, the literature examining the use of melatonin in IBD consists mostly of anecdotal reports, some of which report significant negative outcomes.[78,79] Therefore, currently, the authors do not recommend melatonin treatment for patients with IBD.

SUMMARY AND FUTURE DIRECTIONS

In conclusion, emerging evidence supports sleep and circadian disruption as potential environmental triggers that can worsen IBD disease course. Because sleep and circadian disruption are highly prevalent in both society and IBD patients, there is a need for large placebo-controlled randomized trials to test some of the possible circadian treatment approaches reviewed here. These studies should also focus on the mechanistic pathways between chronotherapeutic treatment approaches and potential positive outcomes, including intestinal permeability, translocation of bacterial endotoxins, intestinal dysbiosis, and proinflammatory cytokines.

REFERENCES

1. Shivashankar R, Tremaine WJ, Harmsen WS, et al. Incidence and prevalence of Crohn's disease and ulcerative colitis in Olmsted County, Minnesota from 1970 through 2010. Clin Gastroenterol Hepatol 2017;15(6):857–63.
2. Peery AF, Crockett SD, Barritt AS, et al. Burden of gastrointestinal, liver, and pancreatic diseases in the United States. Gastroenterology 2015;149(7): 1731–41.
3. Carbonnel F, Jantchou P, Monnet E, et al. Environmental risk factors in Crohn's disease and ulcerative colitis: an update. Gastroenterol Clin Biol 2009; 33(Suppl 3):S145–57.
4. Swanson GR, Gorenz A, Shaikh M, et al. Night workers with circadian misalignment are susceptible to alcohol-induced intestinal hyperpermeability with social drinking. Am J Physiol 2016;311(1):G192–201.
5. Voigt RM, Forsyth CB, Green SJ, et al. Circadian disorganization alters intestinal microbiota. PLoS One 2014;9(5):e97500.
6. Fuller PM, Gooley JJ, Saper CB. Neurobiology of the sleep-wake cycle: sleep architecture, circadian regulation, and regulatory feedback. J Biol Rhythms 2006;21(6):482–93.
7. Emens J, Burgess HJ. Effect of light and melatonin and other melatonin receptor agonists on human circadian physiology. Sleep Med Clin 2015;10:435–53.
8. Scheiermann C, Kunisaki Y, Lucas D, et al. Adrenergic nerves govern circadian leukocyte recruitment to tissues. Immunity 2012;37(2):290–301.
9. Lowrey PL, Takahashi JS. Genetics of circadian rhythms in mammalian model organisms. Adv Genet 2011;74:175–230.
10. Wright KP Jr, Hull JT, Hughes RJ, et al. Sleep and wakefulness out of phase with internal biological time impairs learning in humans. J Cogn Neurosci 2006;18(4): 508–21.
11. Scheer FA, Hilton MF, Mantzoros CS, et al. Adverse metabolic and cardiovascular consequences of circadian misalignment. Proc Natl Acad Sci U S A 2009; 106(11):4453–8.

12. Levandovski R, Dantas G, Fernandes LC, et al. Depression scores associate with chronotype and social jetlag in a rural population. Chronobiol Int 2011;28(9): 771–8.

13. Burgess HJ, Eastman CI. Human tau in an ultradian light-dark cycle. J Biol Rhythms 2008;23(4):374–6.

14. Duffy JF, Cain SW, Chang AM, et al. Sex difference in the near-24-hour intrinsic period of the human circadian timing system. Proc Natl Acad Sci U S A 2011; 108(Suppl 3):15602–8.

15. National Sleep Foundation. 2011 Sleep in America Poll: Communications technology in the bedroom. Available at: https://sleepfoundation.org/sleep-polls. Accessed April 27, 2017.

16. Lucas RJ, Lall GS, Allen AE, et al. How rod, cone, and melanopsin photoreceptors come together to enlighten the mammalian circadian clock. Prog Brain Res 2012;199:1–18.

17. Thapan K, Arendt J, Skene DJ. An action spectrum for melatonin suppression: evidence for a novel non-rod, non-cone photoreceptor system in humans. J Physiol 2001;535:261–7.

18. Moore RY. Neural control of the pineal gland. Behav Brain Res 1996;73:125–30.

19. Klerman EB, Gershengorn HB, Duffy JF, et al. Comparisons of the variability of three markers of the human circadian pacemaker. J Biol Rhythms 2002;17(2): 181–93.

20. Burgess HJ, Fogg LF. Individual differences in the amount and timing of salivary melatonin secretion. PLoS One 2008;3(8):e3055.

21. Benloucif S, Burgess HJ, Klerman EB, et al. Measuring melatonin in humans. J Clin Sleep Med 2008;4(1):66–9.

22. Burgess HJ, Wyatt JK, Park M, et al. Home circadian phase assessments with measures of compliance yield accurate dim light melatonin onsets. Sleep 2015; 38(6):889–97.

23. National Sleep Foundation. 2010 Sleep in America Poll. Available at: https:// sleepfoundation.org/sleep-polls. Accessed April 27, 2017.

24. Winkelman JW. Clinical practice: insomnia disorder. N Engl J Med 2015;373(15): 1437–44.

25. Cowie MR. Sleep apnea: state of the art. Trends Cardiovasc Med 2017;27(4): 280–9.

26. Garcia-Borreguero D, Cano-Pumarega I. New concepts in the management of restless legs syndrome. BMJ 2017;356:j104.

27. Reid KJ, Burgess HJ. Circadian rhythm sleep disorders. Prim Care 2005;32: 449–73.

28. Burgess HJ, Emens JS. Circadian-based therapies for circadian rhythm sleep-wake disorders. Curr Sleep Med Rep 2016;2(3):158–65.

29. Vgontzas AN, Zoumakis E, Bixler EO, et al. Adverse effects of modest sleep restriction on sleepiness, performance, and inflammatory cytokines. J Clin Endocrinol Metab 2004;89(5):2119–26.

30. Parthasarathy S, Vasquez MM, Halonen M, et al. Persistent insomnia is associated with mortality risk. Am J Med 2015;128(3):268–75.e2.

31. Dashti HS, Scheer FA, Jacques PF, et al. Short sleep duration and dietary intake: epidemiologic evidence, mechanisms, and health implications. Adv Nutr 2015; 6(6):648–59.

32. Tan X, Alen M, Cheng SM, et al. Associations of disordered sleep with body fat distribution, physical activity and diet among overweight middle-aged men. J Sleep Res 2015;24(4):414–24.

33. Benedict C, Vogel H, Jonas W, et al. Gut microbiota and glucometabolic alterations in response to recurrent partial sleep deprivation in normal-weight young individuals. Mol Metab 2016;5(12):1175–86.
34. Zhang SL, Bai L, Goel N, et al. Human and rat gut microbiome composition is maintained following sleep restriction. Proc Natl Acad Sci U S A 2017;114(8): E1564–71.
35. Beers TM. Flexible schedules and shift work: replacing the 9-to-5 workday? Monthly Labor Review 2000;33–40.
36. Drake CL, Roehrs T, Richardson G, et al. Shift work sleep disorder: prevalence and consequences beyond that of symptomatic day workers. Sleep 2004;27: 1453–62.
37. Kecklund G, Axelsson J. Health consequences of shift work and insufficient sleep. BMJ 2016;355:i5210.
38. Sookoian S, Gemma C, Fernandez Gianotti T, et al. Effects of rotating shift work on biomarkers of metabolic syndrome and inflammation. J Intern Med 2007; 261(3):285–92.
39. Puttonen S, Viitasalo K, Harma M. Effect of shiftwork on systemic markers of inflammation. Chronobiol Int 2011;28(6):528–35.
40. Heath G, Coates A, Sargent C, et al. Sleep duration and chronic fatigue are differently associated with the dietary profile of shift workers. Nutrients 2016; 8(12):E771.
41. Kantermann T, Sung H, Burgess HJ. Comparing the morningness-eveningness questionnaire and munich chronotype questionnaire to the dim light melatonin onset. J Biol Rhythms 2015;30(5):449–53.
42. Merikanto I, Lahti T, Kronholm E, et al. Evening types are prone to depression. Chronobiol Int 2013;30(5):719–25.
43. Wittmann M, Dinich J, Merrow M, et al. Social jetlag: misalignment of biological and social time. Chronobiol Int 2006;23(1):497–509.
44. Kanerva N, Kronholm E, Partonen T, et al. Tendency toward eveningness is associated with unhealthy dietary habits. Chronobiol Int 2012;29(7):920–7.
45. Roenneberg T, Allebrandt KV, Merrow M, et al. Social jetlag and obesity. Curr Biol 2012;22(10):939–43.
46. Rutters F, Lemmens SG, Adam TC, et al. Is social jetlag associated with an adverse endocrine, behavioral, and cardiovascular risk profile? J Biol Rhythms 2014;29(5):377–83.
47. Parsons MJ, Moffitt TE, Gregory AM, et al. Social jetlag, obesity and metabolic disorder: investigation in a cohort study. Int J Obes (Lond) 2015;39(5):842–8.
48. Keefer L, Stepanski EJ, Ranjbaran Z, et al. An initial report of sleep disturbance in inactive inflammatory bowel disease. J Clin Sleep Med 2006;2(4):409–16.
49. Ranjbaran Z, Keefer L, Farhadi A, et al. Impact of sleep disturbances in inflammatory bowel disease. J Gastroenterol Hepatol 2007;22(11):1748–53.
50. Graff LA, Vincent N, Walker JR, et al. A population-based study of fatigue and sleep difficulties in inflammatory bowel disease. Inflamm Bowel Dis 2011;17(9): 1882–9.
51. Ananthakrishnan AN, Long MD, Martin CF, et al. Sleep disturbance and risk of active disease in patients with Crohn's disease and ulcerative colitis. Clin Gastroenterol Hepatol 2013;11(8):965–71.
52. Ali T, Madhoun MF, Orr WC, et al. Assessment of the relationship between quality of sleep and disease activity in inflammatory bowel disease patients. Inflamm Bowel Dis 2013;19(11):2440–3.

53. Wilson RG, Stevens BW, Guo AY, et al. High C-reactive protein is associated with poor sleep quality independent of nocturnal symptoms in patients with inflammatory bowel disease. Dig Dis Sci 2015;60(7):2136–43.

54. van Langenberg DR, Papandony MC, Gibson PR. Sleep and physical activity measured by accelerometry in Crohn's disease. Aliment Pharmacol Ther 2015; 41(10):991–1004.

55. Burgess HJ, Swanson GR, Keshavarzian A. Endogenous melatonin profiles in asymptomatic inflammatory bowel disease. Scand J Gastroenterol 2010;45(6): 759–61.

56. Preuss F, Tang Y, Laposky AD, et al. Adverse effects of chronic circadian desynchronization in animals in a "challenging" environment. Am J Physiol 2008; 295(6):R2034–40.

57. Tang Y, Preuss F, Turek FW, et al. Sleep deprivation worsens inflammation and delays recovery in a mouse model of colitis. Sleep Med 2009;10(6):597–603.

58. Thaiss CA, Zeevi D, Levy M, et al. Transkingdom control of microbiota diurnal oscillations promotes metabolic homeostasis. Cell 2014;159(3):514–29.

59. Boggild H, Tuchsen F, Orhede E. Occupation, employment status and chronic inflammatory bowel disease in Denmark. Int J Epidemiol 1996;25(3):630–7.

60. Mazzoccoli G, Palmieri O, Corritore G, et al. Association study of a polymorphism in clock gene PERIOD3 and risk of inflammatory bowel disease. Chronobiol Int 2012;29(8):994–1003.

61. Watson NF, Badr MS, Belenky G, et al. Recommended amount of sleep for a healthy adult: a joint consensus statement of the American Academy of Sleep Medicine and Sleep Research Society. J Clin Sleep Med 2015;11(8):931–52.

62. Burgess HJ, Eastman CI. Early versus late bedtimes phase shift the human dim light melatonin rhythm despite a fixed morning lights on time. Neurosci Lett 2004; 356:115–8.

63. Eastman CI, Gazda CJ, Burgess HJ, et al. Advancing circadian rhythms before eastward flight: a strategy to prevent or reduce jet lag. Sleep 2005;28(1):33–44.

64. Burgess HJ, Molina TA. Home lighting before usual bedtime impacts circadian timing: a field study. Photochem Photobiol 2014;90(3):723–6.

65. Chang AM, Aeschbach D, Duffy JF, et al. Evening use of light-emitting eReaders negatively affects sleep, circadian timing, and next-morning alertness. Proc Natl Acad Sci U S A 2015;112(4):1232–7.

66. Landolt HP, Werth E, Borbely AA, et al. Caffeine intake (200 mg) in the morning affects human sleep and EEG power spectra at night. Brain Res 1995;675:67–74.

67. Burke TM, Markwald RR, McHill AW, et al. Effects of caffeine on the human circadian clock in vivo and in vitro. Sci Transl Med 2015;7(305):305ra146.

68. Gallin PF, Terman M, Reme CE, et al. Ophthalmologic examination of patients with seasonal affective disorder, before and after bright light therapy. Am J Ophthalmol 1995;119:202–10.

69. Pail G, Huf W, Pjrek E, et al. Bright-light therapy in the treatment of mood disorders. Neuropsychobiology 2011;64(3):152–62.

70. Terman M, Terman JS. Light therapy for seasonal and nonseasonal depression: efficacy, protocol, safety, and side effects. CNS Spectr 2005;10:647–63.

71. Goel N, Etwaroo GR. Bright light, negative air ions and auditory stimuli produce rapid mood changes in a student population: a placebo-controlled study. Psychol Med 2006;36(9):1253–63.

72. Vetter C, Fischer D, Matera JL, et al. Aligning work and circadian time in shift workers improves sleep and reduces circadian disruption. Curr Biol 2015; 25(7):907–11.

73. Burgess HJ. Using bright light and melatonin to adjust to night work. In: Perlis M, Aloia M, Kuhn B, editors. Behavioral treatments for sleep disorders: a comprehensive primer of behavioral sleep medicine treatment protocols. Elsevier Inc; 2011. p. 159–65.

74. Burgess HJ, Sharkey KM, Eastman CI. Bright light, dark and melatonin can promote circadian adaptation in night shift workers. Sleep Med Rev 2002;6:407–20.

75. Burgess HJ, Revell VL, Molina TA, et al. Human phase response curves to three days of daily melatonin: 0.5 mg versus 3.0 mg. J Clin Endocrinol Metab 2010; 95(7):3325–31.

76. Mei Q, Yu JP, Xu JM, et al. Melatonin reduces colon immunological injury in rats by regulating activity of macrophages. Acta Pharmacol Sin 2002;23(10):882–6.

77. Li JH, Yu JP, Yu HG, et al. Melatonin reduces inflammatory injury through inhibiting NF-kappaB activation in rats with colitis. Mediators Inflamm 2005;2005(4): 185–93.

78. Marquez E, Sanchez-Fidalgo S, Calvo JR, et al. Acutely administered melatonin is beneficial while chronic melatonin treatment aggravates the evolution of TNBS-induced colitis. J Pineal Res 2006;40(1):48–55.

79. Calvo JR, Guerrero JM, Osuna C, et al. Melatonin triggers Crohn's disease symptoms. J Pineal Res 2002;32(4):277–8.

Exercise and Inflammatory Bowel Disease

Insights into Etiopathogenesis and Modification of Clinical Course

Jana G. Hashash, MD, MSc[a,b], David G. Binion, MD[a,*]

KEYWORDS

- Inflammatory bowel disease • IBD • Exercise • Inflammatory disorders
- Physical activity

KEY POINTS

- There is a growing appreciation that regular exercise regimens are essential for patients suffering from chronic inflammatory disorders, including IBD.
- Low- to moderate-intensity exercise for IBD patients in remission and those with mild active disease, improves quality of life of these patients and helps counteract IBD-related complications.
- A regular exercise regimen may also exert a beneficial modifying effect on disease course, improving inflammatory parameters, psychological status and quality of life in patients with IBD.
- Exercise may help counteract IBD-related complications such as improving bone mineral density, immunologic response, psychological health, weight loss, and stress management ability.

INTRODUCTION

Exercise and physical activity are crucial for maintaining health and well-being. A sedentary lifestyle contributes to and complicates a multitude of chronic illnesses, often resulting in multiple comorbidities. Although there are recommendations regarding exercise to maintain health in the general population, there is sparse information regarding exercise and inflammatory bowel disease (IBD). Furthermore, the importance of regular exercise in the optimal management of IBD has not received

[a] Division of Gastroenterology, Hepatology and Nutrition, UPMC Presbyterian Hospital, University of Pittsburgh School of Medicine, University of Pittsburgh, 200 Lothrop Street, Mezzanine Level C Wing PUH, Pittsburgh, PA 15213, USA; [b] American University of Beirut, Box 11-0236 Riad El-Solh, Beirut 1107 2020, Lebanon
* Corresponding author.
E-mail address: binion@pitt.edu

Gastroenterol Clin N Am 46 (2017) 895–905
http://dx.doi.org/10.1016/j.gtc.2017.08.010
0889-8553/17/© 2017 Elsevier Inc. All rights reserved.

attention in guidelines and is often overlooked by practitioners. This review summarizes evidence regarding health benefits of exercise, guidelines regarding exercise in the general population and chronic inflammatory disorder populations, limitations regarding exercise capacity in patients with IBD, the association of lack of exercise with IBD pathogenesis, the role of exercise in beneficially modulating IBD clinical course, and extraintestinal benefits of exercise in patients with IBD.

HEALTH BENEFITS OF EXERCISE: HISTORICAL INFORMATION FROM THE GENERAL POPULATION AND INFLAMMATORY DISORDERS

The 2008 Physical Activity Guidelines for Americans identifies 2 types of physical activity that should be performed on a weekly basis: aerobic and muscle-strengthening exercises.[1] It is recommended that adults perform 150 minutes of moderate physical activity such as brisk walking every week as well as muscle-strengthening activities on at least 2 days of the week to work all major muscle groups including legs, hips, chest, abdomen, shoulders, and arms. If patients choose to perform vigorous-intensity activity (instead of moderate physical activity), such as jogging, running, swimming laps, or playing tennis or basketball, they need 75 minutes per week instead of the 150 minutes.[1] Similarly, these patients should conduct muscle-strengthening activities on at least 2 days of the week to work all major muscle groups.

Regular exercise regimens have been associated with improved cardiovascular status, stamina, and overall well-being. Exercise, which can be limited to as little as 10 minutes of sustained activity per day, has been associated with a decreased lifetime risk of developing ischemic heart disease, hypertension, diabetes, breast cancer, Alzheimer disease, dementia, frailty, and neurodegenerative progression in Parkinson disease.[2–7] Exercise has been shown to decrease serum levels of C-reactive protein (CRP), a biomarker of inflammation and cardiovascular disease risk. In patients with rheumatoid arthritis, exercise programs have uniformly showed benefit regarding improved functional status, emotional status, and quality of life, with no detrimental effects on disease activity.[8–10]

In asthma, a chronic inflammatory disorder of the airways, exercise is a known precipitant of flares in a subset of patients (ie, exercise-induced asthma). Historically, this triggering mechanism prompted recommendations to avoid physical activity in asthmatic children to avoid exertional dyspnea. However, more recent investigation of training programs to promote physical conditioning in children and adolescents with asthma has revealed opposite findings, suggesting that exercise can be safe and well tolerated in most children with asthma, which may potentially improve overall asthma management as well as associated general health benefits.[11] Although exercise did not change the overall occurrence or degree of exercise-induced asthma, physical conditioning was tolerated with the use of a bronchodilator before exercise, which led to improvements in aerobic fitness, quality of life, and psychological status.

EXERCISE AND INFLAMMATORY BOWEL DISEASE

Despite the known beneficial effects of exercise on quality of life and psychological status, which overlap with treatment goals in the management of IBD, there has been limited investigation regarding the role of exercise in IBD care. One of the first recommendations advocating regular exercise for patients with IBD was published by Ball in 1998.[12] This single-investigator article suggested patients with IBD target 20 to 60 minutes of aerobic activity for 2 to 5 days a week in addition to resistance training at least twice per week.[12] The basis for this recommendation came from an extrapolation of exercise guidelines for the general population with the creation of tailored IBD-specific goals, which included improving overall health, preventing muscle weakening, and helping to improve bone mineral density.

The European Crohn's and Colitis Organization's consensus guidelines regarding the management of Crohn disease and ulcerative colitis have identified a beneficial role for exercise in the symptomatic treatment of axial arthropathy associated with IBD, as well as isotonic exercise in patients suffering from reduced bone density.[13] To date, there have been no formal guidelines regarding specific exercise regimens for patients with IBD that target overall improved health, quality of life, and improved psychological status that have been proposed by consensus panels. The reason for this lack of emphasis is likely the result of limited prospective evidence supporting a beneficial role of exercise in the specific IBD patient population.

Patients with IBD with severe disease activity and/or complications from their illness may find exercise challenging. Extraintestinal manifestations of disease, such as arthralgias/arthritis and the common symptoms of diarrhea, fatigue, and tiredness, can limit the ability of a patient with IBD to exercise. Much of the focus regarding medical management of IBD has been on achieving and maintaining control of gut inflammation, management of bowel symptoms, and surveillance regarding the emergence of dysplasia/neoplastic complications. Guidelines regarding management for both Crohn disease and ulcerative colitis have historically not included recommendations regarding sleep hygiene, diet, and exercise, all of which are essential for optimal health. Even patients with IBD who have achieved remission may experience difficulties with exercise, as recent investigation has demonstrated a diminished capacity for muscle function as compared with healthy controls. Wiroth and colleagues[14] showed that muscle strength and endurance, especially in the lower limbs, were decreased in patients with Crohn disease who were in remission when compared with matched healthy controls. The exact etiologic mechanism for this difference in muscle function is not clear, but appeared to be independent of cumulative glucocorticoid use, disease duration or severity, and presence of current inflammation. Similarly, it was shown that patients with IBD have decreased muscle function peak power and reduced peak oxygen uptake.[15]

EXERCISE AS AN ENVIRONMENTAL FACTOR INFLUENCING THE ETIOPATHOGENESIS OF INFLAMMATORY BOWEL DISEASE

Several environmental factors play a critical role in the development and course of IBD. Cigarette smoking is the best-defined environmental risk factor in IBD; it increases the risk for developing Crohn disease and will worsen the clinical trajectory of patients with established disease.[16] Conversely, cigarette smoking has a diametrically opposite effect in ulcerative colitis, whereby it protects against the development of disease and smoking cessation appears to be a risk for the emergence of disease. Given the common association between cigarette smoking and lack of physical fitness, a possible synergy of these 2 environmental factors may play a role in Crohn disease pathogenesis, but this has not been fully explored.

Several studies have investigated whether pre-illness exercise regimens play a protective role against the development of IBD. The results of earlier studies were inconclusive, but the quality of these studies was problematic, as numerous confounding environmental factors made definitive statements problematic.[17–21] More recent retrospective epidemiologic studies have failed to define a protective or causative relationship between pre-illness exercise regimens and the development of IBD.[22,23] Perhaps the strongest prospective study assessing the impact of physical activity on IBD etiopathogenesis was performed by Khalili and colleagues,[24] which used the Nurses' Health Study cohort. The Nurses' Health Study has tracked 121,700 female nurses from 1976, and the Nurses' Health Study II has tracked 116,00 female nurses from 1989 to prospectively assess risk factors for cancer and cardiovascular disease in women's health. These are the largest epidemiologic cohort studies into risk factors for major chronic disease in women ever conducted, and during 3,421,972 person-years of follow-up, there were 284 incident cases of Crohn disease and 363 cases of ulcerative colitis documented.[24] Comparing women with the highest quintile of physical activity with the lowest quintile demonstrated a 44% reduction (hazard ratio 0.56, 95% confidence interval 0.37–0.84) in the risk of developing Crohn disease compared with women with sedentary lifestyles. Physical activity was not associated with risk of ulcerative colitis. Age, smoking, and body mass index in the cohort did not significantly modify the association between physical activity and the risk of ulcerative colitis or Crohn disease. These investigators concluded that in 2 large prospective cohorts of US women, physical activity was inversely associated with risk of Crohn disease but not ulcerative colitis.[24] The impact of physical fitness on the risk of IBD in young men has been assessed by Melinder[25] in a comprehensive epidemiologic study from Sweden. In a study of 240,984 Swedish military conscripts during late adolescence from 1969 to 1976, 986 individuals developed Crohn disease and 1878 were diagnosed with ulcerative colitis. Stratification of recruits by quintiles of physical fitness demonstrated a protective effect of exercise against the development of both forms of IBD. Low fitness in young men was associated with a raised risk of IBD with unadjusted hazard ratios (and 95% confidence intervals) of 1.62 (1.31–2.00) for Crohn disease and 1.36 (1.17–1.59) for ulcerative colitis. Melinder[25] further evaluated this cohort by adjusting for socioeconomic conditions in childhood, physical fitness, body mass index, and erythrocyte sedimentation rate measured during adolescence and subsequent diagnosis of IBD. When results were attenuated by adjustment for prodromal disease activity, there was a reduction in the hazard ratios to 1.32 (1.05–1.66) for Crohn disease and 1.25 (1.06–1.48) for ulcerative colitis. Melinder[25] concluded that the inverse association of physical fitness with IBD risk is consistent with a protective role for exercise; however, these findings were tempered by the fact that evidence of disease activity before diagnosis was present in adolescence, suggesting that some or all of the associations between fitness and IBD may be due to prodromal disease activity reducing exercise capacity and therefore fitness.

In a recent study, Cook and colleagues[26] sought to characterize mechanisms linking the beneficial effects of exercise and IBD by characterizing the impact of exercise on the gut microbiome. Given the increasing appreciation regarding an altered microbiome/intestinal dysbiosis with the emergence of chronic gut inflammation, these investigators evaluated the effects of moderate exercise on the regulation of intestinal immune function. In a series of studies, Woods and colleagues[27] demonstrated that there are differential effects of exercise that are modulated by the psychological context under which the training is performed. The investigators established that the microbiome differed among mice that were sedentary, those that had access to voluntary wheels, and those that were forced to run on a treadmill, which was paralleled by differential in alterations in gut immune function, cytokine production, and oxyradical generation. It was concluded that exercise results in a change in the microbiome, which may be the reason behind its beneficial role in the treatment and prevention of IBD.[27]

CAN EXERCISE MODULATE CLINICAL COURSE IN INFLAMMATORY BOWEL DISEASE?

Exercise has been shown to improve health-related quality of life in patients with chronic diseases, such rheumatoid arthritis, cancer, heart failure, and depression.[28–32]

In humans, it has been shown that low-intensity to moderate-intensity exercise and physical activity for patients with IBD in remission and those with mild active disease improves quality of life of these patients and helps counteract IBD-related complications, without negatively impacting disease activity.[22]

Studies pertaining to the effect of exercise on IBD were mainly conducted in patients with Crohn disease who were either in remission or had mildly active disease. In one study, patients with Crohn disease remained at their same disease status immediately and 6 months after a single 60-minute session of cycling.[33] The quality of life, stress levels, and body mass index and aerobic capacity of patients with Crohn disease improved significantly after a 3-month walking regimen.[34] Similar results with improvements in psychological and physiologic health were demonstrated when a low-intensity walking intervention was introduced to patients with Crohn disease.[35] A study by Jones and colleagues[36] showed that higher levels of exercise were protective against active disease at 6 months among patients with Crohn disease who were in remission. Although a protective effect was seen among patients with ulcerative colitis, this was not statistically significant.[36] In a different study, however, patients with ulcerative colitis were found to experience improvements in their quality of life without interruption of their disease activity when they were subjected to a 10-week 6-hour training program that was composed of moderate exercise as well as stress management, Mediterranean diet, behavioral techniques, and self-care strategies.[37]

Klare and colleagues[38] conducted a prospective randomized controlled trial examining the effects of a 10-week moderate physical activity program on health-related quality of life in patients with IBD. In this study, patients with mild to moderate IBD were recruited and randomized into an intervention group (supervised moderate-intensity running program 3 times a week) or no intervention. Results demonstrated that patients with moderate severity IBD were able to perform symptom-free regular endurance exercise. Although there was a mean increase in quality of life score between before and after the exercise program, this was not significantly different from the mean increase noted in the control group. There was, however, a significant difference in improvements in the social well-being of patients who were enrolled in the exercise intervention program when compared with the control patients. Patients with Crohn disease who had higher exercise levels were less likely to experience a flare of their IBD at 6 months.[39] Also, those patients who exercised had a better mood, maintained their weight, and had fewer bone mineral disturbances.

Exercise was also found to promote healing in colitis models due to protective myokines released from skeletal muscles.[39] It has been demonstrated that a single bout of moderate-intensity exercise in healthy individuals inhibited monocytic intracellular tumor necrosis factor (TNF) production via beta-2 adrenergic activation. This in turn may protect against conditions associated with low-grade inflammation.[40] Similar to healthy human data, TNF expression was decreased in the intestinal lymphocytes of mice undergoing voluntary exercise training.[41]

Cook and colleagues[42] further examined different exercise training intensities in mice. In this study, mice with dextran sulfate sodium–induced colitis were randomized to a sedentary lifestyle, voluntary wheel running, or moderate forced treadmill running. Mice in the longer duration and more intense forced treadmill running group had exacerbated colitis symptoms, inflammation, and higher cytokine expression, whereas mice in the voluntary wheel-running group attenuated inflammatory gene expression and symptoms.[42]

Similar to animal models, despite the positive effects of exercise on disease course, it is important to know that exercise may lead to increase of proinflammatory cytokine release and in turn transiently exacerbate IBD symptoms.

EXTRAINTESTINAL BENEFITS OF EXERCISE IN INFLAMMATORY BOWEL DISEASE

In addition to promoting good health, exercise may help counteract IBD-related complications, such as improving bone mineral density, immunologic response, psychological health, weight loss, and stress management ability. Exercise and physical activity also may help patients cope with and minimize symptoms related to extraintestinal manifestations of IBD. Further research, however, is needed to make recommendations regarding exercise regimens for patients with IBD.

Bone Health

Approximately 40% of patients with Crohn disease have bone mineral density loss, with some reports reaching up to 80%.[43–53] Metabolic bone disease among patients with IBD is multifactorial and could be related to an individual's age or genetic predisposition, precipitated by the inflammatory disease process itself, use of glucocorticoids, malabsorption, weight loss, and lifestyle changes, such as decreased exercise. The inflammation associated with active IBD contributes to high circulating cytokine levels, such as interleukin-1, interleukin-6, and TNF-α. This increase in cytokines in turn augments the normal bone-remodeling process by increasing osteoclastic and decreasing osteoblastic functions.[43] The resulting reduced bone mineral density is observed in patients with IBD, namely patients with Crohn disease, even before the institution of steroid therapy, indicating that the cytokines play a role in altered bone density independent of steroid use.[54] Additionally, it was shown that bone turnover markers normalized in patients with Crohn disease as early as 8 weeks after treatment with anti–TNF-α therapy, regardless of clinical remission, because of its effect on circulating cytokines.[55] Not only do cytokines alter bone morphology, they have been found to negatively affect muscle mass.[56–59]

In healthy individuals, exercise and physical activity improve bone strength by a "muscle-pull" effect that causes an osteogenic stimulus as the muscles undergo a contraction pull on their bony attachments, resulting in a local deformation.[60,61] Another important mechanism in which exercise promotes bone health is via weight-bearing activities that cause a direct compression and more deformation on the bone that similarly results in an osteogenic stimulus. Studies have shown that muscle mass and bone health go hand-in-hand among healthy patients.[62]

Lee and colleagues[43] reported that patients with Crohn disease benefited from high-impact exercises because of their effect on muscle mass, skeletal health, and osteogenic stimuli, and also because they helped increase patients' body weight. The increased weight in turn increases the mechanical loading during activity and will lead to a positive effect on bone health. In a study by Robinson and colleagues,[63] 117 patients with Crohn disease were randomized to a control group or an intervention group that entailed a 12-month low-impact exercise program. Although bone mineral density increased among the intervention group compared with the control group, this increase was not statistically significant. It is possible that if the exercise was more intense, then a significant difference may be achieved. Despite the results, it is noted that among patients with Crohn disease, exercise and physical activity play an important role in preventing and treating disturbed bone mineral density (osteopenia and osteoporosis) and also result in increased muscle mass and muscle strength.

Ankylosing Spondylitis

Ankylosing spondylitis has been closely linked with IBD. One percent to 8% of patients with IBD develop ankylosing spondylitis, and as many as 18% are found to have asymptomatic sacroiliitis that is incidentally diagnosed on imaging.[64] Studies have shown that exercise plays an important role in improving joint flexibility of patients with ankylosing spondylitis, specifically the spinal column, and that exercise further increases muscle strength and leads to less joint pain.[65–67]

Psychological Benefit of Exercise

Exercise has been shown to help in stress reduction, which subsequently positively impacts IBD symptoms and overall quality of life.[68,69] Different exercises have been investigated, including walking, running, swimming, and yoga, all of which have had a significant impact on stress reduction. Stress itself is a trigger for active disease, so elimination and minimization of stress may play a role in prolonging periods of disease remission among patients with IBD. Stress reduction also decreases symptoms of anxiety and leads to improved quality of life.[70]

Immune Response

Low-intensity and moderate-intensity exercise has been shown to improve the immune system.[71] High-intensity exercises and prolonged periods of exercise, however, tend to negatively impact the immune system. By exercising in moderation, an individual's immune system is naturally boosted, subsequently leading to a "healthier" body.

Maintaining Normal Weight

In the past, patients with IBD were thought to be underweight and cachectic; however, more recently, with the obesity epidemic, up to 40% of patients with IBD are found to be obese.[72] Obesity is a proinflammatory state, and exercise helps individuals lose weight that in turn aids in the reduction of proinflammatory cytokines that are associated with obesity. Seminerio and colleagues[73] showed that obesity was more commonly encountered among patients with ulcerative colitis rather than patients with Crohn disease. Additionally, obese patients were found to have comorbid conditions, such as diabetes mellitus, hypertension, and hyperlipidemia, and these patients had a poor quality of life and elevated biochemical inflammatory markers (CRP). The poor quality of life and elevated CRP, however, were not independently correlated with obesity.[73] Additionally in that study, obesity was not found to be a predictor of high health care utilization. Results of the study by Seminerio and colleagues[73] were different from prior literature that demonstrated that obese patients with Crohn disease had higher hospitalization rates than normal-weight patients with Crohn disease.[74] Older literature demonstrated that obese patients with Crohn disease were more likely to have anoperineal complications within a shorter time frame, require surgery within a shorter time frame, and had higher instances of active disease.[74,75] Similarly, poor outcomes were noted among obese patients with ulcerative colitis, especially in terms of worse surgical outcomes with higher chance of pelvic sepsis and perioperative morbidity when compared with nonobese patients with ulcerative colitis.[76] The effect of obesity on IBD medications has not been clearly investigated, but it has been noted that obese patients have rapid clearance of biologic agents and, as a result, have suboptimal response to therapy. Exercise helps obese patients reach their ideal weight, thus limiting complications from the obesity, decreasing the proinflammatory state, and also improving response to therapy, particularly biologic therapy.

SUMMARY

Regular exercise is essential for maintaining a healthy lifestyle, improving physical endurance, preventing frailty, and improving quality of life and psychological status. There is a growing appreciation that regular exercise regimens are essential for patients suffering from chronic inflammatory disorders, including IBD. Although data are limited, an emerging signal suggests that regular exercise early in life may help to prevent the development of Crohn disease. Mechanistic studies suggest benefits of moderate exercise on both mucosal immune function and maintaining a healthy gut microbiome. Maintaining a regular exercise regimen also may exert a beneficial modifying effect on disease course, improving inflammatory parameters, psychological status, and quality of life in patients with IBD.

REFERENCES

1. Available at: https://health.gov/paguidelines/guidelines/adults.aspx. Accessed June 14, 2017.
2. Goodwin VA, Richards SH, Taylor RS, et al. The effectiveness of exercise interventions for people with Parkinson's disease: a systematic review and meta-analysis. Mov Disord 2008;23(5):631-40.
3. Crizzle AM, Newhouse IJ. Is physical exercise beneficial for persons with Parkinson's disease? Clin J Sport Med 2006;16(5):422-5.
4. Earhart GM, Falvo MJ. Parkinson disease and exercise. Compr Physiol 2013;3(2): 833-48.
5. Lautenschlager NT, Cox KL, Flicker L, et al. Older adults at risk for Alzheimer disease: a randomized trial. JAMA 2008;300(9):1027-37.
6. Rolland Y, Pillard F, Klapouszczak A, et al. Exercise program for nursing home residents with Alzheimer's disease: a 1-year randomized, controlled trial. J Am Geriatr Soc 2007;55(2):158-65.
7. Taylor RS, Brown A, Ebrahim S, et al. Exercise-based rehabilitation for patients with coronary heart disease: systematic review and meta-analysis of randomized controlled trials. Am J Med 2004;116(10):682-92.
8. Minor MA, Hewett JE, Webel RR, et al. Efficacy of physical conditioning exercise in patients with rheumatoid arthritis and osteoarthritis. Arthritis Rheum 1989; 32(11):1396-405.
9. de Jong Z, Munneke M, Zwinderman AH, et al. Is a long-term high-intensity exercise program effective and safe in patients with rheumatoid arthritis? Results of a randomized controlled trial. Arthritis Rheum 2003;48(9):2415-24.
10. Stenström CH, Minor MA. Evidence for the benefit of aerobic and strengthening exercise in rheumatoid arthritis. Arthritis Rheum 2003;49(3):428-34.
11. Lucas SR, Platts-Mills TA. Physical activity and exercise in asthma: relevance to etiology and treatment. J Allergy Clin Immunol 2005;115(5):928-34.
12. Ball E. Exercise guidelines for patients with inflammatory bowel disease. Gastroenterol Nurs 1998;21:108-11.
13. Harbord M, Annese V, Vavricka SR, et al. The first European evidence-based consensus on extra-intestinal manifestations in inflammatory bowel disease. J Crohns Colitis 2016;10:239-54.
14. Wiroth JB, Filippi J, Schneider SM, et al. Muscle performance in patients with Crohn's disease in clinical remission. Inflamm Bowel Dis 2005;11:296-303.
15. Ploeger HE, Takken T, Wilk B, et al. Exercise capacity in pediatric patients with inflammatory bowel disease. J Pediatr 2011;158:814-9.
16. Cosnes J. Smoking, physical activity, nutrition and lifestyle: environmental factors and their impact on IBD. Dig Dis 2010;28:411-7.
17. Marri SR, Buchman AL. The education and employment status of patients with inflammatory bowel diseases. Inflamm Bowel Dis 2005;11:171-7.

18. Sonnenberg A. Occupational distribution of inflammatory bowel disease among German employees. Gut 1990;31:1037–40.
19. Persson P-G, Leijonmarck CE, Bernell O, et al. Risk indicators for inflammatory bowel disease. Int J Epidemiol 1993;22:268–72.
20. Boggild H, Tuchsen F, Orhede E. Occupation, employment status and chronic inflammatory bowel disease in Denmark. Int J Epidemiol 1996;25:630–7.
21. Klein I, Reif S, Farbstein H, et al. Preillness non dietary factors and habits in inflammatory bowel disease. Ital J Gastroenterol Hepatol 1998;30:247–51.
22. Narula N, Fedorak RN. Exercise and inflammatory bowel disease. Can J Gastroenterol 2008;22(5):497–504.
23. Halfvarson J, Jess T, Magnuson A, et al. Environmental factors in inflammatory bowel disease: a co-twin control study of a Swedish-Danish twin population. Inflamm Bowel Dis 2006;12:925–33.
24. Khalili H, Ananthakrishnan AN, Konijeti GG, et al. Physical activity and risk of inflammatory bowel disease: a prospective study from the Nurses' Health Study cohorts. BMJ 2013;347:f6633.
25. Melinder C. Physical fitness in adolescence and subsequent inflammatory bowel disease risk. Clin Transl Gastroenterol 2015;6:e121.
26. Cook MD, Allen JM, Pence BD, et al. Exercise and gut immune function: evidence of alterations in colon immune cell homeostasis and microbiome characteristics with exercise training. Immunol Cell Biol 2016;94(2):158–63.
27. Woods JA, Allen JM, Berg Miller ME, et al. Exercise alters the gut microbiome and microbial metabolites: implications for colorectal cancer and inflammatory bowel disease. Abstracts/Brain, Behavior, and Immunity 2015;49:e1–50.
28. Zou LY, Yang L, He XL, et al. Effects of aerobic exercise on cancer-related fatigue in breast cancer patients receiving chemotherapy: a meta-analysis. Tumour Biol 2014;35:5659–67.
29. Courneya KS, Segal RJ, Mackey JR, et al. Effects of exercise dose and type on sleep quality in breast cancer patients receiving chemotherapy: a multicenter randomized trial. Breast Cancer Res Treat 2014;144:361–9.
30. Pina IL, Apstein CS, Balady GJ, et al. Exercise and heart failure: a statement from the American Heart Association Committee on Exercise, Rehabilitation, and Prevention. Circulation 2003;107:1210–25.
31. Edemann F, Gelbrich G, Dungen HD, et al. Exercise training improves exercise capacity and diastolic function in patients with preserved ejection fraction: results of the Ex-DHF (Exercise training in Diastolic Heart Failure) pilot study. J Am Coll Cardiol 2011;58:1780–91.
32. Cooney GM, Dwan K, Greig CA, et al. Exercise for depression. Cochrane Database Syst Rev 2013;(9):CD004366.
33. D'Inca R, Varnier M, Mestriner C, et al. Effect of moderate exercise on Crohn's disease patients in remission. Ital J Gastroenterol Hepatol 1999;31:205–10.
34. Loudon CP, Carroll V, Butcher J, et al. The effects of physical exercise on patients with Crohn's disease. Am J Gastroenterol 1999;94:697–703.
35. Ng V, Millard W, Lebrun C, et al. Low-intensity exercise improves quality of life in patients with Crohn's disease. Clin J Sport Med 2007;17:384–8.
36. Jones PD, Kappelman MD, Martin CF, et al. Exercise decreases risk of future active disease in inflammatory bowel disease patients in remission. Inflamm Bowel Dis 2015;21(5):1063–71.
37. Elsenbruch S, Langhorst J, Popkirowa K, et al. Effects of mind-body therapy on quality of life and neuroendocrine and cellular immune functions in patients with ulcerative colitis. Psychother Psychosom 2005;74:277–87.

38. Klare P, Nigg J, Nold J, et al. The impact of a ten-week physical exercise program on health-related quality of life in patients with inflammatory bowel disease: a prospective randomized controlled trial. Digestion 2015;91:239–47.

39. Bilski J, Mazur-Bialy A, Brzozowski B, et al. Can exercise affect the clinical course of inflammatory bowel disease? Experimental and clinical evidence. Pharmacol Rep 2016;68(4):827–36.

40. Dimitrov S, Hulteng E, Hong S. Inflammation and exercise: inhibition of monocytic intracellular TNF production by acute exercise via b2-adrenergic activation. Brain Behav Immun 2017;61:60–8.

41. Hoffman-Goetz L, Pervaiz N, Guan J. Voluntary exercise training in mice increases the expression of antioxidant enzymes and decreases the expression of TNF-a in intestinal lymphocytes. Brain Behav Immun 2009;23:498–506.

42. Cook MD, Martin SA, Williams C, et al. Forced treadmill exercise training exacerbates inflammation and causes mortality while voluntary wheel training is protective in a mouse model of colitis. Brain Behav Immun 2013;33:46–56.

43. Lee N, Radford-Smith G, Taaffee DR. Bone loss in Crohn's disease: exercise as a potential countermeasure. Inflamm Bowel Dis 2005;11:1108–18.

44. Ardizzone S, Bollani S, Bettica P, et al. Altered bone metabolism in inflammatory bowel disease: there is a difference between CD and ulcerative colitis. J Intern Med 2000;247:63–70.

45. Habtezion A, Silverberg MS, Parkes R, et al. Risk factors for low bone density in CD. Inflamm Bowel Dis 2002;8:87–92.

46. Robinson RJ, al-Azzawi F, Iqbal SJ, et al. Osteoporosis and determinants of bone density in patients with CD. Dig Dis Sci 1998;43:2500–6.

47. Dinca M, Fries W, Luisetto G, et al. Evolution of osteopenia in inflammatory bowel disease. Am J Gastroenterol 1999;94:1292–7.

48. Jahnsen J, Falch JA, Aadland E, et al. Bone mineral density is reduced in patients with CD but not in patients with ulcerative colitis: a population based study. Gut 1997;40:313–9.

49. Bjarnason I, Macpherson A, Mackintosh C, et al. Reduced bone density in patients with inflammatory bowel disease. Gut 1997;40:228–33.

50. Staun M, Tjellesen L, Thale M, et al. Bone mineral content in patients with CD. A longitudinal study in patients with bowel resections. Scand J Gastroenterol 1997; 32:226–32.

51. Pigot F, Roux C, Chaussade S, et al. Low bone mineral density in patients with inflammatory bowel disease. Dig Dis Sci 1992;37:1396–403.

52. Schoon EJ, van Nunen AB, Wouters RS, et al. Osteopenia and osteoporosis in CD: prevalence in a Dutch population-based cohort. Scand J Gastroenterol Suppl 2000;232:43–7.

53. Schulte C, Dignass AU, Mann K, et al. Reduced bone mineral density and unbalanced bone metabolism in patients with inflammatory bowel disease. Inflamm Bowel Dis 1998;4:268–75.

54. Ghosh S, Cowen S, Hannan WJ, et al. Low bone mineral density in CD, but not in ulcerative colitis, at diagnosis. Gastroenterology 1994;107:1031–9.

55. Franchimont NPV, Collette J, Vermiere S, et al. Rapid improvement of bone metabolism after infliximab treatment in CD. Aliment Pharmacol Ther 2004;20:607–14.

56. Visser M, Pahor M, Taaffe DR, et al. Relationship of interleukin-6 and tumor necrosis factor-alpha with muscle mass and muscle strength in elderly men and women: the Health ABC Study. J Gerontol A Biol Sci Med Sci 2002;57:M326–32.

57. Roubenoff R, Roubenoff RA, Cannon JG, et al. Rheumatoid cachexia: cytokine-driven hypermetabolism accompanying reduced body cell mass in chronic inflammation. J Clin Invest 1994;93:2379–86.
58. Schols AM, Buurman WA, Staal van den Brekel AJ, et al. Evidence for a relation between metabolic derangements and increased levels of inflammatory mediators in a subgroup of patients with chronic obstructive pulmonary disease. Thorax 1996;51:819–24.
59. Anker SD, Ponikowski PP, Clark AL, et al. Cytokines and neurohormones relating to body composition alterations in the wasting syndrome of chronic heart failure. Eur Heart J 1999;20:683–93.
60. Frost HM. On our age-related bone loss: insights from a new paradigm. J Bone Miner Res 1997;12:1539–46.
61. Frost HM. Muscle, bone, and the Utah paradigm: a 1999 overview. Med Sci Sports Exerc 2000;32:911–7.
62. Burr DB. Muscle strength, bone mass, and age-related bone loss. J Bone Miner Res 1997;12:1547–51.
63. Robinson RJ, Krzywicki T, Almond L, et al. Effect of a low-impact exercise program on bone mineral density in CD: a randomized controlled trial. Gastroenterology 1998;115:36–41.
64. Bernstein CN, Blanchard JF, Rawsthorne P, et al. The prevalence of extraintestinal diseases in inflammatory bowel disease: a population-based study. Am J Gastroenterol 2001;96:1116–22.
65. Ince G, Arpel T, Durgun B, et al. Effects of multimodal exercise program for people with ankylosing spondylitis. Phys Ther 2006;86:924–35.
66. Lim HJ, Moon YI, Lee MS. Effects of home-based daily exercise therapy on joint mobility, daily activity, pain, and depression in patients with ankylosing spondylitis. Rheumatol Int 2005;25:225–9.
67. Fernandez-de-Las-Penas C, Alonso-Blanco C, Alguacil-Diego IM, et al. One-year follow-up of two exercise interventions for the management of patients with ankylosing spondylitis: a randomized controlled trial. Am J Phys Med Rehabil 2006;85:559–67.
68. Lykouras D, Karkoulias K, Triantosb C. Physical exercise in patients with inflammatory bowel disease. J Crohns Colitis 2017;11(8):1024.
69. Brown JD. Staying fit and staying well: physical fitness as a moderator of life stress. J Pers Soc Psychol 1991;60:555–61.
70. DiLorenzo TM, Bargman EP, Stucky-Ropp R, et al. Long-term effects of aerobic exercise on psychological outcomes. Prev Med 1999;28:75–85.
71. Brolinson PG, Elliott D. Exercise and immune system. Clin Sports Med 2007;26:311–9.
72. Singh S, Dulai PS, Zarrinpar A, et al. Obesity in IBD: epidemiology, pathogenesis, disease course and treatment outcomes. Nat Rev Gastroenterol Hepatol 2017;14(2):110–21.
73. Seminerio JL, Koutroubakis IE, Ramos-Rivers C, et al. Impact of obesity on the management and clinical course of patients with inflammatory bowel disease. Inflamm Bowel Dis 2015;21(12):2857–63.
74. Blain A, Cattan S, Beaugerie L, et al. Crohn's disease clinical course and severity in obese patients. Clin Nutr 2002;21:51–7.
75. Hass DJ, Brensinger CM, Lewis JD, et al. The impact of increased body mass index on the clinical course of Crohn's disease. Clin Gastroenterol Hepatol 2006;4:482–8.
76. Efron JE, Uriburu JP, Wexner SD, et al. Restorative proctocolectomy with ileal pouch anal anastomosis in obese patients. Obes Surg 2001;11:246–51.

The Practical Pros and Cons of Complementary and Alternative Medicine in Practice

CrossMark

Integrating Complementary and Alternative Medicine into Clinical Care

Rachel W. Winter, MD, MPH, Joshua R. Korzenik, MD*

KEYWORDS

- Complementary and alternative medicine • Inflammatory bowel disease
- Psychosocial care • Health care delivery • CAM safety and efficacy

KEY POINTS

- Complementary and alternative medicine (CAM) has its limitations with regard to the need for better and more robust data, particularly because most studies in CAM for inflammatory bowel disease (IBD) are small, short-term, and do not address drug interactions with IBD medications.
- IBD care is gradually expanding to address other concerns that can affect health outcomes, including diet, psychosocial care, exercise, stress management, and sleep, among other areas.
- A movement toward increased patient autonomy is driving many of the choices of medications and other approaches to include CAM as an option for disease management.
- Physicians should expand their knowledge in CAM to be able to fully address their patients' needs and expectations.

The widespread use of complementary and alternative medicine (CAM) relies on an expectation or belief that the conventional calculus of risk and benefit used to select most standard medications, whether an anti-tumor necrosis factor (anti-TNF) agent or mesalamine, can be tilted toward the same or greater benefit with less risk through nonconventional approaches. CAM therapies may also rely on different theories of health and possibly a different conception of care that incorporates a more inclusive

Disclosure Statement: The authors have no disclosures to report.
Division of Gastroenterology, Hepatology and Nutrition, Brigham and Women's Hospital, Crohn's and Colitis Center, Harvard Medical School, 850 Boylston Street, Chestnut Hill, Boston, MA 02467, USA
* Corresponding author.
E-mail address: jkorzenik@bwh.harvard.edu

Gastroenterol Clin N Am 46 (2017) 907–916
http://dx.doi.org/10.1016/j.gtc.2017.08.013
0889-8553/17/© 2017 Elsevier Inc. All rights reserved.

or holistic set of concerns. This article discusses a broad overview of the promise and limitations of CAM with regard to the philosophic issues and their practical use, as well as more far reaching implications that CAM embodies in terms of delivery of care for people with inflammatory bowel disease (IBD). Although the promise is great, and CAM has been embraced by many patients and providers, the barriers to successful use are considerable and need to be well understood.

Patients with IBD and their providers are often frustrated with available medications due to concerns about adverse events or because of inadequate efficacy. The alternatives offered by CAM may answer these needs. However, a difficulty with many CAM studies and approaches is that the data are often promising but weak. The large methodologically rigorous multicenter randomized controlled trials (RCTs), which are the gold standard for trials registered with the US Food and Drug Administration (FDA), do not have a counterpart in CAM trials. Some of the therapies, such as an herbal preparation, should be able to be studied with similar clinical trials methods as a new potential biologic for IBD, whereas other interventions, such as Reiki, dietary interventions, or energy healing, would require less conventional clinical trial designs. In addition, most of the published trials relied on to support the use of CAM are small, single-center studies. When the applicability of large multicenter studies to a particular subject cohort is assessed, the relevance of even these large trials is often tenuous.[1] Few CAM trials are followed up with larger multicenter studies with rigorous endpoints and most do not meet accepted research standards. Longer term use of these CAM therapies in IBD is also not frequently studied and extrapolation from short-term trials is relied on. The safety of many of these approaches is not entirely known.

Even with development and growth of funding through governmental support, such as the National Center for Complementary and Integrative Health, the grants available for CAM are dwarfed by the costs shouldered by large pharmaceutical companies for a phase 3 program in IBD. Government funding for complementary and integrative health in IBD in particular has been limited and has focused more on small but promising pilot studies.[2,3] Furthermore, the funding for the development of alternative approaches has not been a priority in the larger pharmaceutical industry approaches, though some areas, such as microbial-based therapeutic and potential probiotics, are receiving considerable industry support.

A further issue is that negative larger trial results might be ignored in clinical practice if smaller studies are positive. A medication example is the use of omega-3 or fish oil fatty acids in Crohn disease. A small high-profile study was positive for maintenance of remission with only 39 subjects in the fish oil group and a similarly sized placebo group.[4] Two larger trials with 188 and 189 subjects in active treatment and parallel placebo groups were negative but this therapy is still widely used.[5] Although a case can still be made for the use of fish oil, the data are certainly contradictory. Other interventions, such as the specific carbohydrate diet, are tried widely in IBD despite the lack of RCTs among the IBD patient population. Although some patients report a benefit and open-labeled series have been published, robust data are lacking.[6,7] A more difficult question is what level of data should be required to determine efficacy of these therapies and to influence real-world decisions. Limited data and inadequate trials make it difficult for patients to select, or for practitioners to recommend, a specific diet for IBD, and often decisions are made based on guidance from anecdotes or open-labeled series. Furthermore, the increasing awareness of limitations of RCTs and the growth of patient-shared data through networks such as http://www.patientslikeme.com and www.crohnology.com offer alternative sources of data to guide choices.

If an approach is deemed very safe, the level of supportive data required to prove its efficacy might arguably be less, particularly if the therapy is being added to other medications and is not relied on as sole therapy. However, although likely safe, the absence of larger trials in IBD, even for herbal therapies, raises an important concern. Herbal therapies are not regulated by the FDA and some may have alternative side effects, such as liver toxicity. For those supplements shown to be safe in other diseases or for other indications, it is uncertain whether the safety profile translates to IBD. For example, curcumin, possibly the best researched of any herbal therapies, with more than 10,000 citations in PubMed, has only a small number of studies that are RCTs in humans, and only a few in IBD. Long-term trials in IBD are lacking. With so few studies and without long-term trials, it is often difficult to determine an accurate assessment of safety or efficacy for this supplement, as well as others. In addition, recommending these therapies to subpopulations of patients, such as pregnant or breastfeeding women or children, can pose additional challenges. There are often limited data in these patient subgroups for widely used conventional medications, less for CAM approaches, and even less in herbal therapies and the IBD patient. Because herbal medications are not regulated, interactions of supplements with prescribed medications are inadequately studied as well.

DOES COMPLEMENTARY AND ALTERNATIVE MEDICINE IMPLY A DIFFERENT APPROACH TO INFLAMMATORY BOWEL DISEASE CARE?

The prodigious amount of information and clinical guidance in articles elsewhere in this issue provide a thorough review of alternate approaches to care for IBD patients. Many therapies or approaches that started out in an alternative realm have been eventually adopted by conventional medicine after publication of additional studies and supportive data. Acupuncture is a prime example of CAM that has been embraced widely in the medical field. Probiotics and fecal transplants are rapidly being included as standard of care, even if the data supportive of specific probiotics are still lacking in IBD. Curcumin, for which data is perhaps most supportive of a benefit, could easily be adopted into this model and widely used in treating patients with IBD.

An herbal therapy may more easily fit into the prevailing biologic paradigm of using a medication to treat a particular biochemical pathway to reduce inflammation and symptoms. Even if an alternative medication, whether complementary or as a possible replacement for another conventional immunosuppressant, such as curcumin, may have effects that reduce TNF levels. However, many of the therapies discussed in this issue, such as mindfulness or acupuncture, imply a different conception of disease and of restoring health. Even within pathophysiology, the care model for patients with IBD might be adapted to meet other needs that affect patient outcomes. The implications for care of the IBD patient are that there are a broader set of concerns that should be included in addressing a patient's health care. The ideas presented in this issue focusing on diet, exercise, psychosocial care, and other aspects of health implicitly endorse a different model of care in which physicians and patients are involved in discussing an extended set of topics to treat disease, in addition to conventional therapy.

Developing a model of care that incorporates many of these approaches is a substantial challenge and requires a team of motivated individuals. Furthermore, there are many ways of bringing these ideas together. This article reviews several approaches that are being developed and trialed. Although the quality improvement model can certainly address several of these areas, these efforts, at least initially, have focused particularly on process measures and how to deliver optimally what is considered conventional and standard care. In addition to those models for improving patient outcomes, efforts are being undertaken at many sites around the country to develop a model of health care that promotes slightly different goals and a shift in patient involvement.

THE IMPORTANCE OF A COMPREHENSIVE APPROACH

The older model of care, which has dominated until recently, has viewed the physician as the high priest, with the interaction between the physician and the patient focused on obtaining information for appropriate testing or treatment. This model has been rapidly evolving to include other elements critical to health. Although CAM does not necessarily imply a wholesale change in how medical care is conceived and delivered, it may involve a shift in care. With expansion of the conception of care to be more holistic, the physician becomes integrated into a broader team, which coordinates a set of other practitioners.

Several other issues, especially psychosocial issues, may affect how a patient perceives her or his illness or may contribute to morbidity from that illness. Depression and anxiety are prevalent among patients with IBD and have been shown to increase significantly during relapse of disease. Depression is twice as prevalent in the IBD population compared with the general population.[8] Mikocka-Walus and colleagues[9] showed baseline rates of 29% to 35% of anxiety and depression among subjects with IBD during remission and increased rates during relapse. Of these, 80% of patients reported anxiety and 60% reported depression during relapse. Similarly, studies from the Nurses' Health Study reported that women with recent depression symptoms had an increased risk of subsequent diagnosis of Crohn disease and a retrospective study also showed that psychosocial issues, such as depression and anxiety, are also common reasons for hospitalization among patients with IBD and that disease severity is not the only significant factor affecting rates of hospitalization (Brigham and Women's Hospital study).[10,11] Addressing these issues, in addition to treating intestinal inflammation, is critical in caring for a patient with IBD. Knowing this information, how can clinicians successfully integrate addressing psychosocial issues into the care plan for patients with IBD?

WHAT MODELS EXIST FOR INTEGRATION?

Although many recognize the importance of providing comprehensive care to patients with IBD, integrating CAM into an allopathic medical practice can be challenging. This article discusses a few models currently being explored at centers around the world.

Two models at IBD centers in the United States have been shown to effectively incorporate psychosocial services into the IBD clinic experience. These models differ in their infrastructure but both aim to create a comprehensive program, including medical care, social work, and psychiatric care.

At the University of Pittsburgh, the IBD Specialty Medical Home has been created. This model is a patient-centered model designed to optimize medical, surgical, and psychiatric care of a patient, and to decrease the burden of multiple appointments with various providers on different days.[12] The University of Pittsburgh has created a unique model that integrates visits for medical therapy for IBD with visits that address additional needs specific to patients with IBD, including a focus on how stress, anxiety, depression, and pain can exacerbate symptoms of IBD, and the role nutrition plays in IBD. This model, which was designed in collaboration with the University of Pittsburgh Medical Center health plan, has resulted in improved adherence to medications, increased quality of life of patients, and decreases in unnecessary use of health care.[12]

At Brigham and Women's Hospital, the CIRCLE program was recently initiated. This program is a comprehensive program with expertise from an IBD social worker, psychiatrist, nutritionist, IBD nurse educator, and stress management nurse practitioner, in addition to the medical caregivers. Like the medical home, this program was initially designed for patients identified as high-end users. The lead social worker works with the physicians, patient, and CIRCLE team to design an individual program catered to each patient's specific needs and interests. Although this program is fairly new, preliminary data have shown it to be effective in reducing rates of hospitalization, as well as decreasing depression and anxiety scores among patients with these diagnoses.[11]

Preliminary data from these programs have shown them to be effective in both addressing psychosocial needs of patients and increasing quality of life. However, integrating alternative medicine into a traditional medically focused clinic can be challenging and may not always be feasible. In addition, there are often services from which patients may greatly benefit, such as tai chi, acupuncture, and so forth, that cannot be integrated in the physical space at a medical clinic. At many institutions, separate centers have been established to offer alternative medicine methods. In Boston, Massachusetts, centers focusing on CAM have been established at both Brigham and Women's Hospital and Massachusetts General Hospital. The IBD centers in Boston often work closely with these centers to provide additional services for patients and to create a comprehensive program to address their disease and needs.

The Osher Center for Integrative Medicine at Harvard Medical School and Brigham and Women's Hospital offers a variety of services, including acupuncture, chiropractic care, therapeutic massage, and programs in mindfulness-based stress reduction, tai chi, and yoga. Researchers at the Osher Center have shown the benefit of an integrative medicine program among patients with low back pain, showing a decrease in pain and symptom bothersomeness, in addition to improved functional status, among patients who participated in the program.[13] Anecdotally, similar results have been seen among the authors' patients who have been referred to the center. The Benson-Henry Institute for Mind Body Medicine at Massachusetts General Hospital has similar program offerings, including a stress management and resiliency program, mind-body programs, tai chi, and yoga. Research at the Benson-Henry Institute has shown a dramatic decrease in health care use among patients who complete a Relaxation Response Resiliency Program.[14]

In Europe, centers that have more extensive integration of alternative approaches and practices for IBD care have been developed, including The Center for Integrative Gastroenterology, Kliniken Essen-Mitte, and the Integrative and Internal Medicine Chair at the University of Duisburg-Essen. The Essen-Mitte Clinic is a well-established clinic and rated as one of the best in the country that offers integrative care for IBDs. The treatment concept for IBD patients encompasses a 14-day stay on site in which patients are assessed and an individual, multimodal treatment concept is worked up, which is covered completely by all health insurance companies in Germany. The department has 54 inpatient beds, 12 of which are dedicated to gastroenterology. In addition, an associated large outpatient clinic provides continuity of care with these alternative approaches. The center provides comprehensive diagnostic facilities for IBD with a special research focus in noninvasive diagnostic procedures. Even though the Kliniken Essen-Mitte is not a part of the university hospital campus, they are adjacent to the university hospital and care is integrated. The Essen unit is heavily focused on research in cooperation with the university hospital with productive research inclusive of yoga, leeches, and Ayurveda, among others.[15,16]

The general therapeutic concept includes a variety of options, from inpatient treatment to outpatient care, as well as a semiresidential daycare clinic to facilitate lifestyle modifications to support health and well-being. A lifestyle modification program was implemented more than 14 years ago and has evolved since its inception. The study center was chosen for its diverse experience of recruiting subjects to diagnostic and clinical studies and its established research infrastructure. The center has published more than 50 trials to date, recruiting thousands of subjects. It is well-equipped, with a study coordinator, study physicians, a medical technical assistant, a study nurse, and several research fellows, as well as doctoral candidates, and it is experienced in conducting self-initiated, funded, or commissioned research. The department is well-connected to and well-respected within the IBD community, and strongly connected to its related self-help organizations. It has an exceptional reputation within integrative medicine and extensive experience in studying diagnostic tools in IBD, various pharmacologic treatments, and the effects of lifestyle interventions, offering it routinely to both inpatients and outpatients. This unique program in IBD has the support of insurance companies, enabling it to be independent and successful.

WHAT ARE THE CHALLENGES IN INTEGRATING COMPLEMENTARY AND ALTERNATIVE MEDICINE?

The practical use of CAM in an individual has its own limitations. This interest in CAM is partly driven as a consumer movement, fueled by increasing access to information through the Internet. Few insurance companies are willing to cover the costs of CAM approaches. The profile of individuals interested in using CAM tends to be predominantly female, more educated, and living in cities. Whether users of CAM consist of a wealthier group of individuals is less clear but certainly the lack of insurance support means those who use CAM must have the ability to absorb the costs. With the increasing use of CAM and research showing its benefits not only on health but also on overall cost of care, insurance support for these therapies may change. Some states, such as Washington State, have mandated reimbursement of CAM practitioners.[17] In addition, many insurance plans or health maintenance organization groups are beginning to include CAM in their available resources. However, until there is additional support for CAM, cost and reimbursement remain an issue.

Further barriers include the lack of knowledge and awareness among health care providers. Additional barriers to integrating CAM in a traditional medical practice include

1. Patients may see CAM as an alternative to conventional medicine rather than adjunctive therapy.

    Alternative therapy has the potential to greatly improve the quality of life and decrease morbidity among patients with IBD, and there are emerging data that some supplements, such as curcumin, may help to treat inflammation.[18,19] However, CAM should not be seen as a substitute for conventional medical therapy for IBD but rather as adjunctive therapy. In one study, subjects who used CAM for IBD were shown to have lower rates of adherence to medical therapy.[20] It is very likely that these alternatives to conventional medical therapy can improve quality of life and decrease disease morbidity, but they should complement, and be used in conjunction with, medical therapy. By discussing these therapies with patients, referring them to affiliated CAM centers and promoting their use, it is likely that adherence to both conventional and alternative therapy can increase, resulting in greater overall results for patients and for the health care system.

2. Cost.

    As previously mentioned, currently, there is limited, if any, insurance coverage for CAM. Participation in programs or use of CAM can come at a great cost to patients and may not be financially feasible for many patients. Supplements, such as turmeric, vitamins, and other supplements, can be expensive, especially if recommended for long-term therapy. In addition, CAM can be time-consuming. Classes such as yoga and tai chi, and appointments with social workers, nutritionists, and stress management specialists, require time to be set aside by patients to attend these sessions. However, there may be a tradeoff because there may be a shift in how patients use their time. If participation in CAM reduces their health care use, patients may spend more time attending CAM appointments but less time at other clinic appointments, emergency department visits, and in the hospital as an inpatient. In addition, as technology improves and programs are developed to provide at home services, including video visits, online programs, and apps, the time patients spend at appointments may be further decreased, enabling them to participate in programs at their convenience.

3. Insufficient data.

The data supporting the use of CAM are limited. Most studies are small or uncontrolled, which can make it more difficult to prove their efficacy. Additionally, larger studies sometimes conflict with smaller studies and it is difficult to perform RCTs in CAM. Many of the therapies or programs are not regulated or standardized, making larger studies more challenging. Although there are few adverse side effects of CAM, participating in programs or attending classes can be time-consuming. There are few risks to taking additional vitamins, though the FDA does not regulate vitamins and herbs, and thus there is always slight uncertainly regarding the ingredients of a product. A lack of data showing the efficacy of CAM may make it more challenging for care providers to strongly advocate its use.

4. Physician knowledge about and comfort with CAM.

Physicians are rarely the source informing patients about CAM. When patients who use CAM, whether for general health or specifically for IBD, were polled, most did not hear about CAM from their providers but rather from friends, a naturopath, or the Internet.[20] Traditionally, medical training has not included education on alternative medicine. Although some medical schools are now incorporating classes to educate students about CAM or recommending that students try tai chi, yoga and massage therapy, among others, a physician's knowledge of CAM may be limited and generated mostly from his or her own personal experience or from anecdotes from patients. As a result, physicians may not be comfortable discussing therapies with which they are not familiar and they may not recommend treatments that are not substantiated by RCTs or large studies. Although some hospitals have affiliated centers for CAM, many gastroenterologists may not be aware of their services or may not work at a practice that is associated with a CAM center, making the recommendation and referral process more difficult. In addition, although physicians may be knowledgeable regarding certain subsets of CAM, such as dietary recommendations for patients with IBD, their comfort level with other therapies may not be as extensive. More alternative approaches, such as energy healing, are even further outside the realm of most practitioners and less likely to be brought into a discussion.

5. Transparency.

Care providers may be hesitant to discuss CAM therapies about which they are less familiar. Also, inquiry about use of CAM among patients may not be in a provider's common repertoire of questions. Similarly, patients may be reluctant to initiate conversation about or to discuss their use of alternative approaches to therapy because of a perception of disapproval from their physician. A patient may perceive a physician's lack of discussion about alternative treatment in IBD as disapproval of CAM. Patients also may not share their use of CAM if not directly asked because they may not recognize the role of CAM in treating their IBD, may not remember to mention it, or may be uncertain about their care provider's opinion regarding their use of CAM.

WHAT ARE THE BENEFITS OF INTEGRATING COMPLEMENTARY AND ALTERNATIVE MEDICINE?

Despite potential roadblocks in proving efficacy of various CAM therapies, referring patients, and advocating for the use of CAM and/or cost of services or supplements not covered by insurance, there are many benefits to CAM. Patients who are enrolled in comprehensive programs at IBD centers have reported better quality of life and decreased health care costs. Similar results have been seen when studying the patient population at integrative medicine centers. Additional advantages of integration of CAM with conventional therapy include

1. Better overall health for patients

   Although the data are limited, small studies have shown benefit in integrating CAM, both with regard to quality of life and health care use. One small study of 48 subjects, 29 of whom had a diagnosis of IBD, showed improvement in quality of life and alterations in gene expression after participating in a 9-week relaxation response–based, mind-body group intervention.[21] This program integrated several techniques, including breathing, yoga, and cognitive reappraisal skills, among others, to elicit a daily relaxation response. As previously mentioned, the University of Pittsburgh has shown increased quality of life and medication adherence and decreased health care use among patients enrolled in the Specialty Medical Home, and Brigham and Women's Hospital has shown decreased scores of anxiety and depression and decreased hospitalization among patients enrolled in a comprehensive outpatient program.[11,12]

2. Reduced health care use

   In addition to increased quality of life and decreased morbidity from IBD, patient use of CAM can also result in decreased health care costs, because these therapies are often less expensive than clinic and emergency department visits. Although not specific to IBD, a retrospective study evaluating the effect of the Relaxation Response Resiliency Program at the Benson-Henry Institute showed a dramatic improvement in health care use among patients who completed the program. Among the 4452 patients who received this program within the study period, total use decreased by 43%. This included decreases in clinical encounters and emergency department visits, in addition to laboratory tests, procedures, and imaging tests ordered.[14] Enrollment of a larger percentage of IBD patients in similar programs could result in substantial reduction in cost of care for these patients.

3. Patient autonomy to participate in care, choose programs that may be beneficial to them.

   Patient involvement in the choice of medications and health care decisions is implicit in CAM. The increased involvement can lead to more engagement and activation in other elements of their care, whether diet, sleep, exercise, or adherence to medication.

4. CAM integrates therapies that are low risk with good safety profiles.

   As previously discussed, the safety, although likely with many of the herbal approaches or other interventions, has often not been rigorously studied, particularly for longer term treatment and in IBD in particular. A blanket assumption of safety cannot be made without better studies, even if the risk for many of these therapies seems small.

SUMMARY

CAM seems to many clinicians to be a step away from conventional therapies and approaches without adequate data. Some of the ideas, although in need of further study in IBD, also rely on data in IBD, that diet, sleep, exercise, psychosocial care, and stress management may improve patient outcomes. Health and disease are determined by numerous factors and addressing some of them is likely to bring about better health. The typical IBD patient spends only a few hours a year with his or her IBD health care providers. Consequently, most of the time, patients are responsible for their own care. As patient autonomy grows, there is a parallel movement to include other aspects of health care, including CAM, into IBD care. Ultimately, these issues bring up the larger questions: what is health, what is required to achieve and maintain healing for those with IBD, and who is the healer?

REFERENCES

1. Ha C, Ullman TA, Siegel CA, et al. Patients enrolled in randomized controlled trials do not represent the inflammatory bowel disease patient population. Clin Gastroenterol Hepatol 2012;10:1002–7.
2. Onken JE, Greer PK, Calingaert B, et al. Bromelain treatment decreases secretion of pro-inflammatory cytokines and chemokines by colon biopsies in vitro. Clin Immunol 2008;126:345–52.
3. Jedel S, Hoffman A, Merriman P, et al. A randomized controlled trial of mindfulness-based stress reduction to prevent flare-up in patients with inactive ulcerative colitis. Digestion 2014;89:142–55.
4. Belluzzi A, Brigmola C, Campierei M, et al. Effect of an enteric-coated fish-oil preparation on relapses in Crohn's disease. N Engl J Med 1996;334(24):1557–60.
5. Feagan BG, Sandborn WJ, Mittmann U, et al. Omega-3 free fatty acids for the maintenance of remission in Crohn disease: the EPIC randomized controlled trials. JAMA 2008;299(14):1690–7.
6. Chinonyelum O, Ghassan W, Lee D, et al. Specific carbohydrate diet for pediatric inflammatory bowel disease in clinical practice within an academic IBD center. Nutrition 2016;32(4):418–25.
7. Kakodkar S, Farooqui AJ, Mikolaitis SL, et al. The specific carbohydrate diet for inflammatory bowel disease: a case series. J Acad Nutr Diet 2015;115(8):1226–32.
8. Walker JR, Ediger JP, Graff LA, et al. The Manitoba IBD cohort study: a population-based study of the prevalence of lifetime and 12-month anxiety and mood disorders. Am J Gastroenterol 2008;103(6):1989–97.
9. Mikocka-Walus AA, Turnbull DA, Moulding NT, et al. Controversies surrounding the comorbidity of depression and anxiety in inflammatory bowel disease patients: a literature review. Inflamm Bowel Dis 2007;13:225–34.
10. Ananthakrishnan AN, Khalili H, Pan A, et al. Association between depressive symptoms and incidence of Crohn's disease and ulcerative colitis: results from the Nurses' Health Study. Clin Gastroenterol Hepatol 2013;11(1):57–62.

11. Korzenik JR, Hosmer-Kirby C, Collins E, et al. A study of a novel pilot program to address the psychosocial needs of IBD patients: possible impact on disease outcome and reduction of healthcare utilization. San Diego, California, May 21–24, 2016.

12. Regueiro MD, McAnallen SE, Greer JB, et al. The inflammatory bowel disease specialty medical home. Inflamm Bowel Dis 2016;22(8):1971–80.

13. Eisenberg DM, Buring JE, Hrbek AL, et al. A Model of Integrative Care for Low-Back Pain. J Altern Complement Med 2012;18(4):354–62.

14. Stahl JE, Dossett ML, Lajoie AS, et al. Relaxation response and resiliency training and its effect on healthcare resource utilization. PLoS One 2015;1–14. http://dx.doi.org/10.1371/journal.pone.0140212.

15. Cramer H, Schäfer M, Schöls M, et al. Randomised clinical trial: yoga vs written self-care advice for ulcerative colitis. Aliment Pharmacol Ther 2017;1–11. http://dx.doi.org/10.1111/apt.14062.

16. Lauche R, Kumar S, Hallmann J, et al. Efficacy and safety of ayurvedic herbs in diarrhhoea-predominant irritable bowel syndrome: a randomised controlled cross-over trial. Complement Ther Med 2016;26:171–7.

17. Lafferty WE, Tyree PT, Bellas AS, et al. Insurance coverage and subsequent utilization of complementary and alternative medical (CAM) providers. Am J Manag Care 2006;12(7):397–404.

18. Cheifetz AS, Gianotti R, Luber R, et al. Complementary and alternative medicines used by patients with inflammatory bowel diseases. Gastroenterology 2017;152: 415–29.

19. Lang A, Salomon N, Wu JCY, et al. Curcumin in combination with mesalamine induces remission in patients with mild-to-moderate ulcerative colitis in a randomized controlled trial. Clin Gastroenterol Hepatol 2015;13:1444–9.

20. Nguyen GC, Croitoru K, Silverberg MS, et al. Use of complementary and alternative medicine for inflammatory bowel disease is associated with worse adherence to conventional therapy: the COMPLIANT study. Inflamm Bowel Dis 2016;22(6): 1412–7.

21. Kuo B, Bhasin M, Jacquart J, et al. Genomic and clinical effects associated with a relaxation response mind-body intervention in patients with irritable bowel syndrome and inflammatory bowel disease. PLoS One 2015;1–26. http://dx.doi.org/10.1371/journal.pone.0123861.

UNITED STATES POSTAL SERVICE®

Statement of Ownership, Management, and Circulation (All Periodicals Publications Except Requester Publications)

1 Publication Title	2 Publication Number		3 Filing Date
GASTROENTEROLOGY CLINICS OF NORTH AMERICA	000 – 279		9/18/17

4 Issue Frequency	5 Number of Issues Published Annually	6 Annual Subscription Price
MAR, JUN, SEP, DEC	4	$330.00

7 Complete Mailing Address of Known Office of Publication (Not printer) (Street, city, county, state, and ZIP+4®)

ELSEVIER INC.
230 Park Avenue, Suite 800
New York, NY 10169

Contact Person
STEPHEN R. BUSHING

Telephone (include area code)
215-239-3688

8 Complete Mailing Address of Headquarters or General Business Office of Publisher (Not printer)

ELSEVIER INC.
230 Park Avenue, Suite 800
New York, NY 10169

9 Full Names and Complete Mailing Addresses of Publisher, Editor, and Managing Editor (Do not leave blank)

Publisher (Name and complete mailing address)

ADRIANNE BRIGIDO, ELSEVIER INC.
1600 JOHN F KENNEDY BLVD. SUITE 1800
PHILADELPHIA, PA 19103-2899

Editor (Name and complete mailing address)

KERRY HOLLAND, ELSEVIER INC.
1600 JOHN F KENNEDY BLVD. SUITE 1800
PHILADELPHIA, PA 19103-2899

Managing Editor (Name and complete mailing address)

PATRICK MANLEY, ELSEVIER INC.
1600 JOHN F KENNEDY BLVD. SUITE 1800
PHILADELPHIA, PA 19103-2899

10 Owner (Do not leave blank. If the publication is owned by a corporation, give the name and address of the corporation immediately followed by the names and addresses of all stockholders owning or holding 1 percent or more of the total amount of stock. If not owned by a corporation, give the names and addresses of the individual owners. If owned by a partnership or other unincorporated firm, give its name and address as well as those of each individual owner. If the publication is published by a nonprofit organization, give its name and address.)

Full Name	Complete Mailing Address
WHOLLY OWNED SUBSIDIARY OF REED/ELSEVIER, US HOLDINGS	1600 JOHN F KENNEDY BLVD. SUITE 1800 PHILADELPHIA, PA 19103-2899

11 Known Bondholders, Mortgagees, and Other Security Holders Owning or Holding 1 Percent or More of Total Amount of Bonds, Mortgages, or Other Securities. If none, check box ► ☐ None

Full Name	Complete Mailing Address
N/A	

12 Tax Status (For completion by nonprofit organizations authorized to mail at nonprofit rates) (Check one)
The purpose, function, and nonprofit status of this organization and the exempt status for federal income tax purposes:

☒ Has Not Changed During Preceding 12 Months
☐ Has Changed During Preceding 12 Months (Publisher must submit explanation of change with this statement)

13 Publication Title	14 Issue Date for Circulation Data Below
GASTROENTEROLOGY CLINICS OF NORTH AMERICA	JUNE 2017

15 Extent and Nature of Circulation			Average No. Copies Each Issue During Preceding 12 Months	No. Copies of Single Issue Published Nearest to Filing Date
a. Total Number of Copies (Net press run)			441	299
b. Paid Circulation (By Mail and Outside the Mail)	(1)	Mailed Outside-County Paid Subscriptions Stated on PS Form 3541 (Include paid distribution above nominal rate, advertiser's proof copies, and exchange copies)	150	125
	(2)	Mailed In-County Paid Subscriptions Stated on PS Form 3541 (Include paid distribution above nominal rate, advertiser's proof copies, and exchange copies)	0	0
	(3)	Paid Distribution Outside the Mails Including Sales Through Dealers and Carriers, Street Vendors, Counter Sales, and Other Paid Distribution Outside USPS®	117	89
	(4)	Paid Distribution by Other Classes of Mail Through the USPS (e.g. First-Class Mail®)	0	0
c. Total Paid Distribution (Sum of 15b (1), (2), (3), and (4))		►	267	214
d. Free or Nominal Rate Distribution (By Mail and Outside the Mail)	(1)	Free or Nominal Rate Outside-County Copies included on PS Form 3541	87	85
	(2)	Free or Nominal Rate In-County Copies included on PS Form 3541	0	0
	(3)	Free or Nominal Rate Copies Mailed at Other Classes Through the USPS (e.g. First-Class Mail)	0	0
	(4)	Free or Nominal Rate Distribution Outside the Mail (Carriers or other means)	0	0
e. Total Free or Nominal Rate Distribution (Sum of 15d (1), (2), (3) and (4))		►	87	85
f. Total Distribution (Sum of 15c and 15e)		►	354	299
g. Copies not Distributed (See instructions to Publishers #4 (page #3))		►	87	0
h. Total (Sum of 15f and g)		►	441	299
i. Percent Paid (15c divided by 15f times 100)		►	75.42%	71.57%

* If you are claiming electronic copies, go to line 16 on page 3. If you are not claiming electronic copies, skip to line 17 on page 3.

16 Electronic Copy Circulation	Average No. Copies Each Issue During Preceding 12 Months	No. Copies of Single Issue Published Nearest to Filing Date
a. Paid Electronic Copies ►	0	0
b. Total Paid Print Copies (Line 15c) + Paid Electronic Copies (Line 16a) ►	267	214
c. Total Print Distribution (Line 15f) + Paid Electronic Copies (Line 16a) ►	354	299
d. Percent Paid (Both Print & Electronic Copies) (16b divided by 16c × 100) ►	75.42%	71.57%

☒ I certify that 50% of all my distributed copies (electronic and print) are paid above a nominal price.

17 Publication of Statement of Ownership

☒ If the publication is a general publication, publication of this statement is required. Will be printed in the DECEMBER 2017 issue of this publication.

☐ Publication not required.

18 Signature and Title of Editor, Publisher, Business Manager, or Owner

STEPHEN R. BUSHING - INVENTORY DISTRIBUTION CONTROL MANAGER

Date 9/18/17

I certify that all information furnished on this form is true and complete. I understand that anyone who furnishes false or misleading information on this form or who omits material or information requested on the form may be subject to criminal sanctions (including fines and imprisonment) and/or civil sanctions (including civil penalties).

PS Form 3526, July 2014 (Page 3 of 4) PSN: 7530-01-000-9931 PRIVACY NOTICE: See our privacy policy on www.usps.com

PS Form 3526, July 2014 (Page 1 of 4 (see instructions page 4)) PSN: 7530-01-000-9931 PRIVACY NOTICE: See our privacy policy on www.usps.com

Moving?

Make sure your subscription moves with you!

To notify us of your new address, find your **Clinics Account Number** (located on your mailing label above your name), and contact customer service at:

Email: journalscustomerservice-usa@elsevier.com

800-654-2452 (subscribers in the U.S. & Canada)
314-447-8871 (subscribers outside of the U.S. & Canada)

Fax number: 314-447-8029

Elsevier Health Sciences Division
Subscription Customer Service
3251 Riverport Lane
Maryland Heights, MO 63043

*To ensure uninterrupted delivery of your subscription, please notify us at least 4 weeks in advance of move.

ELSEVIER

Printed and bound by CPI Group (UK) Ltd, Croydon, CR0 4YY

03/10/2024

01040390-0006